Clinical Aphasiology
Volume 22

Clinical Aphasiology
Volume 22

Editor

Margaret L. Lemme, PhD
University of Wisconsin
Madison, Wisconsin

Editorial Board

Jennifer Horner, PhD
Duke University Medical Center
Durham, North Carolina

Michael L. Kimbarow, PhD
Rehabilitation Institute of Michigan
Wayne State University
Detroit, Michigan

Linda A. Nicholas, MS
Aphasia Research
VA Medical Center
Minneapolis, Minnesota

Connie A. Tompkins, PhD
University of Pittsburgh
Pittsburgh, Pennsylvania

pro·ed

8700 Shoal Creek Boulevard
Austin, Texas 78757-6897

Printed in the United States of America
LC 86–647891

ISBN 0–89079–595–9

8700 Shoal Creek Boulevard
Austin, Texas 78757-6897

1 2 3 4 5 6 7 8 9 10   98 97 96 95 94

CONTENTS

PREFACE

We are beginning a decade in which many traditional paradigms in health care and speech-language pathology will undergo change. Our legislators have committed to focus both government and public attention on research, treatment, and rehabilitation of the brain, declaring the 1990s "The Decade of the Brain." Concepts of paradigm change and focus on research, treatment, and rehabilitation of the communicative sequelae of brain injury are not new to clinical aphasiologists. Since the early 1970s, these specialists in speech-language pathology have met annually at the Clinical Aphasiology Conference. This conference has provided clinicians and researchers engaged in the clinical management and investigation of persons with acquired neurologic speech-language disorders an opportunity to present their recent investigations and to engage in discussion with colleagues having similar interests. Subsequently, *Clinical Aphasiology* (formerly *Proceedings of the Clinical Aphasiology Conference*) has presented the current concepts, clinical knowledge, and prevailing logic underlying the management of adult neurogenic communication disorders.

While the data, analytic concerns, conceptualizations, modes of analysis, substantive findings, and theoretical conclusions of the research vary from those of earlier studies, there are also important continuities in the clinical aphasiology literature. Increasingly since the mid-1980s, the interest and scope of practice of clinical aphasiologists have embraced right-hemisphere communication disorders, cognitive-communicative disorders secondary to traumatic brain injury, communication impairments related to dementia, and cognitive-linguistic performance in normal elderly adults. The infusion of theory and empirical findings from normal adult communicative function and related language disorders has both enriched the clinical literature and refined theories of brain-language behavior and efficacious clinical-management procedures.

Clinical Aphasiology, Volume 22 contains a collection of original manuscripts presented at the 1992 Clinical Aphasiology Conference, Durango, Colorado. The standard of primary publication is supported by a two-tiered peer-review system and protected by policies that prohibit multiple submission and duplicate publication. Initially, conference proposals were blind-reviewed by a five-member program committee and rated in terms of scientific and clinical merit, contribution to knowledge, potential for stimulating useful discussion, and relevance to clinical management of people with acquired neurologic language disorders. Priority was given to papers dealing directly with clinical issues. Following the conference, manuscripts were reviewed again by five members of an editorial board before being accepted or rejected for publication in this volume.

This volume is divided into eight major sections. The conference keynote, "Right Hemisphere and Verbal Communication: Conceptual, Methodological, and Clinical Issues," written by invitation by Yves Joanette and Pierre Goulet, introduces the first major section. Additional contributions to right-hemisphere function and deficits include investigations of the effects of visual and inferential complexity on picture description, categorization skills, verbal learning, and first-encounter conversations in right-hemisphere-damaged adults.

In the second section, neurodiagnostic techniques are used to investigate and develop an understanding of attention deficit in adult aphasia. Principles and methods of diagnosis and assessment are introduced in the third section, which offers: evidence for reliability in a prognosis profile and in measures of connected speech in aphasia; assessment of generalization and of narrative discourse; and evaluation from different clinical perspectives for varied patient populations. Continuing with evaluation, section four considers the validity of limb apraxia testing, while section five focuses on apraxia of speech and includes theoretical and treatment issues. The sixth section contains feature analysis for treatment and differential cognitive performance of traumatically brain-injured patients.

Many researchers suggest that a complete theory of treatment, including a set of assumptions about the nature of language function, aphasia, and recovery, provides a rationale for treatment and enables a clinician to identify *what* is being treated and *why* a particular procedure is selected. Yet a review by Horner and Loverso indicated most clinical treatment for adult aphasia is not theoretically based. Section seven, Theory-Driven Treatment Considerations for Aphasia, is divided into two subsections and revisits this topic. A trilogy of papers, presented in a special conference session, Theory-Driven Therapy: From Occult Art to Science or the Other Way Around, explores what theory-driven treatment can and cannot be expected to accomplish, considers a cognitive neuropsychological orientation to aphasia treatment, and pragmatically examines application of theory-driven therapy in the management of aphasic adults. The second subsection highlights linguistic theory as a framework for aphasia treatment and presents a specific approach for treatment of aphasic sentence-production deficits. Continuing with treatment considerations, the last major section of this volume features the effects of context variables, cueing, and multimodality training in aphasic patients.

As editor, it is my pleasure to conclude this preface by acknowledging my sincere appreciation to those who, in one way or another, have contributed to the development of this book. This volume would have been impossible without the assistance of many unidentified aphasic patients, many clinician-researchers, and the officers of the 1992 Clinical Aphasiology Conference (CAC). First, I offer a special thanks and acknowledgment to our adult speech-language-disordered patients, who endure multiple probes and repeated testing in the service of clinical progress and increased quality communicative treatment. Second, a sincere thank you goes to the illustrious contributors to this volume. The literature in clinical aphasiology is built by single contributions that fill a space previously empty, and each contribution must be robust enough to bear the weight of contributions to come. Additionally, thanks to the officers of the 1992 CAC: Linda E. Nicholas, conference chairperson; Felice L. Loverso, program chairman; program committee members—Marilyn Selinger, Donald Robin, Joseph Duffy, Reg Warren, and Richard Peach; Lee Ann Golper, treasurer; and local arrangements—Thomas Prescott, Donna Bottenburg, Beth Henderson, Kathy Walker, and Russel Davis. Finally, this volume was completed because of the clinical and research expertise, patience, and support so generously given by the members of the editorial board: Jennifer Horner, Mike Kimbarow, Linda Nicholas, and Connie Tompkins. They carefully reviewed, evaluated, and offered important editorial contributions to each manuscript, thus strengthening this volume substantially. Also, Tinney Kees, who volunteered editorial service and provided specific suggestions, is due special thanks. Final thanks go to the PRO-ED editor, Gerry Wallace, the production manager, Alan Grimes, and his coworker, Tracy Sergo, for their assistance and troubleshooting.

This volume is a product of some of the expertise and energy found in clinical aphasiology today. The hope is that this volume will lead to even more energy, continuing development, and refinement of the prevailing ideas concerning research, theory, and rehabilitation of communicative disorders subsequent to brain injury. Knowing that clinicians must always function with at least two levels in mind—theory and treatment—this volume is dedicated to clinicians, to clinical-researchers, and to the graduate student clinicians who follow.

M. L. L.

CONTRIBUTING AUTHORS

Adamovich, Brenda L. B.
East Carolina University School of
Medicine,
Pitt County Memorial Hospital, and
Regional Rehabilitation Center
P.O. Box 6028
Greenville, NC 27834-6028

Bayles, Kathryn A.
Center for Neurogenic
Communication Disorders
University of Arizona
Speech and Hearing Sciences Bldg.
Tucson, AZ 85721

Beeson, Pelagie M.
Center for Neurogenic
Communication Disorders
University of Arizona
Speech and Hearing Sciences Bldg.
Tucson, AZ 85721

Belanger, Steven
Vanderbilt Rehabilitation Center
Newport Hospital
Friendship Street
Newport, RI 02840

Boada, Richard
University of Pittsburgh
1101 Cathedral of Learning
Pittsburgh, PA 15260

Brookshire, Robert H.
Speech Pathology Section (127A)
VA Medical Center
1 Veterans Drive
Minneapolis, MN 55417

Buoyer, Frances G.
Speech and Language Pathology
Program
Department of Surgery, Box 3887
Duke University Medical Center
Durham, NC 27710

Burton, Wendy
Racho Los Amigos Medical Center
Downey, CA 90242

Byng, Sally
Department of Clinical
Communication Studies
City University
Northampton Square
London EC1V 0HB

Clarkson, Janine V.
Communication Disorders
Department
Gaylord Hospital
P.O. Box 400
Wallingford, CT 06492

Coelho, Carl A.
Communication Disorders
Department
Gaylord Hospital
P.O. Box 400
Wallingford, CT 06492

Dawson, Deborah V.
Division of Biometry
Department of Community and
Family Medicine
Duke University Medical Center
Durham, NC 27710

DeMarco, Salvatore
East Carolina University
Department of Speech-Language &
Auditory Pathology
Greenville, NC 27858

Doyle, Patrick
VA Medical Center (117A)
Highland Drive
Pittsburgh, PA 15260

Dronkers, Nina
VA Medical Center
150 Muir Road
Martinez, CA 94553

Duffy, Joseph
Mayo Clinic, Speech Pathology, E-8A
200 First Street, SW
Rochester, MN 55902

Duffy, Robert J.
University of Connecticut
Department of Communication
Sciences
850 Bolton Road, U-85
Storrs, CT 06268

Elia, Deanne
University of Connecticut
Department of Communication
Science
850 Bolton Road
Storrs, CT 06268

Eller, Mary Ann
Speech and Language Pathology
Program
Department of Surgery, Box 3887
Duke University Medical Center
Durham, NC 27710

Folkins, John W.
Department of Speech Pathology &
Audiology
University of Iowa
Iowa City, IA 52242

Freed, Donald B.
Communication Disorders & Sciences
Division of Special Education &
Rehabilitation
University of Oregon
Eugene, OR 97403-1211

Golper, Lee Ann
Speech Pathology (126)
VA Medical Center
800 Zorn Avenue
Louisville, KY 40206

Goulet, Pierre
Laboratoire Théophile-Alajouanine
C.H. Côte-des-Neiges
4565 Chemin de la Reine-Marie
Montreal H3W 1W5

Hageman, Carlin
Department of Communicative
Disorders
Communication Arts Center (238)
University of Northern Iowa
Cedar Falls, IA 50614-0356

Hashi, Michiko
Department of Communicative
Disorders
University of Wisconsin–Madison
1975 Willow Drive
Madison, WI 53706

Holland, Audrey L.
Department of Speech and Hearing
Sciences
University of Arizona
Tucson, AZ 85721

Horner, Jennifer
Speech and Language Pathology
Program
Department of Surgery, Box 3887
Duke University Medical Center
Durham, NC 27710

Hough, Monica Strauss
East Carolina University
Dept. of Speech, Language &
Auditory Pathology
Greenville, NC 27858

Hutchinson, Thomas A.
Clinical and Special Needs
Riverside Publishing Company
P.O. Box 1970
Iowa City, IA 52244

Jackson, Amy
VA Medical Center
Speech-Language Pathology (117A)
Highland Drive
Pittsburgh, PA 15260

Joanette, Yves
Laboratoire Théophile-Alajouanine
C.H. Côte-des-Neiges
4565 Chemin de la Reine-Marie
Montreal H3W 1W5

Kennedy, Mary R. T.
19514 34th Avenue, NE
Seattle, WA 98155

Liles, Betty Z.
Department of Communication
Sciences
University of Connecticut
Storrs, CT 06268

Marshall, Robert
VA Medical Center (126P)
2710 Veterans Hospital Road SW
Portland, OR 97207

Massaro, Maryellen
Head-Injury Day Treatment
Harmarville Rehabilitation Center
Box 11460–Guys Run Road
Pittsburgh, PA 15260-0460

McNeil, Malcolm R.
Communication Disorders
University of Pittsburgh
1101 Cathedral of Learning
Pittsburgh, PA 15260

Moon, Jerald B.
Department of Speech Pathology/
Audiology
University of Iowa
Iowa City, IA 52242

Myers, Penelope
2705 Bamber Lane, SW
Rochester, MN 55902

Newhoff, Marilyn
University of Georgia
Communication Disorders
Aderhold Hall
Athens, GA 30602

Nicholas, Linda
VA Medical Center–Minneapolis
Aphasia Research
1 Veterans Drive (127A)
Minneapolis, MN 55417

Oleyar, Karen
VA Medical Center
Speech-Language Pathology (117A)
Highland Drive
Pittsburgh, PA 15260

Jon Pabst, Mary
Wake County Schools
Greenville, NC 27858

Peach, Richard K.
Rush-Presbyterian-St. Luke's Medical
Center
Department of Communication
Disorders & Sciences
1653 W. Congress Parkway
Chicago, IL 60612

Peterson, Connie
Racho Los Amigos Medical Center
Downey, CA 90242

Phillips, David S.
Department of Public Health
Oregon Health Sciences Universities
Portland, OR 97207

Prescott, Thomas E.
VA Medical Center–Denver
1055 Clermont Street (126)
Denver, CO 80220

Purdy, Mary H.
88 Robbins Drive
Wethersfield, CT 06268

Rapcsak, Steven Z.
VA Medical Center
Tucson, AZ 85721

Robin, Donald
Department of Speech Pathology/
Audiology
University of Iowa
Iowa City, IA 52242

Rubens, Alan B.
Department of Neurology
University of Arizona
Tucson, AZ 85721

Rubin, Scott
Communication Disorders
University of Georgia
Athens, GA 30602

Selinger, Marilyn
VA Medical Center–Denver
1055 Clermont Street (126)
Denver, CO 80220

Shapiro, Lewis
Department of Psychology
Florida Atlantic University
P.O. Box 3091
Boca Raton, FL 33431-0991

Southwood, Helen
Department of Biocommunications
University of Alabama
Birmingham, AL 35203

Spencer, Kristie A.
University of Pittsburgh
1101 Cathedral of Learning
Pittsburgh, PA 15260

Strand, Edythe
University of Washington
Speech and Hearing Sciences
1417 42nd Street NE (JG-15)
Seattle, WA 98105

Thompson, Cynthia K.
Northwestern University
Communication Sciences and
Disorders
Speech and Language Disorders
2299 Sheridan Road
Evanston, IL 60208-3066

Tompkins, Connie A.
University of Pittsburgh
1101 Cathedral of Learning
Pittsburgh, PA 15260

Wambaugh, Julie L.
VA Medical Center
Speech-Language Pathology (117A)
Highland Drive
Pittsburgh, PA 15260

Watt, James H.
University of Connecticut
Department of Communication
Sciences
850 Bolton Road, U-85
Storrs, CT 06268

Wertz, Robert T.
VA Medical Center–Martinez
Audiology/Speech Pathology (126)
Martinez, CA 94553

Clinical Aphasiology, Vol. 22, 1994, pp. 1–23

Right Hemisphere and Verbal Communication: Conceptual, Methodological, and Clinical Issues

Yves Joanette and Pierre Goulet

This paper is a version of a conference keynote that was intended to provoke a collective debate about some of the issues concerning the effects of right brain damage (RBD) on the verbal communication abilities of right-handers. It should probably have been kept oral, but this version will at least allow a larger number of people to enter the discussion. Still, it should be read with the ears more than with the eyes. Moreover, the reader should be aware that this material is not meant to be a data-driven contribution to the field. It simply reflects some of the authors' present thoughts. Thus, some readers may feel that there are too many questions and not sufficient answers, or that some of the ideas put forward are not supported by the appropriate experimental demonstration, and they will be right. The wealth of unanswered questions is immense. The ideas introduced here have been favored by some convergence of facts, but their final demonstration has yet to come.

Moving from historical perspectives to clinical issues, we will mention eight different but complementary aspects of the problem. These points are not the only possible topics; rather, they are taken here only as examples of the kinds of questions we think should be discussed more explicitly. Some of these questions are of purely epistemological value, others are very practical, and most of them relate to some conceptual or methodological problems. But all of them are crucial for anyone who is interested in better understanding and helping those individuals with a nonaphasic verbal communication deficit following right brain damage.

THE FALL AND RISE OF THE RIGHT HEMISPHERE

After hesitating for many centuries between Aristotle and Hippocrates, between the heart and the brain (and thereafter, between the cavities of the brain and its substance), science finally convinced itself that language and other cognitive activities were based in the convolutions of the brain, along with some of the subcortical structures. After the regularity of the brain's convolutions was finally discovered and coupled with the conviction that the different aspects of human activities could be conceived atomistically, the essence of modern neuropsychology was laid down through one of the first of a series of excesses, the phrenological approach. Franz Joseph Gall, his pupils, and his colleagues thus proposed in the early 19th century a notion that still lies at the core of modern conceptions about the neurobiological bases of intellectual activities, namely, that discrete components of the brain are responsible for discrete components of what we now call cognitive functions. But for all those centuries, whatever the conceptions proposed, *both* halves of the brain—or of the heart!—were thought to contribute equally. No distinction was made whatsoever between the relative contributions of the right and the left hemispheres to an individual's cognitive functions.

However, at the same time that phrenological proposals were being popularized in northern France, a clever and observant surgeon in southern France came to some clinical conclusions that would change the way both hemispheres would be regarded. This surgeon was Marc Dax. From 1800 to 1834 he had to treat a series of patients who had lost the ability to speak after suffering brain lesions (some of them from saber blows). In a paper given in Montpellier in 1836, Dax first presented the principle that the brain's hemispheres make asymmetrical contributions to language. Even though Dax's claim was never published in his lifetime, it was the origin of modern conceptions about the brain's asymmetry vis-à-vis language functions. According to Ombredane (1951), it was the discussions around the official recognition of Marc Dax's paper by the *Académie de médecine de Paris* that forced Broca to take his position. Approximately three weeks after Dax's paper was authenticated in May 1865, Broca popularized the asymmetry concept on June 15, 1865, in an address to the *Société d'anthropologie* in Paris.

The essence of Dax's oral and Broca's written contributions is that articulated language is essentially a product of the left hemisphere. Although most of those who refer to this period insist that the privileged role of the left hemisphere for language was thus unveiled, it must be realized that it was not the role but its privileged status that was new; in part, Dax and Broca simply restated the left hemisphere's long-known contribution to language. The real revolution was that the right hemisphere *lost* its presumed contribution to language. Thus, the end of the 19th century should be remembered as the period during which the right hemisphere lost its postulated contribution to language whereas the left hemisphere kept its presumed abilities. For nearly a century researchers would deny the right hemisphere any role in language functions, the few exceptions being some sporadic and ill-received contributions, such as those of Huglings-Jackson (1879).

The right hemisphere blackout in language functions lasted until the mid-20th century. At that point, some other trailblazing clinicians, as clever and observant as Dax had been, suggested that right hemisphere lesions, although usually not the origin of an aphasia proper, nonetheless could cause limitations in right-handed patients' communicating abilities. Pioneers such as MacDonald Critchley (1962), Jon Eisenson (1962), and Ed Weinstein (1964) thus came up with the notion that an acquired right hemispheric lesion could produce communication problems. The terms delineating those problems were clumsy, though, such as Eisenson's (1962) notion of the "super-ordinary" aspects of language. Nonetheless, the right hemisphere was more and more suspected of having some capacities for some aspects of verbal processing. Thus, a century after its exclusion and only some 30 years ago, the right hemisphere was again recognized as playing a role in language.

It is now well known that an acquired lesion to a nondominant right hemisphere, though not responsible for an aphasia, can be at the root of some impairments in the ability to communicate. Apart from those at the prosodic level, impairments have been reported potentially to involve the processing of the semantic aspects of words and text-level abilities, as well as the adequacy between language and context (for reviews, see Code, 1987; Joanette, Goulet, & Hannequin, 1990; Myers, 1984, 1986). Most of the conceptual frameworks needed to describe these problems were not available when the term *aphasia* was coined, which probably explains why the impairments were not recognized as aphasic. Also, these impairments were so mild as to sometimes escape notice by clinicians. Thus, most authors, past and present, have referred to these problems as *nonaphasic*. Labeling these problems as either aphasic or nonaphasic, however, is essentially an arbitrary decision. We will refer to them as *verbal communication deficits*, because they usually involve more than the traditional components of linguistic functioning (e.g., phonology, morphology, syntax) and frequently include text-level processes (see Joanette & Brownell, 1990) as well as pragmatic aspects of language.

As we near the dawn of the 21st century, the left hemisphere is conceived to be necessary but not sufficient for normal communication ability. Numerous studies and clinical reports have clearly demonstrated that the integrity of the right hemisphere is also needed. The question now is to identify clearly the components of communication for which the integrity of the right hemisphere is needed. In doing so, though, numerous problems arise in terms of the available conceptual frameworks or methodologies. At the same time, the clinical approach to these problems suffers because this field is still young. Consequently, our purpose in this chapter is not to provide an overview of the current teaching and knowledge about the verbal communication deficits in right-brain-damaged (RBD) right-handers; some of us already have provided the literature with such comprehensive reviews. Rather, the goal here is to raise questions about some of the current conceptual, methodological, and clinical issues in the field. The first six sections will treat intermingled conceptual and methodological issues, and the last two sections will deal with clinical issues. In doing so, we hope to generate discussion and a collective effort toward understanding the effective contribution of the right hemisphere to verbal communication.

AN INTEGRATED MODEL OF VERBAL COMMUNICATION: WHERE TO LOOK

One of the first problems with the research on and clinical approaches to the impairments reported among RBD patients is the limit inherent to the conceptual framework used to refer to these impairments. There is no available conceptual framework that can situate, in an integrated manner, each of the aspects of the communicative impairments found among RBD patients.

It has been stressed already that the kinds of impairments exhibited by RBD patients can affect one or another of the cognitive components allowing for verbal communication. The term *verbal communication*—or its equivalents, such as *communicative abilities*—refers to a series of cognitive abilities that permit exchange of information between two or more individuals in a given context. The concept of *verbal communication* includes, linguistic abilities, among other things, even though the impairments found among RBD patients do not mainly affect the linguistic skills *per se*.

The concept of *verbal communication* is useful in referring in a general manner to the impairments among RBD patients, but it lacks theoretical support. Indeed, to our knowledge, there is no theoretical framework sufficiently integrated and complete to cover all the possible levels of impairments found in RBD patients. For example, Garrett's (1984) model has been frequently cited in many neurolinguistic studies on aphasia. This model contains a series of representation levels allowing for language production, from the message level to the motor control level. Unfortunately, the content of each of these levels is not always clearly detailed. Moreover, many of the different communicative deficits reported among RBD patients are found at the message level. Thus, the message level corresponds in fact to a whole area of communication, a condition that prevents it from being useful for our purpose.

Authors interested in text-level processes have proposed other possible theoretical frameworks. For example, Frederiksen's (1990) model is more explicit than Garrett's. Frederiksen treats Garrett's message level as numerous levels of representation of the message, his model has its own limitations. Among other things, it fails to integrate the communicative context sufficiently to account for the role of shared knowledge in discourse production. Also, this model is oriented toward some types of discourse production and comprehension, but it overlooks conversational discourse and abilities such as topic shifts and topic maintenance.

Other models, such as Ellis and Beattie's (1986) model, seem to incorporate more of the context and thus palliate some of the previously mentioned limitations. The Ellis and Beattie model remains a very general sketch of verbal and nonverbal communication, however, and does not allow for an operationalization of the different components included, overtly or covertly.

In conclusion, none of these models offers a satisfactory integrated, specific theoretical framework that allows systematic exploration of the verbal communication deficits among RBD patients. (Of course, that was not the initial goal of these conceptual frameworks.) Given that no specific theoretical framework exists, the concept of *verbal communication* itself is ill-defined and lacks theoretical support. This concept essentially denotes a domain of cognitive abilities that depends on the contribution of specific linguistic components (e.g., syntactic processes) and other cognitive components (e.g., inference-making processes). The expression remains useful with regard to the kind of difficulties RBD patients have, but the fact that it corresponds to nothing in particular must be kept in mind. It is hoped that studies aimed at elaborating an integrated conceptual framework for verbal communication will soon be available.

VERBAL COMMUNICATION OR GENERAL INTELLECTUAL DEFICITS? A CIRCULAR QUESTION

An issue frequently raised in the literature concerns the linguistic specificity of the communicative impairments that RBD patients exhibit. Indeed, authors such as Gainotti, Caltagirone, & Miceli (1979) have proposed that, at least for lexico-semantic deficits, RBD impairments could reflect diminished intellectual functioning. This suggestion was made after these authors noted that those RBD patients who had lower IQs were the ones with communicative deficits, as measured at the lexico-semantic level. However, as will be suggested, this is a very difficult question to tackle; indeed, it may turn out to be a false question.

The suggested IQ deficit in RBD patients leads to the following questions: What is intelligence, and is it possible to appreciate general intellectual functioning apart from verbal communicative abilities? The first of these two questions lies at the heart of a longstanding debate in psychology. However, we must remember that there is no such thing, in cognitive models, as an *intellectual module*. In other words, the concept of general intellectual functioning is a clinical concept that is either the overall reflection in each cognitive component of some deeply nested intellectual abilities or potential or, conversely, the summation of all the cognitive potential and abilities found in a given individual. The current clinical appreciation of intelligence relies heavily on linguistic abilities. In fact, most of the standardized tests of intellectual functioning (e.g., WAIS, Wechsler, 1955) are heavily loaded on language that is either appreciated directly (e.g., vocabulary) or used as a tool by which to appreciate other cognitive abilities (e.g., similarities). This brings us to the second point: If, as many would have it, the kind of communication problems seen among RBD patients involves more than merely linguistic abilities and should incorporate aspects of cognition (e.g., the ability to make inferences), it has to be realized that many of the same abilities could be appreciated in so-called general intellectual abilities.

In sum, the attribution of the impairments that RBD patients have in verbal communication to an altered general intellectual functioning is very difficult to explore experimentally. Depending on the relevant concept of intelligence, the attribution might even be tautologous. Indeed, not only is language, and verbal communication in general, highly involved in the appreciation of general intellectual functioning, but the kind of impairments RBD patients have extends beyond—or underlies—the limits of linguistic abilities *per se*. These impairments probably reflect impaired cognitive abilities that are the basis of an individual's intellectual functioning. Thus, it is not certain that the intellectual-functioning hypothesis could account for all types of verbal communication deficits. Trying to dissociate these two notions is probably circular. Instead, we need to identify the cognitive abilities that are indeed necessary for good verbal communication.

THE SEMANTIC PROCESSING OF WORDS: HOW TO LOOK AND WHAT TO LOOK FOR

One of the most productive research areas regarding the right hemisphere's effective contribution to verbal communication pertains to the semantic processing of words (see Chapter 4 in Joanette, Goulet, & Hanne-quin, 1990, for an up-to-date review). It is well known that a right hemisphere lesion can result in an inability to access or to process certain kinds of words adequately. This inability converges with the wealth of data coming from the split-brain and the normal subject literature about the capabilities of the right hemisphere. These studies demonstrated that the right hemisphere has its optimal potential for automatically activated, concrete, picturable, and frequent substantives. However, it is still to be discovered whether the effects of right hemispheric lesions can be described by reference to this potential. Though interest in the effects of right hemispheric lesions on lexico-semantic abilities generates more and more research questions, our impression is that there are a number of methodological and conceptual limitations that should be discussed for those contributions to be even more relevant. The following are examples of these issues.

The Representation–Access Debate: The Priming Paradigm Disillusion

A persistent question in aphasiology, and one that is present in the RBD literature, is whether the lexico-semantic difficulties of a patient are due to a representation or an access problem.[1] In other words, does the problem stem from some weakened lexico-semantic network, or is it to be attributed to limitations in the mechanisms that provide access to the presumed semantic network? Trying to sort out these two possibilities is not an easy task, but cognitive psychology has contributed some answers to this question over the last decade, for example, provided Milberg and Blumstein's (1981) seminal work in aphasia using what is known as the priming paradigm. Although this particular contribution lacked the methodological sophistication to distinguish between automatic and controlled priming conditions (Posner & Snyder, 1975), others *can* differentiate these two notions, which can contribute significantly to the access/representation debate. For instance, according to Siéroff (1991), automatic semantic priming essentially informs us about the quality of the representation, whereas controlled semantic priming depends on both the quality of the representation *and* the quality of the access mechanisms. Thus, this was the better paradigm with which to study the nature of the lexico-semantic impairment among RBD patients. This paradigm has been used in only

---

1. At the time this paper was written, the representation–access dichotomy was still popular. Since then, the field has evolved toward a rephrasing of this dichotomy along an activation continuum.

two studies with RBD patients, however, one by Gagnon, Goulet, and Joanette (1989) and another one by Tompkins (1990).

The use of lateralized priming in normal subjects can shed light on the use of the priming paradigm with RBD patients. After studying right and left hemifield automatic and controlled semantic-priming conditions with undergraduate students, Chiarello, Senehi, and Nuding (1987) suggested that, whereas right hemifield (left hemisphere) presentations were associated with efficient automatic *and* controlled priming effects, left hemifield (right hemisphere) presentations were associated with automatic, but not controlled, priming. In a study of automatic and controlled priming in left- and right-brain-damaged patients, Gagnon et al. (1989) came up with nonconvergent results. Gagnon et al. (1989) showed that both automatic *and* controlled priming conditions were unaffected in both left-brain-damaged (LBD) mild aphasics and RBD patients. However, using a third task—a semantic judgment task that required even more effort—they showed that both LBD and RBD patients were impaired. Assuming that the priming condition this study investigated was in fact controlled, the results suggest that, contrary to the conclusions of Chiarello et al. (1987), normal access to the semantic network requires the integrity of both the left and the right hemisphere.

However these priming studies might contribute to the representation/access debate in the RBD literature, there are a number of problems with the priming paradigm itself. First, not every researcher has determined the presence of circumstances sufficient to distinguish automatic from controlled priming conditions. An automatic priming condition is characterized by some benefits in the related condition (e.g., the existence of a semantic relation) in the absence of any costs from the unrelated condition (see Siéroff, 1991, for a review). In controlled priming, more benefits are expected in the related condition, but they are accompanied by costs in the unrelated condition. Most aphasia studies have not adequately checked for the presence of such effects. Thus, many authors simply propose the experimental setup that *should* yield such distinctive priming conditions without verifying, through a cost-benefit analysis, whether these conditions are respected, such as was done in the Gagnon et al. (1989) study. As for the two studies reported in the RBD literature, neither Tompkins (1990) nor Gagnon et al. (1989) obtained costs in a priming paradigm that was supposedly of a controlled type. These results raise further questions: Did this result reflect an experimental setup that did not induce a properly controlled type of priming, or is the absence of costs also characteristic of controlled priming? If it is the latter case, the theory behind priming conditions should be revised.

But this is only part of the issue. Another part is the problem inherent to the method used to verify the automatic or controlled nature of the priming condition. Indeed, the cost-benefit analysis can be done only if related and unrelated primes are compared with what is referred to as a *neutral* prime (e.g., XXXX, BLANK, or a nonword). However, the neutral status of these "neutral" primes is an object of debate. Even more problematic is the fact that most of the reference studies of the priming paradigm have been done on undergraduate students. It is not at all certain that the normal mature or aged population performs on those tasks in the same way as undergraduates do.

Thus, it becomes apparent that the priming paradigm can offer an interesting solution to disentangle the representation/access debate. Nonetheless, a number of preliminary studies are needed to obtain a theoretically and pragmatically valid experimental paradigm with a normal subject population that will be representative of the brain-damaged patients about whom we would like to increase our knowledge.

Oral Naming: What to Look For

One of the lexico-semantic production tasks frequently proposed to RBD patients—either for direct evaluation of their performance or because they were a control group in a study of LBD patients—is the oral-naming, verbal fluency, or lexical evocation task (also labeled the FAS test or the Category test). Typically, this task requires the subject to produce words orally using a given selection criterion within a certain amount of time, usually 1 or 2 minutes. The criteria used are either formal (e.g., the letter *B*) or semantic (e.g., names of animals).

Oral-naming tasks are useful in determining whether the right hemisphere contributes to the lexical or the semantic aspects of lexical semantics in production and, consequently, in knowing how to characterize the effects of a right hemisphere lesion. For example, Joanette and Goulet (1986), as well as Laine and Niemi (1988), claimed that only semantic, but not formal, criteria were associated with diminished oral-naming performance among RBD patients. Even though there were nonconvergent results in the literature (Joanette et al., 1990), this result was still in line with the numerous studies done with normal subjects using divided-field presentations. The results also converged with split-brain studies showing that the right hemisphere is capable of processing some semantic aspects of words but is much less capable of handling their formal aspects. Up to this point, everything seemed clear, but some recent results could challenge this interpretation in a dramatic manner.

Sabourin, Goulet, and Joanette (1988) showed that, regardless of the semantic or formal nature of the criteria, RBD patients exhibited significantly lower performance only if the criteria were highly productive, not when they were moderately or slightly productive. The criteria's productivity was defined as the normal subject's ability, for a given criterion, to generate words associated to it. In this study, two semantic and two formal criteria were used for each of three levels of productivity. Obviously, this result, if confirmed, would put a focus on a different set of interests about the nature of the right hemisphere's contribution to lexical semantics. It certainly shows how much our knowledge about the nature of the right hemisphere's contribution to lexical semantics is constrained by the current methodological as well as conceptual limits of our era. This is probably just the evolution of science, but we might want to be aware of it.

Is the Concreteness Effect Due to Concreteness?

In addition to the problems about the type of activation involved and the role that the right hemisphere plays in lexical semantics, another problem lies in the nature of the words that are best processed by the right hemisphere. That is, for a given kind of activation, and for a given type of contribution, the question is whether the right hemisphere has a preference for certain word types that could be characterized semantically. If one looks at the normal subject and the split-brain literature, the most frequently documented difference between the right and the left hemispheres' capabilities concerns concreteness effects. It is known that, whereas the left hemisphere can process both concrete and abstract nouns, the right hemisphere can process only concrete ones. Concreteness is certainly not the only lexical characteristic that may point to a difference between the two hemispheres, but it is the one that has generated the most studies (Joanette et al., 1990).

Only a few studies have investigated the concreteness effect among RBD and LBD patients. However, numerous studies have used lateralized presentation of concreteness in normal subjects to document each hemisphere's potential. Results of these studies are controversial, because some studies indicated that the right hemisphere can process concrete words, whereas others did not (Searleman, 1977). The reason for this discrepancy may be that there are methodological differences between the studies, including subject selection, but another explanation might find its source in psycholinguistics and the literature of cognitive psychology. Indeed, the question is whether concreteness by itself is the determining factor; whether it is a composite factor expressing other more basic features; whether it is intimately linked with other features to the point that its independent existence could be threatened; or whether concreteness is a genuine elementary factor but one that generates methodological problems because it is difficult to control for linked factors. The latter questions have been recently raised by Schwanenflugel, Harnishfeger, and Stowe (1988), who, when looking at normal subjects' performance in central vision, compared concreteness to imagery, frequency, semantic association, and meaningfulness, as well as to context availability. These authors found that context availability accounted most for the "concreteness" effect. Given the importance of the concreteness effect in understanding the contribution of the right hemisphere to lexical semantics, as well as to the effects of a right hemisphere lesion on lexico-semantic abilities, we need to undertake a series of studies to see what is (or are) the factor (or factors) that most suitably accounts for it. The question is still open, but the results obtained by Schwanenflugel et al. are certainly sufficient to question the legitimacy of the concreteness effects with regard to the right hemisphere.

In sum, the question regarding the concreteness effect is whether the concepts invoked are adequate. Although there may well be common lexical characteristics of the words that are best processed by the right hemisphere, concreteness might not be one of them. Again, this is how science evolves, but let us be reminded of it!

INFERENCING DEFICITS AMONG RIGHT-BRAIN-DAMAGED SUBJECTS: THE RIGHT RABBIT TO CHASE?

One of the most recurrent hypotheses about RBD patients' difficulties at the text level has been that they have a problem with inferencing abilities (for a review, see Joanette et al., 1990). Indeed, authors of numerous studies—many due to the original contributions of Hiram Brownell, Howard Gardner, and their colleagues in Boston—have proposed an inferencing deficit as a possible explanation for RBD individuals' impaired abilities at the text level. These studies looked at abilities such as understanding metaphors (Winner & Gardner, 1977), understanding indirect speech acts (Weylman et al., 1986), organizing the content of sentences (Delis, 1980), extracting the moral of a story (Wapner et al., 1981), inferring actors' attitudes (Cicone et al., 1980), or incorporating nonexplicit information in narratives (Joanette et al., 1986). However, the existence of an inferencing deficit has only been *suggested* by these studies, **not** *demonstrated*.

A certain number of studies did look at inferencing abilities *per se*, that is, the ability to produce new information by mentally manipulating other pieces of readily available information. These studies looked at either *pragmatic* inferencing or *logical* inferencing. The former refers to an inference for which at least one of the premises is previously known to the subject (usually part of semantic memory), whereas the latter is based entirely on new information or premises.

Only a few published studies have looked at logical inferencing abilities among RBD patients (e.g., Caramazza, Gordon, Zurif, & De Luca, 1976; Read, 1981). The results of these studies are not easy to interpret, though, given the problems they raise. For example, in the Caramazza et al. (1976) study, the authors conclude that RBD subjects have difficulties solving syllogisms because they have difficulties with the spatially based processes the authors claim to be necessary to accomplish the task. However, only the linguistic, determinants of the syllogisms have been investigated. In fact, Caramazza et al.'s results show that RBD subjects have difficulties when the adjective of the question is not the same as the adjective of the premise, that is, the so-called congruency of the predicates.

Searching for a way to cope with these problems, Joanette and Goulet (1987a) looked at the logical-inferencing performance of a group of RBD subjects compared to the performance of a group of normal age-, sex-, and education-matched controls. Logical inferencing was evaluated through the use of three-term two-relation syllogisms similar to the following: "John is taller than Paul, and Paul is taller than Bill. Who is the tallest?" To control for all possible determinants, both linguistic and spatial determinants of syllogism resolution were controlled for in the preparation of the stimuli. Thus, linguistic determinants such as the congruence and markedness of the comparators were considered. Syllogisms were also constructed in such a way that spatial determinants were controlled for. Thus, some syllogisms were *end anchored* (e.g., "Jane is taller than Linda, and Rachel is shorter than Linda"), whereas others were *center anchored* (e.g., "Linda is shorter than Jane, and Linda is taller than Rachel"). The results showed no difference whatsoever between RBD subjects' and normal control subjects' performances. For one or two types of syllogisms, however, there was a tendency for normal controls to perform at chance level, so one should interpret these results prudently. Nevertheless, the performances of the RBD subjects reflected a hierarchy in the spatial and linguistic determinants used to construct the syllogisms. Thus, the RBD subjects' performances were not simply random. In any case, these results, taken together with the ones previously cited in the literature, call into question the claim that RBD patients suffer from an inferencing deficit. Better controlled studies are needed to answer this question.

Convergent results were obtained for pragmatic inferencing. It must first be noted that a certain number of studies in the literature have been looking at such inferencing abilities among RBD patients (Brookshire & Nicholas, 1984; Brownell, Potter, Birhle, & Gardner, 1986; Goodenough et al., 1982; McDonald & Wales, 1986; Tompkins & Mateer, 1985). However, the results of these different studies are inconsistent and, taken together, inconclusive. In another study (Joanette & Goulet, 1987b), we looked at the pragmatic-inferencing abilities of a group of 30 RBD subjects compared to those of a group of normal age-, sex-, and education-matched controls. Pragmatic inferencing was studied in the context of sentences, a short text, and within produced narratives on the basis of iconographic material in which not all information was explicit. The details of the respective methods cannot be discussed here, but the results are very much convergent: There was no difference whatsoever between RBD subjects' and normal controls' performances. This series of convergent results is, by itself, in convergence with those obtained in the previously mentioned logical-inferencing study (Joanette & Goulet, 1987a).

In sum, from our experience with logical and pragmatic inferencing in RBD subjects, and from the literature that looked specifically at logical or pragmatic inferencing abilities among RBD subjects, it is certainly difficult to conclude that an inferencing deficit characterizes patients with a right hemisphere lesion. If, as it seems, this result is to be ascertained by future studies, reasons remain to be found that can account for RBD subjects' lower performances when faced with text-level tasks such as humor, sarcasm, or other previously mentioned abilities. Certainly, inferencing *per se* does not seem to be the only source of the problem. If this conclusion were to be confirmed by future studies, then what is the source of RBD patients' difficulties? One possible line of exploration is the concept of plausibility metrics put forward by Gardner, Brownell, Wapner, and Michelow (1983). In trying to understand a text, a listener regularly has to choose between many different possible meanings and submit these meanings to an evaluation of the relative *plausibility* of each in view of the specific context in which the verbal material has been provided. One example of this is the understanding of indirect speech acts. A given sentence such as *"The door is open"* can yield an incredibly large number of meanings, from the most literal to the most figurative. Just think of this sentence told at 10:00 A.M. by the person who is responsible for opening a museum and the same sentence expressed by a White House spokesperson after a Yeltsin-Bush meeting on denuclearization. Thus, plausibility evaluation and choosing the most plausible meaning are everyday necessities in verbal communication. However, the need for plausibility evaluation is not restricted to text-level processes; indeed, many of the experimental conditions used in research ask for such a plausibility evaluation. For example, Lesser (1974) asked RBD subjects to choose the best picture associated with a word in a study meant to aid in understanding lexico-semantic abilities.

A very large number of the tasks that have been reported in the literature as possible indicators of an inferencing impairment are also tasks in which the need for plausibility evaluation is high. For instance, in Brownell et al.'s (1986) study of backward inferencing, the results reported could be alternatively explained by difficulties in evaluating the relative plausibility of the different meanings. In this study, short texts induced first one inference in the subject and then another, forcing the subject to revise the first inference. To answer the experimenters' questions, subjects had to state whether a given more-or-less-plausible affirmation was the most convenient by reference to the initial set of sentences. Among these possibilities were the initial and the revised inferences. According to Brownell et al. (1986), RBD subjects performed less capably than did normal control subjects, choosing the revised inference significantly less frequently. At first glance, this result could indicate that RBD subjects had difficulties inferencing, as the title of the paper suggests. Looking at the RBD subjects' performances, however, the authors reported that RBD subjects did not choose the revised inference mainly because the first inference was maintained. In other words, the problem could also arise from a difficulty in choosing the right inference or from an inability to reject the first inference. Thus, one possibility is that RBD subjects had both inferences available to them but that the evaluation of the relative plausibility of these two inferences provided the context of the task, and the text was so limited that the first inference was chosen much more frequently. This possible explanation still has to be explored systematically, though, before the whole literature on the subject shifts from inferencing to plausibility in accounting for the verbal communication problems in RBD patients. In any case, it would be most surprising if there were only one possible cause to all the text-level verbal communication impairments found among RBD patients.

In fact, another avenue that will certainly be explored further is linked with the fact that RBD patients are impaired mostly on those aspects of verbal communication that could be characterized as the most difficult ones. In other words, when sufficiently precise and integrated conceptual frameworks are implemented, it may turn out that the aspects of verbal communication for which RBD patients have problems correspond to more effortful processes or to less common representations. One example of this pertains to the presumed specific impairments RBD subjects have with the metaphorical meaning of sentences or words (e.g., Brownell, Potter, & Michelow, 1984). In a recent study that looked at the ability of RBD patients to process the literal meanings of words (e.g., *pupil* as a part of the eye, or *warm* as a cue temperature), the secondary nonmetaphorical meanings (e.g., *pupil* as a student), and the secondary metaphorical meanings (e.g., *warm* as a cue on the nature of the relationship with someone), Gagnon (1992) suggested that it was nearly impossible to come up with a task in which the secondary nonmetaphorical meanings of words were precisely equivalent to the secondary metaphorical ones. Indeed, the strength of the association between a given word and its secondary nonmetaphorical meanings is only rarely equivalent to the strength of its association with any metaphorical meanings. Such a limitation could explain why RBD patients are said to have specific problems with the metaphorical meanings of texts or words: The integrity of the two hemispheres might be more important when the task is more complex, a simple bit of reasoning that makes simple sense. Applying this principle to the inferencing problem, one could argue that maybe part of the problems RBD subjects have is because to infer is more complex than not to infer, and that different types of inferences in different contexts may ask for greater contributions than other types and other contexts.

In conclusion, it is not certain that the text-level impairments documented among RBD patients are best understood as an inferencing impairment. In fact, inferencing may not be the issue. Plausibility evaluation appears to be a potentially interesting avenue to explore further, but even this might not be the answer. Ultimately, we need a more precise and integrated understanding of these text-level processes to eliminate the possibility that we may be facing a simple complexity hierarchy according to which the more complex the task is, the more the two hemispheres participate.

THE QUESTION OF THE CONTROL GROUPS: AN UNSOLVED ENIGMA

When we study how a right hemisphere brain lesion affects a right-hander's verbal communication abilities, there are at least two basic questions that require an equal number of control groups. The first question is whether a right hemisphere lesion affects verbal communication. For this purpose, verbal communication abilities are evaluated by reference to the performance of a group of normal control subjects matched according to all the factors thought to influence performance (e.g., age, sex, handedness, education). This procedure has been followed by many researchers in the field and has provided interesting results, despite the fact that not all the factors that might influence performance have been adequately controlled for in all studies (e.g., hospitalization).

However, strategies to address the second question are much less easy to implement. This question relates to the specificity of the right hemisphere's contribution and is typically expressed by asking whether the impairments in a given verbal communication ability are specific to RBD patients or whether they are present in any brain-lesioned patient. To answer this second question adequately requires a second control group, this one made up of non-RBD brain-lesioned subjects; given that there are only two hemispheres, the control subjects must be LBD patients. This is where the problems begin. Which LBD patients should be included in such a study? The first of many possibilities is to choose LBD patients with aphasia. The problem here is that the aphasia usually prevents those patients from executing the experimental task. The alternative is to rely on a group of mildly aphasic LBD patients. Now the problem is that this group might not be comparable with the RBD group, because the sizes and the localizations of the lesions might differ. Another possibility would be to gather a group of nonaphasic LBD patients with lesions equivalent in size. The problem here is that most of the RBD patients will have perisylvian lesions, whereas the nonaphasic LBD patients will have lesions of the frontal or the occipital poles. But let us imagine that someone is very patient and stubborn and does indeed find a certain number of nonaphasic or very mildly aphasic patients with similarly sized left hemisphere lesions in the perisylvian area. This would take time and effort, but it could be done. This time, however, the problem lies in the representatives of this group. Indeed, such a group inevitably will include individuals with a very unexpected and maybe deviant functional organization of the brain as regards language. It could be, for instance, that many of these individuals would develop an aphasia following a right hemisphere lesion, thus realizing a crossed aphasia (Joanette, 1989).

In other words, it may be easy to identify a control group for a study that assesses the presence of a deficit, but to identify one in a study that addresses the specificity question is much more difficult. In fact, it is our impression that no such ideal group exists. It may thus be necessary to look for convergences of results from many different control groups, including subjects whose deficits have a more general involvement of the brain, such as in dementia of the Alzheimer's type.

WILL THE REAL RBD PATIENT WITH VERBAL COMMUNICATION DEFICITS PLEASE STAND UP?

One question only rarely discussed in the literature is whether *all* RBD patients exhibit verbal communication deficits. Every clinician knows that this is not the case; anyone who has had the opportunity to evaluate a series of patients with a right hemisphere lesion can testify that not all RBD patients appear to have verbal communication impairments. Nonetheless, this reality has only rarely been echoed in studies of the verbal communication deficits among RBD patients. Indeed, in most studies, RBD patients are amalgamated in an experimental group not chosen with regard to the presence of such deficits. Thus, according to chance, some RBD groups of subjects may contain a higher proportion of communication-impaired subjects than others, which may account for some of the inconsistency in the literature.

In a previous study, Joanette, Goulet, and Daoust (1991) skimmed the RBD literature to document this question, highlighting two complementary sets of information. The first set of information consisted of 64 studies that pertained to more or less the same aspects of verbal communication; for example, 17 studies were about the performance of RBD subjects on an oral-naming task. Of those 64 studies, approximately half reported the presence of an impairment among RBD patients, whereas the other half did not conclude that such an impairment existed. In other words, if patients in these studies are indeed representative of the RBD population, one could infer that approximately half of all RBD patients present verbal communication deficits.

A second set of information comes from nine studies that distinguished between "impaired" and "nonimpaired" RBD patients. Indeed, some authors have looked at their group of RBD patients and tried to distinguish between those that performed more poorly than the controls and those that did not. The proportion of impaired RBDs was reported as highly variable. However, if one looks at the median, the figure is not incompatible with the 50% identified by Joanette et al. (1991). It is also somewhat comparable to the figure reported by Deal, Deal, Wertz, Kitselman, and Dwyer (1979). Indeed, these authors previously suggested that approximately two-thirds of RBD patients had communicative deficits, as measured by the *Porch Index of Communicative Ability*. Our clinical impression is that the figure is probably somewhat similar with regard to the proportion of LBD patients who show signs of an aphasia. If this latter impression were confirmed by a study, it could be concluded that the likelihood of a left hemisphere lesion producing an aphasia is roughly equal to the likelihood of a right hemisphere lesion producing verbal communication deficits—which also makes simple sense.

The subsequent question, of course, concerns the characteristics of those RBD patients with a verbal communication deficit. Why do some patients show such impairments and not others? Some years ago, one of the authors of this chapter participated in a study that provided some tentative answers (Joanette, Lecours, Lepage & Lamoureux, 1983). In this study, RBD patients' abilities were documented on a number ($N = 42$) of mostly traditional linguistic tasks. Results indicated three factors associated with the intensity of overall impairment ("none," "mild," and "severe," even though the most severe were still quite discrete clinically): first, the presence of a cortical lesion (versus a subcortical lesion, i.e., one involving the basal ganglia and thalamus); second, a family history of left-handedness; and third, a low level of education. These three factors are determined by the brain, genetics, and the environment, respectively. The first one— presence of a cortical lesion—is somewhat reassuring, if not unexpected. Even though a lesion affecting the subcortical structure can probably produce verbal communication impairments among RBD patients, just as it can produce an aphasia when the left hemisphere is involved, this finding testifies that cortical lesions are still more relevant. The second factor—familial left-handedness—is in convergence with many papers in the literature (e.g., Hécaen, de Agostini, & Monzon-Montes, 1981) that show familial left-handedness in right-handers to be associated with a lesser degree of left hemisphere lateralization for language. Consequently, a right hemisphere lesion may thus result in more important deficits. Finally, the third factor—education—is also convergent with the current literature on the relationship of education and the degree of the brain's functional organization for language. Indeed, according to Lecours et al. (1988), there is a tendency for less-educated individuals to exhibit a lesser degree of brain lateralization for language. Thus, if the right hemisphere makes a relatively more important contribution to language among less educated individuals, it is logical to note a more important effect of a right hemisphere lesion among those less educated individuals. This is what was found in that third factor. In addition, other factors have been suggested in the literature. As was previously mentioned, Gainotti et al. (1979) have suggested that RBD patients with communication impairments are those with a diminished intellectual functioning; we have already discussed this contribution as potentially circular. For Weinstein (1964), RBD patients with a communicative impairment would be those showing anosognosia. Even though this observation might be correct, the exact link between this clinical sign and the presence of a verbal communication deficit is still to be clearly understood.

As can be seen, not all RBD patients present a verbal communication deficit: The inclusion criterion—the presence of a right hemisphere lesion—is not sufficient to obtain a homogeneous group. Using this criterion appears more and more like trying to understand aphasia by studying groups of LBD patients, whether they are aphasic or not! It thus seems important to identify those subjects **with** a verbal communication impairment and to concentrate on those. This field could thus probably benefit from single-case studies, as is the case for the aphasia field. Given the problems in identifying those patients beforehand, an alternative way of facing this problem is to include a *post hoc* subgrouping analysis in each study. For example, Joanette, Goulet, Ska, and Nespoulous (1986) have used a hierarchical clustering technique to sort the subgroups of RBD patients with and without a given impairment. The exercise becomes interesting when one also includes normal control subjects in this process, because that allows for the identification of those normal controls who would behave like impaired RBD patients. The fact that not all RBD patients show a verbal communication impairment also has important clinical consequences. Indeed, it becomes more and more important to identify which patient has a problem before considering whether to offer some support.

PATTERN(S) OF VERBAL COMMUNICATION DEFICITS AMONG RBD PATIENTS: SINGULAR OR PLURAL?

The last aspect of the question of the verbal communication deficits among RBD patients that will be discussed here follows the preceding question logically. Indeed, if one is now convinced that not all RBD patients exhibit such a deficit, what about the pattern of verbal communication deficits among those who *are* impaired? In other words, is there only one pattern of impairments among all those who are affected? As one can imagine, there have been few contributions on this topic. The only indications known to us come from the previously cited study by Joanette et al. (1991). In this study the authors used three different tasks that tackled the word level (oral naming, or ON), sentence level (sentence completion, or SC), and text level (narrative production, or NP), respectively. Using a cutoff point based on the performance of the normal controls, results showed that of a total of 33 patients, 4 of them were affected on all three abilities, whereas 9 were not affected. However, the most interesting results come from the other 20 RBD subjects: These subjects showed that all possible patterns were possible and that opposite patterns could be shown to exist. Thus, 3 RBD subjects showed no impairment on ON and NP along with an impaired SC, whereas 6 subjects exhibited the reverse pattern, showing impairments on ON and NP with an intact SC. All three opposite patterns were found.

The next step is to look for the causes for these contrastive patterns. One possibility is that they reflect some kind of interindividual differences present before the occurrence of the lesion that result in distinctive expression of a similar lesion in different individuals. These interindividual differences could in turn result from genetic as well as environmental factors, some of them still to be unveiled.

However, another possibility is that these distinctive patterns are the expression of the extent and the localization of the lesion in the right hemisphere, presuming that the right hemisphere does contribute distinctively to verbal communication abilities. Hints for this possibility are found in the Joanette et al. (1983) study in which 42 RBD patients were classified according to the nature of the language deficits, that is, according to their pattern of impairments. A *post hoc* analysis indicated that two factors were at the source of these distinctive patterns: the extent of the lesion, and its pre- versus retrorolandic localization. Given that these two factors are linked, this result reduplicated for the right hemisphere what is probably the most universal characteristic about the relation between the left hemisphere and the different types of aphasia—namely, that an aphasia following a prerolandic lesion usually differs from an aphasia following a retrorolandic lesion.

Even though this study's results have to be further documented, they suggest that when the right hemisphere contributes to verbal communication, it does so distinctively. One of the biggest challenges of our field is to discover exactly how the right hemisphere is organized for verbal communication. Given that more than 100 years of contributions did not allow us to obtain satisfying answers with regard to the left hemisphere and language, this may be quite a challenge.

CONCLUSION: WHAT IS LEFT IN THE RIGHT HEMISPHERE, OR WHAT IS RIGHT IN THE LEFT HEMISPHERE?

The series of conceptual, methodological, and clinical issues that should be addressed with regard to the verbal communication deficits among right-brain-damaged patients is certainly not limited to the list of topics discussed in the present paper. This list was simply a start-up to which many other points could have been added, like the question of the evaluation and the treatment of those verbal communication deficits. But the present list may be sufficient to demonstrate clearly that the field is far from being able to produce all the answers it would like to produce. This conclusion is important for those interested in research opportunities because it opens a large number of avenues still to be explored. It is also of the utmost importance for determining the clinical approach to be used with these patients, for prudence must be taken in evaluating, labeling, and treating them.

But maybe the most serious issue to which this conclusion will provide any answer is the usefulness of the concept of a right hemisphere verbal communication deficit. Up to now, no particular aspect of verbal communication other than prosody has been unequivocally demonstrated to be affected following a right hemisphere lesion. Worse, there are indications that in some cases, nonaphasic LBD subjects can present some of the signs reported following a right hemisphere lesion. It may be that, by focusing on the RBD subjects' verbal communication deficits, we are focusing on one particular example of a "nonaphasiogenic" acquired brain lesion that affects one or many of the cognitive components necessary for normal verbal communication. We might do better to consider our subjects of interest to be those patients with one form or another of these verbal communication deficits, usually following a right hemisphere lesion, but not in all cases. Because it has been shown that the right hemisphere's integrity is needed for some of the more linguistic components of language, and that prosody depends on both left- and right-hemisphere-based processes, it might be suggested that we abandon the concept of a right hemisphere syndrome and replace it with the concept of a verbal communication syndrome that includes aphasia when the impairment mostly affects the properly linguistic abilities. This is not to say that all patients would be the same, but it might help all of us to consider these communicative impairments to be on a single continuum of verbal communication. Such a continuum would be under the constraints of many factors, including the localization of the lesion, both inter- and intra-hemispherically speaking. However, what is right is left to be discovered.

REFERENCES

Broca, P. (1865). Sur la faculté du langage articulé [On the faculty of speech]. *Bulletin de la société d'anthropologie, 6*, 337–393.

Brookshire, R. H., & Nicholas, L. E. (1984). Comprehension of directly and indirectly stated main ideas and details in discourse by brain-damaged and non-brain damaged listeners. *Brain and Language, 21*, 21–36.

Brownell, H. H., Potter, H. H., Birhle, A. M., & Gardner, H. (1986). Inference deficits in right-brain-damaged patients. *Brain and Language, 27*, 310–321.

Brownell, H. H., Potter, H. H., & Michelow, D. (1984). Sensitivity to lexical denotation and connotation in brain-damaged patients: A double dissociation? *Brain and Language, 22*, 253–265.

Caramazza, A., Gordon, J., Zurif, E. B., & De Luca, D. (1976). Right-hemispheric damage and verbal problem solving behavior. *Brain and Language, 3*, 41–46.

Chiarello, C., Senehi, J., & Nuding, S. (1987). Semantic priming with abstract and concrete words: Differential asymmetries may be post-lexical. *Brain and Language, 31*, 43–60.

Cicone, M., Wapner, W., & Gardner, H. (1980). Sensitivity to emotional expressions and situations in organic patients. *Cortex, 16*, 145–158.

Code, C. (1987). *Language aphasia and the right hemisphere*. Chichester: Wiley.

Critchley, M. (1962). Speech and speech-loss in relation to duality of the brain. In V. B. Mountcastle (Ed.), *Interhemispheric relations and cerebral dominance* (pp. 208–213). Baltimore: Johns Hopkins University Press.

Dax, M. (1836). Lésions de la moitié gauche de l'encéphale coïncidant avec l'oubli des signes de la pensée (Read at the Southern Conference held at Montpellier in 1836). *Gazette Hebdomadaire de Médecine et de Chirurgie, 2ème série, 2*, 259–262.

Deal, J., Deal, L., Wertz, R. T., Kitselman, K., & Dwyer, C. (1979). Right hemisphere PICA percentile: Some speculations about aphasia. In R. H. Brookshire (Ed.), *Clinical Aphasiology Conference proceedings* (pp. 30–37). Minneapolis: BRK Publisher.

Delis, D. C., Wapner, W., Gardner, H., & Moses, J. A. (1983). The contribution of the right hemisphere to the organization of paragraphs. *Cortex, 19*, 43–50.

Eisenson, J. (1962). Language and intellectual modifications associated with right cerebral damage. *Language and Speech, 5*, 49–53.

Ellis, A., & Beattie, G. (1986). *The psychology of language and communication*. New York: Guilford.

Frederiksen, C. H., Bracewell, R. J., Breuleux, A., & Renaud, A. (1990). The cognitive representation and processing of discourse: Function and dysfunction. In Y. Joanette & H. H. Browell (Eds.), *Discourse ability and brain damage: Theoretical and empirical perspectives* (pp. 69–110). New York: Springer Verlag.

Gagnon, L. (1992). Appréciation du sens métaphorique chez des sujets cérébrolésés droits. Unpublished master's thesis, Université de Montréal.

Gagnon, J., Goulet, P., & Joanette, Y. (1989). Activation automatique et contrôlée du savoir lexico-sémantique chez les cérébrolésés droits. *Langages, 24,* 95–111.

Gainotti, G., Caltagirone, C., & Miceli, G. (1979). Semantic disorders of auditory language comprehension in right-brain-damaged patients. *Journal of Psycholinguistic Research, 8,* 13–20.

Gardner, H., Brownell, H. H., Wapner, W., & Michelow, D. (1983). Missing the point: The role of the right hemisphere in the processing of complex linguistic materials. In E. Perecman (Ed.), *Cognitive processing in the right hemisphere* (pp. 169–191). New York: Academic.

Garrett, M. (1984). In D. Caplan, A. R. Lecours, & A. Smith (Eds.), *Biological perspectives on language* (pp. 172–193). Cambridge: MIT Press.

Goodenough-Trépanier, C., Powelson, J., & Zurif, E. (1982). Bridging in right-hemisphere patients. Paper presented at the Academy of Aphasia Annual Meeting, Lake Mohonk.

Hécaen, H., de Agostini, M., & Monzon-Montes, A. (1981). Cerebral organization in left-handers. *Brain and Language, 12,* 261–284.

Huglings-Jackson, J. (1879). On affections of speech from disease of the brain. *Brain, 2,* 203–222.

Joanette, Y. (1989). Aphasia in left-handers and crossed aphasia. In F. Boller & J. Grafman (Eds.), *Handbook of neuropsychology* (Vol. 2, pp. 173–184). Amsterdam: Elsevier.

Joanette, Y., & Brownell, H. (Eds.). (1990). *Discourse ability and brain damage: Theoretical and empirical perspectives.* New York: Springer-Verlag.

Joanette, Y., & Goulet, P. (1987a). Syllogistic reasoning in right-brain-damaged right-handers: Preliminary results. Paper presented at the Annual Meeting of the Academy of Aphasia, Phoenix.

Joanette, Y., & Goulet, P. (1987b). Inference deficits in right-brain-damaged right-handers: Absence of evidence. *Journal of Clinical and Experimental Neuropsychology, 9,* 271.

Joanette, Y., & Goulet, P. (1986). Criterion-specific reduction of verbal fluency in right-brain-damaged right-handers. *Neuropsychologia, 24,* 875–879.

Joanette, Y., Goulet, P., & Daoust, H. (1991). Incidence et profils des troubles de la communication verbale chez les cérébrolésés droits. *Revue de Neuropsychologie, 1,* 3–28.

Joanette, Y., Goulet, P., & Hannequin, D. (1990). *Right hemisphere and verbal communication.* New York: Springer-Verlag.

Joanette, Y., Goulet, P., Ska, B., Nespoulous, J. L. (1986). Informative content of narrative discourse in right-brain damaged right-handers. *Brain and Language, 29,* 81–105.

Joanette, Y., Lecours, A. R., Lepage, Y., Lamoureux, M. (1983). Language in right-handers with right-hemisphere lesions: A preliminary study including anatomical, genetic, and social factors. *Brain and Language, 20,* 217–248.

Laine, M., & Niemi, J. (1988). Word fluency production strategies of neurological patterns: Semantic and phonological clustering. *Journal of Clinical and Experimental Neuropsychology, 10,* 28.

Lecours, A. R., Mehler, J., Parente, M. A., et al. (1988). Illiteracy and brain damage: 3. A contribution to the study of speech and language disorders in illiterates with unilateral brain damage (initial testing). *Neuropsychologia, 26,* 575–589.

Lesser, R. (1974). Verbal comprehension in aphasia: An English version of three Italian tests. *Cortex, 10,* 247–263.

McDonald, S., & Wales, R. (1986). An investigation of the ability to process inferences in language following right hemisphere brain damage. *Brain and Language, 29*, 68–80.

Milberg, W., & Blumstein, S. E. (1981). Lexical decision and aphasia: Evidence for semantic processing. *Brain and Language, 14*, 371–385.

Myers, P. (1986). Right hemisphere communication impairment. In R. Chapey (Ed.), *Language intervention strategies in adult aphasia* (pp. 444–461). Baltimore: Williams & Wilkins.

Myers, P. (1984). Right hemisphere impairment. In A. Holland (Ed.), *Language disorders in adults* (pp. 177–208). San Diego: College-Hill.

Ombredane, A. (1951). *L'Aphasie et l'élaboration de la pensée explicite*. Paris: Presses Universitaires de France.

Posner, M. I., & Snyder, C. R. R. (1975). Facilitation and inhibition in the processing of signals. In P. M. A. Rabbit & S. Dornic (Eds.), *Attention and performance* (pp. 669–682). New York: Academic.

Read, D. E. (1981). Solving deductive reasoning problems after unilateral temporal lobectomy. *Brain and Language, 12*, 92–100.

Sabourin, L., Goulet, P., & Joanette, Y. (1988). La disponibilité lexicale chez les cérébrolésés droits. *Canadian Psychology/Psychologie canadienne, 29*, 2a.

Schwanenflugel, P. S., Harnishfeger, K. P., & Stowe, R. W. (1988). Context availability and lexical decisions for abstract and concrete words. *Journal of Memory and Language, 27*, 499–520.

Searleman, A. (1977). A review of right hemisphere linguistic capabilities. *Psychological Bulletin, 84*, 503–528.

Siéroff, E. (1991). Introduction à l'attention sélective: définitions et propriétés. *Revue de Neuropsychologie, 2*, 3–28.

Tompkins, C. A. (1990). Knowledge and strategies for processing lexical metaphor after right or left hemisphere brain damage. *Journal of Speech and Hearing Research, 33*, 307–316.

Tompkins, C., & Mateer, C. A. (1985). Right hemisphere appreciation of prosodic and linguistic indications of implicit attitude. *Brain and Language, 24*, 185–203.

Wapner, W., Hamby, S., & Gardner, H. (1981). The role of the right hemisphere in the apprehension of complex linguistic materials. *Brain and Language, 14*, 15–33.

Wechsler, D. (1955). *Wechsler Adult Intelligence Scale, Manual*. New York: Psychological Corporation.

Weinstein, E. A. (1964). Affections of speech with lesions of the non-dominant hemisphere. *Research Publications of the Association for Research in Nervous and Mental Disease, 42*, 220–228.

Weylman, S. T., Brownell, H. H., & Gardner, H. (1986). Comprehension of indirect requests by organic patients. Presented at the Annual Meeting of the Academy of Aphasia, Nashville, October

Winner, E., & Gardner, H. (1977). The comprension of metaphor in brain-damaged patients. *Brain, 100*, 717–723.

Clinical Aphasiology, Vol. 22, 1994, pp. 25–34

The Effects of Visual and Inferential Complexity on the Picture Descriptions of Non-Brain-Damaged and Right-Hemisphere-Damaged Adults

Penelope S. Myers and Robert H. Brookshire

Many of the descriptions of communication impairments associated with right hemisphere damage (RHD) come from studies in which patients have been asked to talk about complex pictorial stimuli. Investigators have found that RHD subjects have problems in interpreting or drawing inferences from pictorial materials such as (1) line drawings depicting metaphors and idioms (Myers & Linebaugh, 1981; Winner & Gardner, 1977); (2) cartoons depicting humorous situations (Bihrle, Brownell, & Powelson, 1986; Dagge & Hartje, 1985); (3) scenes portraying indirect requests (Hirst, LeDoux, & Stein, 1984; Foldi, 1987); (4) pictures presenting emotions conveyed through facial expression and body language (Borod, Koff, Lorch, & Nicholas, 1986; Cicone, Wapner, & Gardner, 1980); and (5) scenes depicting stories and events (Joanette, Goulet, Ska, & Nespoulous, 1986; Mackisack, Myers, & Duffy, 1987; Myers, 1979; Rivers & Love, 1980).

There are at least two competing explanations for these deficits. One is that they arise from a general inference deficit across modalities. Another is that they arise from a modality-specific problem in visual perception.

RHD is said to be associated with a variety of visual perceptual deficits, such as problems in recognizing pictured objects. These deficits surface when objects are embedded, incomplete, or rotated (Layman & Green, 1988; Warrington & James, 1967; Warrington & Taylor, 1973), and they may contribute to impairments in picture interpretation. Because pictures are two-dimensional, objects in these scenes are often depicted as embedded or incomplete to give depth to the picture. The more objects in the picture, the more likely objects will be depicted as embedded.

Left-sided neglect may also contribute to RHD patients' perceptual deficits by inhibiting their attention to left-side detail, and perhaps to contextual information anywhere in the stimulus array. For these reasons, RHD patients may have difficulty interpreting pictured scenes because they have problems perceiving what is in the pictures.

On the other hand, a common feature of the pictorial stimuli used in studies of RHD communication deficits is that their meanings tend to be implied rather than directly stated. That is, one must draw inferences about the pictorial stimuli to express their meanings fully. Evidence of inference deficits has been found in studies using verbal stimuli (Brownell, Potter, Bihrle, & Gardner, 1986; Molloy, Brownell, & Gardner, 1989; Weylman, Brownell, Roman, & Gardner, 1989) and may be a factor in studies using pictorial stimuli.

The issue of the relative influence of visuoperceptual and inferential deficits on the picture description impairments of RHD patients remains unresolved because few studies have controlled for visual complexity in their stimuli, and fewer have manipulated the inferential complexity of pictured scenes. The purpose of this study was to investigate the effects of visual and inferential complexity on the picture descriptions of RHD and non-brain-damaged (NBD) adults by manipulating the visual and inferential complexity of pictured stimuli within the same task. We asked whether communication deficits in response to pictured scenes result from a modality-specific problem with visual input or from a more general problem with inferring implied meaning. The results reported here are part of a larger study investigating the effects of visual and inferential complexity on RHD subjects' pictured scene interpretation.

METHOD

Subjects were 24 adults with unilateral right hemisphere damage (RHD) caused by a cerebrovascular accident and 30 non-brain-damaged (NBD) adults. RHD subjects had a mean age of 64 years (S.D. 12.73; 41–85 years), and a mean education level of 12.8 years (S.D. 3.81; 8–21 years). They were at least 1 month post onset. NBD subjects had a mean age of 78 years (S.D. 5.85; 66–88 years), and a mean education level of 14.2 years (S.D. 3.00; 8–21 years). All subjects were right-handed.

The stimuli were eight colored photographs of Norman Rockwell illustrations differing from one another in visual and inferential complexity. Visually complex (VC) pictures contained from 14 to 57 visually distinguishable objects; visually simple (VS) pictures contained from 2 to 10 objects. Inferentially simple (IS) pictures conveyed straightforward activities requiring little interpretation, whereas inferentially complex (IC) pictures required a greater number of inferences for accurate interpretation.

There were four sets of two pictures, representing the following four categories: (1) visually complex/inferentially complex; (2) visually simple/inferentially complex; (3) visually complex/inferentially simple; and (4) visually simple/inferentially simple.

The eight pictures came from a set of 32 Norman Rockwell illustrations. A series of validation trials with normal judges yielded the set of eight, two in each of the four categories. Eight of 10 judges independently agreed on the categorization of each of these eight pictures.

In the experimental task, subjects were asked to "tell what is happening" in each of the eight pictures. They were verbally cued to the left if they failed to mention any left-side information. Pictures were presented one at a time in four random orders counterbalanced across subjects. A training task was administered prior to the experimental task. The subjects were asked to describe from one to four pictures, depending on how quickly they learned the task. To participate in the study, subjects had to describe actions, as well as objects, in two consecutive training pictures.

Responses were tape-recorded and orthographically transcribed. A list of concepts (accurate and inaccurate) generated for each picture by the RHD and NBD subjects was compiled by the first author. The main concept measure came from the work of Nicholas (Brookshire & Nicholas, 1994; Nicholas & Brookshire, 1993) on discourse production in adults with brain damage. Each distinguishable idea contained in the transcripts was considered a concept. Any concept mentioned by at least two subjects was entered into the list. The total number of concepts per picture ranged from 12 to 27.

Those concepts identified by at least 30% of the NBD subjects were labeled "major concepts." To determine the proportion of major concepts identified for a given picture by a given subject, the number of major concepts mentioned by that subject in response to that picture was divided by the total number of major concepts for that picture.

Point-to-point agreement between the first author and a second speech-language pathologist on the presence or absence of specific concepts was calculated on randomly selected picture descriptions representing 10% of the sample. Point-to-point agreement on the presence or absence of specific concepts was 97% for both subject groups.

The effect of neglect on the proportion of major concepts mentioned was examined by dividing the RHD group into two subgroups. In addition to performing the experimental task, all subjects were given three tests of neglect—copying a simple scene, four line bisections, and a line cancellation task. Each subjects' scores on the neglect tests were combined to create an individual composite neglect score. RHD subjects with low neglect scores were placed in a "low neglect" (RHD/LN) group, and RHD subjects with high neglect scores were placed in a "high neglect" (RHD/HN) group. The low neglect group comprised 14 subjects with a mean neglect score of 6.8 and a range of 0–13; the high neglect group comprised 10 subjects with a mean score of 61.1 and a range of 14–159.

RESULTS

Subjects' responses to the eight pictures were divided among four conditions, with responses to four pictures in each condition: (1) visually simple; (2) visually complex; (3) inferentially simple; and (4) inferentially complex (see Table 1). In each condition one variable (e.g., visual complexity) was held constant while the other changed (e.g., inferential complexity). Thus, for example, the stimuli in the visually simple condition included both inferentially simple and inferentially complex pictures that were visually simple.

A groups by conditions repeated measures analysis of variance was calculated on the proportion of major concepts mentioned by the NBD, RHD/LN, and RHD/HN groups in the four conditions. The results yielded a significant main effect for groups ($F_{2,51}$ = 15.69; p. < .001); a significant main effect for conditions ($F_{3,153}$ = 36.58; p. < .001); and a significant groups by conditions interaction ($F_{6,153}$ = 3.72, p. = .002).

Effects of Conditions

To determine whether the conditions (visual or inferential complexity) affected the proportion of major concepts mentioned by subjects, t-tests were calculated for each group on the differences (a) between the proportion of concepts mentioned by subjects in response to visually simple and

Table 1. Picture Types in Each of Four Picture Conditions

Condition	Picture Types
Visually simple (**VS**)	**VS**IS (pictures 7 and 8)
	VSIC (pictures 3 and 4)
Visually complex (**VC**)	**VC**IS (pictures 5 and 6)
	VCIC (pictures 1 and 2)
Inferentially simple (**IS**)	VSIS (pictures 7 and 8)
	VCIS (pictures 5 and 6)
Inferentially complex (**IC**)	VSIC (pictures 3 and 4)
	VCIC (pictures 1 and 2)

Note: VSIS = Visually simple/inferentially simple; VSIC = Visually simple/inferentially complex; VCIS = Visually complex/inferentially simple; VCIC = Visually complex/ inferentially complex.

visually complex pictures and (b) between the proportion of major concepts mentioned by subjects in response to inferentially simple and inferentially complex stimuli. The familywise error rate for multiple comparisons was adjusted by setting the Type I (alpha) error rate at .004 (.05/12; the Bonferroni technique). There was no significant effect of visual complexity on the performance of any of the three groups (NBD: $t(29) = 1.34$, $p > .10$; RHD/LN: $t(13) = 0.23$, $p > .10$; RHD/HN: $t(9) = -1.31$, $p > .10$). In contrast, all three groups mentioned a significantly smaller proportion of major concepts in response to inferentially complex stimuli than in response to inferentially simple stimuli (NBD: $t(29) = 4.65$, $p < .001$; RHD/LN: $t(13) = 5.84$, $p < .001$; RHD/HN: $t(9) = 5.90$, $p < .001$; see Figure 1).

Effects of Groups

To examine the role of the group effect in the interaction, the simple effects of groups (NBD, RHD/LN, RHD/HN) within conditions (VS, VC,

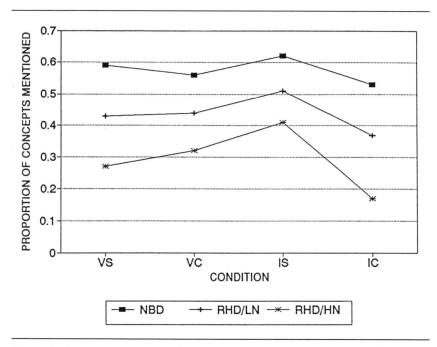

Figure 1. Average proportion of major concepts mentioned by non-brain-damaged (NBD), right-hemisphere-damaged with low neglect (RHD/LN), and right-hemisphere-damaged with high neglect (RHD/HN) subjects in the visually simple (VS), visually complex (VC), inferentially simple (IS), and inferentially complex (IC) conditions.

Table 2. Proportion of Major Concepts Produced by High Neglect (RHD/HN), Low Neglect (RHD/LN), and Non-Brain-Damaged (NBD) Groups

Condition	Significant Differences*
Visually simple	RHD/HN < RHD/LN < NBD
Visually complex	RHD/HN < NBD
Inferentially complex	RHD/HN < RHD/LN < NBD
Inferentially simple	RHD/HN < NBD

*$p < .05$.

IS, IC) were evaluated by means of a one-way analysis of variance for each of the four conditions. These analyses yielded significant group differences in all four conditions [(VS: $F_{2,51} = 17.65$; $p < .001$), (VC: $F_{2,51} = 9.04$; $p < .001$), (IS: $F_{2,51} = 7.82$; $p < .001$); and (IC: $F_{2,51} = 21.62$; $p < .001$)]. Post hoc Tukey HSD tests revealed that in all four conditions the RHD/HN group produced a significantly smaller proportion of major concepts than did the NBD group ($p < .05$; see Table 2). The RHD/HN group also produced a significantly smaller proportion of major concepts than did the RHD/LN group, but only in two conditions—visually simple and inferentially complex ($p < .05$). The RHD/LN group differed significantly from the NBD group in these same two conditions ($p < .05$), but not in the other two. This seemingly odd result, in which the visually *simple* condition appears to have an effect, turns out not to be so odd when one considers the effect of the inferentially complex pictures within the visually simple condition.

The effect of inferential complexity within the visually simple condition can be seen in the accuracy of subjects' inferences as depicted in Figure 2. Space does not permit a discussion of this measure, but the y-axis of the graph shows the percent of subjects' inaccurate inferences (IWIT) in response to the pictures in this condition. RHD subjects produced far more inaccurate inferences in response to visually simple/inferentially complex (VSIC) pictures than they did in response to visually simple/inferentially simple (VSIS) pictures. The VSIC pictures were among the most difficult for subjects to interpret, perhaps because they had so few visual cues or so little visual redundancy. The differences in performance accuracy clearly implicate inferential rather than visual complexity as the reason for the findings in the visually simple condition. Subjects, especially RHD subjects, had much more difficulty interpreting the two inferentially complex pictures than the two inferentially simple pictures that made up the visually simple condition.

To further evaluate the effects of neglect on the production of major concepts, the five major concepts for each picture that were mentioned

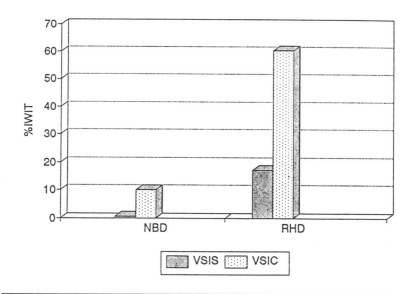

Figure 2. Effects of inferential complexity on visually simple pictures as demonstrated by percent of inference errors (%IWIT) made by non-brain-damaged (NBD) and right-hemisphere-damaged (RHD) subjects in response to visually simple/inferentially simple (VSIS) and visually simple/inferentially complex (VSIC) pictures.

most frequently by the NBD subjects were identified, and the correlation between the proportion of these concepts mentioned by each subject in the RHD group and his or her neglect score was calculated. The resulting Pearson correlation coefficient was −.60, suggesting that neglect has a moderate negative relationship to the proportion of major concepts mentioned by subjects in the RHD group. In other words, subjects with high neglect tended to mention a smaller proportion of major concepts than did subjects with low neglect.

DISCUSSION

The results of this study suggest that visual complexity has little effect on subjects' descriptions of complex pictured scenes. Both NBD and RHD subjects mentioned essentially the same number of major concepts in response to visually simple pictures as they did in response to visually complex pictures.

On the other hand, inferential complexity consistently affected subjects' performance. Both RHD and NBD subjects produced a significantly smaller proportion of major concepts in response to inferentially complex pictures than they did in response to the inferentially simple pictures. (A possible qualifier deserves mention. This study did not operationalize and measure how many main concepts were explicitly represented in the pictures, and how many were inferred.)

The RHD group as a whole tended to generate fewer major concepts in all conditions than the NBD group did, which suggests that RHD subjects are less able than NBD subjects to interpret and describe pictures. The high neglect RHD group produced significantly fewer major concepts in all conditions than the NBD group did, which was not the case for the low neglect RHD group. Subjects with high neglect performed similarly to subjects with less neglect, but they tended to be more impaired. There was also a moderate to strong correlation between subjects' neglect scores and the number of major concepts they produced, suggesting that the production of concepts may be associated with the severity of RHD subjects' neglect.

In addition, other measures too lengthy to report here demonstrated that both the RHD and NBD subjects were highly accurate in identifying pictured elements but that RHD subjects, particularly those with high neglect scores, were significantly impaired relative to NBD subjects in inferential accuracy. These findings suggests that RH subjects did not have difficulty recognizing isolated items in the pictures but that they did have trouble interpreting what they saw within the context of a given picture.

In general, the results of this study suggest that the impaired communication of RHD patients describing pictured scenes is more strongly related to the inferential than to the visual complexity of the pictured stimuli and that inference deficits are a more powerful explanation than visuoperceptual deficits for the observed impairments. Consequently, pictured scenes and pictured story sequences seem to be appropriate stimulus materials for testing RHD patients, despite the fact that RHD may be associated with visuoperceptual deficits. The results also suggest that manipulating the level of inferential complexity within pictured scenes may be a useful strategy for measuring at least some of the communication deficits exhibited by this population.

The results of this study also have implications for how RHD communication impairments are conceptualized. Some RHD patients seem to have inference deficits, regardless of the modality of stimulus input, verbal or visual. And in the visual modality, these deficits seem to be independent of visuoperceptual impairments. These results lend weight to the notion of an underlying or central inference deficit suggested by Myers (1991).

ACKNOWLEDGMENTS

The authors wish to thank the following institutions for providing subjects for this study: the National Rehabilitation Hospital and The George Washington University Medical Center, Washington, D.C.; Mount Vernon Hospital, Mount Vernon, Virginia; Healthsouth Rehab Center, Baltimore, Maryland; North Memorial Medical Center and the VA Medical Center, Minneapolis, Minnesota; and the Mayo Clinic, Rochester, Minnesota. The authors also wish to thank Anna L. Starratt, Elise Fitzpatrick, and Ruth Kozan for their efforts in recruiting non-brain-damaged subjects for the study.

REFERENCES

Bihrle, A. M., Brownell, H. H., & Powelson, J. A. (1986). Comprehension of humorous and nonhumorous materials by left and right brain-damaged patients. *Brain and Cognition, 5,* 399–411.

Borod, J. C., Koff, E., Lorch, M. P., & Nicholas, M. (1986). The expression and perception of facial emotion in brain-damaged patients. *Neuropsychologia, 24,* 169–180.

Brookshire, R. H., & Nicholas, L. E. (1994). Test-retest stability of measures of connected speech in aphasia. In M. L. Lemme (Ed.), *Clinical Aphasiology, Vol. 22* (pp. 119–133) Austin, TX: PRO-ED.

Brownell, H. H., Potter, H., Bihrle, A., & Gardner, H., (1986). Inference deficits in right brain-damaged patients. *Brain and Language, 27,* 310–321.

Cicone, M., Wapner, W., & Gardner, H. (1980). Sensitivity to emotional expressions and situations in organic patients. *Cortex, 16,* 145–158.

Dagge, M., & Hartje, W. (1985). Influence of contextual complexity on the processing of cartoons by patients with unilateral lesions. *Cortex, 21,* 607–616.

Foldi, N. S. (1987). Appreciation of pragmatic interpretation of indirect commands: Comparison of right and left hemisphere brain-damaged patients. *Brain and Language, 31,* 88–108.

Hirst, W., LeDoux, J., & Stein, S. (1984). Constraints on the processing of indirect speech acts: Evidence from aphasiology. *Brain and Language, 23,* 26–33.

Joanette, Y., Goulet, P., Ska, B., & Nespoulous, J-L. (1986). Informative content of narrative discourse in right-brain-damaged right-handers. *Brain and Language, 29,* 81–105.

Layman, S., & Green, E. (1988). The effect of stroke on object recognition. *Brain and Cognition, 7,* 87–114.

Mackisack, E. L., Myers, P. S., & Duffy, J. R. (1987). Verbosity and labeling behavior: The performance of right hemisphere and non-brain-damaged adults on an inferential picture description task. In R. H. Brookshire (Ed.), *Clinical aphasiology, Vol. 17* (pp. 143–151). Minneapolis: BRK.

Molloy, R., Brownell, H. H., & Gardner, G. (1989). Discourse comprehension by right hemisphere stroke patients: Deficits of prediction and revision. In

Y. Joanette (Ed.), *Discourse ability and brain damage: Theoretical and empirical perspectives* (pp. 113–130). New York: Springer-Verlag.

Myers, P. S. (1979). Profiles of communication deficits in patients with right cerebral hemisphere damage. In R. H. Brookshire (Ed.), *Clinical aphasiology, Vol. 4* (pp. 38–46). Minneapolis: BRK.

Myers, P. S. (1991) Inference failure: The underlying impairment in right hemisphere communication disorders. In T. E. Prescott (Ed.), *Clinical aphasiology, Vol. 20* (pp. 167–180). Austin, TX: PRO-ED.

Myers, P. S., & Linebaugh, C. W. (1981). Comprehension of idiomatic expressions by right-hemisphere-damaged adults. In R. H. Brookshire (Ed.), *Clinical aphasiology, Vol. 6* (pp. 254–262). Minneapolis: BRK.

Nicholas, L. E., & Brookshire, R. H. (1993). A system for quantifying the informativeness and efficiency of the connected speech of adults with aphasia. *Journal of Speech and Hearing Research, 36,* 338–350.

Rivers, D., & Love, R. (1980). Language performance on visual processing tasks in right hemisphere lesion cases. *Brain and Language, 10,* 348–366.

Warrington, E. K., & James, M. (1967). Disorders of visual perception in patients with localized cerebral lesions. *Neuropsychologia, 5,* 82–93.

Warrington, E. K., & Taylor, A. M. (1973). The contribution of the right parietal lobe to object recognition. *Cortex, 9,* 152–164.

Weylman, S. T., Brownell, H. H., Roman, M., & Gardner, H. (1989). Appreciation of indirect requests by left- and right-brain-damaged patients: The effects of verbal context and conventionality of wording. *Brain and Language, 36,* 580–591.

Winner, E., & Gardner, H. (1977). The comprehension of metaphor in brain-damaged patients. *Brain, 100,* 719–727.

Clinical Aphasiology, Vol. 22, 1994, pp. 35–51

Categorization Skills in Right Hemisphere Brain Damage for Common and Goal-Derived Categories

Monica Strauss Hough, Mary Jon Pabst, and Salvatore DeMarco

This study investigated the access and organization of common and goal-derived categories in adults with right hemisphere brain damage using a word fluency task. Common categories are groups of natural object concepts, such as vegetables and fruit, that have a graded structure (Rosch, 1975; Rosch & Mervis, 1975). In such a structure, not all members represent the category equally well; some members will be better examples than others and thus will more typically represent the category. Grossman (1981) observed that right hemisphere brain-damaged (RBD) adults performed similarly to non-brain-damaged (NBD) subjects in regard to the number of items produced and sensitivity to graded structure for common categories on an exemplar generation task. The RBD subjects, however, produced many clusters of items related to the target category. These consisted of atypical items whose referents held less obvious features in common. That is, the examples tended to be less representative and were not from the central portion of the semantic field. Joanette and Goulet (1986) found that RBD subjects named significantly fewer items, as well as fewer acceptable items, on exemplar generation than did normal controls; however, the typicality of responses within a category was not analyzed. Joanette, Goulet, and LeDorze (1988) found no significant differences between RBD patients and NBD controls in the number or pattern of errors produced on a semantic generation task. However, the RBD subjects produced fewer exemplars after the first 30 seconds of the task than did the NBD subjects. During the first 30 seconds, the RBD adult may be able to produce many exemplars because production is more automatic; that is, the exemplars are strongly linked to the superordinate. After the first 30 seconds, subjects may have to organize the activation of specific semantic information to produce more exemplars. This may be a less automatic process.

Barsalou (1983, 1987) investigated the structure of goal-derived categories. These categories, such as "things to inventory in a store," are constructed for use in specialized, goal-oriented contexts. They possess graded structures but are not as established in memory as common categories because people have had less experience with them. Minimal research has been conducted on RBD adults' knowledge of goal-derived categories. Because these categories may involve a construction process different from that of common categories, RBD adults may have difficulty using them. Specifically, producing goal-derived category exemplars appears to require an organizational strategy to achieve dimensions of the category goal; many diverse concepts and ideas are integrated under one category label. Given the nature of the organizational deficits observed in RBD adults when confronted with a variety of stimuli (Joanette, Goulet, & Hannequin, 1990; Myers, 1986), it may be expected that they will display impairment in generating examples for goal-derived categories. Furthermore, because they have difficulty in attending to critical information (Hough & Pierce, in press; Myers, 1990), RBD adults may fail to respond to the entire referential field of a category, thereby producing more atypical or out-of-set responses.

In the present study, the primary concern was the brain-damaged subjects' sensitivity to graded structure, particularly for goal-derived categories. The number of total and correct category responses, mean typicality ratings, and proportion of responses per typicality range were examined. An analysis of error types and a time production analysis also were conducted.

METHOD

Subjects

Ten adults who suffered right hemisphere brain damage as the result of a single cerebrovascular accident (CVA) and 10 NBD adults participated in the study. Subject characteristics and clinical test data are presented in Table 1. The groups did not differ significantly on age ($t = 1.80$; $p > .09$) or education ($t = 1.04$; $p > .30$). No RBD subject was less than two months post CVA. All subjects were right-handed by self-report. Unilateral neglect, identified through neurologic examination, was reported in 2 of the 10

Table 1. Subject Characteristics and Clinical Test Data

	Subjects	
Characteristics	Right Hemisphere	Non-Brain-Damaged
Age		
Range	45–79	44–75
Mean	65.80	60.80
SD	11.80	9.12
Years of Education		
Range	6–18	4–16
Mean	9.50	10.20
SD	3.66	3.68
Months post CVA		
Range	2–10	
Mean	5.30	
SD	3.30	
BNT		
Range	25-55	37–59
Mean	40.20	51.80
SD	9.99	6.63
TAWF		
Range	69–113[a]	75–111
Mean	85.00	96.2
SD	14.18	13.78
WAB Quotients		
AQ		
Range	93.8–97.7	
Mean	95.6	
SD	1.50	
CQ		
Range	81.2–95.8	
Mean	90.3	
SD	3.92	

Note: BNT = *Boston Naming Test* scores; TAWF = *Test of Adolescent/Adult Word Finding;* WAB = *Western Aphasia Battery;* AQ = Aphasia Quotient; CQ = Cortical Quotient.
[a]Standard scores.

subjects with right hemisphere brain damage. All brain-damaged subjects were administered the *Western Aphasia Battery* (Kertesz, 1982) to rule out the presence of aphasia and to determine overall cognitive involvement. The *Boston Naming Test* (Kaplan, Goodglass, & Weintraub, 1983) and the *Test of Adolescent/Adult Word Finding* (German, 1990) were administered to examine word retrieval abilities in both groups.

Table 2. Category Labels

Common Categories
Furniture
Fruit
Weapons
Sports
Clothing
Goal-derived Categories
Things to take on a camping trip
Things to take from one's house during a fire
Things to inventory at a store
Things that can float
Things that have a smell

Materials

Five goal-derived and five common categories were presented to each subject. Category labels are presented in Table 2. The common categories were 5 of the 10 categories for which Rosch (1975) has established typicality norms. The goal-derived categories had typicality norms developed by Hough (1988) with NBD middle-aged adults. In determining the typicality of an exemplar, a rating of 1 indicates that a member is the best example of a category, whereas a rating of 7 refers to the most unusual exemplar within a category.

Procedure

Subjects were asked to generate as many examples as possible for each category. No preset time limit was established; subjects took as much time as they needed and signaled the examiner when they had completed. However, exemplar production was timed to allow a breakdown of number and type of category response per time interval. Category labels were provided both auditorily and visually. All responses were hand-recorded and audiotaped.

RESULTS

Separate two-way ANOVAs were conducted on the mean number of total responses and the mean number of accurate responses on the common and goal-derived categories for both groups. Mean performance for both

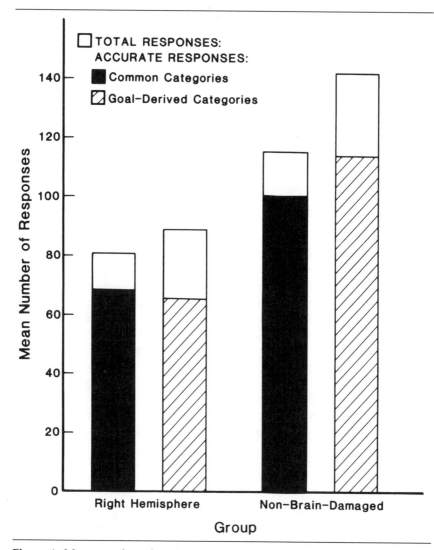

Figure 1. Mean number of total and accurate responses on the common and goal-derived categories for the right hemisphere and non-brain-damaged groups.

analyses is presented in Figure 1. The same pattern of performance was observed for both the total and the accurate responses. The NBD group produced significantly more total [F (1,18) = 13.15; p < .01] and accurate responses [F (1,18) = 19.12; p < .0004] than the RBD group for both category types. The NBD group produced significantly more total [F (1,18) = 4.72; p < .05] and accurate responses [F (1,18) = 5.60; p < .03] for the goal-derived than for the common categories, whereas the RBD subjects showed no significant differences between the two types of categories.

Subject responses also were evaluated in regard to typicality using Rosch's (1975) and Hough's (1988) norms for the common and goal-derived categories, respectively. Only in-set responses were evaluated. An ANOVA conducted on the mean typicality ratings data revealed significant differences only between category types [F (1,18) = 37.33; $p < .0001$]. Overall typicality means and standard deviations for the common and goal-derived categories were 2.2 ± .1 and 2.5 ± .2, respectively. Regardless of group, mean typicality ratings were significantly higher for the goal-derived categories than for the common ones.

The number of in-set subject responses within a particular typicality range was determined to obtain an additional perspective on subjects' appreciation of category centrality. The typicality ranges chosen were similar to those used by Grossman (1981) and Hough (1988). A repeated measures 2 Arcsin ($\sqrt{p}$) (Daniel, 1987) ANOVA with post hoc contrastive analyses (multiple comparison testing) (Kirk, 1982) on significant effects and interactions was conducted on the responses per typicality range. Significant findings were observed for typicality range, F (5,108) = 170.20; $p < .0001$; group × typicality range, F (5,108) = 2.79, $p < .02$; category type × typicality range, F (5,108) = 26.01, $p < .0001$; and group × category type × typicality range, F (5,108) = 2.38, $p < .03$. The data representing the significant three-way interaction are presented in mean proportions in Table 3. The primary significant findings pertained to typicality ranges 1 and 4: For the RBD group, significantly more common category exemplars fell within typicality range 1 than did goal-derived category exemplars, whereas a significantly higher number of goal-derived category exemplars fell within

Table 3. Mean Proportion of Responses per Typicality Range for the Goal-Derived and Common Categories

| | *Group* | | | |
| | RH BD+ | | NBD++ | |
Ranges	Common	Goal-Derived	Common	Goal-Derived
1.00–1.49	.352(.03)*	.216(.03)	.316(.05)	.261(.02)
1.50–1.99	.171(.03)	.161(.04)	.183(.03)	.173(.03)
2.00–2.99	.252(.04)	.255(.04)	.264(.03)	.270(.03)
3.00–3.99	.077(.02)	.202(.03)	.079(.02)	.140(.04)
4.00–4.99	.075(.02)	.088(.02)	.087(.02)	.091(.01)
5.00–7.00	.064(.03)	.061(.01)	.089(.02)	.070(.01)

* Standard deviations are in parentheses.
+ Right hemisphere brain-damage.
++ Non-brain-damaged.

Range 4 ($p < .01$). Although the NBD group showed a pattern of exemplar production throughout typicality ranges similar to the RBD group's, significant differences between the two category types for typicality ranges 1 and 4 were not observed.

Subject errors were identified and analyzed for both types of categories. The observed error types, their operational definitions, and examples are presented in Table 4. Interjudge percentage of agreement for identifying error types was 92%. Errors were analyzed in a three-way repeated measures ANOVA with contrastive analyses on significant effects and interactions. Only the following four error types were statistically analyzed: out-of-set related responses, out-of-set unrelated responses, hierarchically off responses, and repetitions. There were too few functionally off and jargon responses to subject to a formal analysis. Significant findings were observed for error type, $F (3,54) = 23.29, p < .0001$; category type, $F (1,18) = 23.41, p < .0001$; group × error type, $F (3,54) = 4.13, p < .03$; and error type × category type, $F (3,54) = 5.54, p < .008$. A trend toward significance was observed for the three-way interaction ($p < .065$) (group × category type × error type). This interaction was examined further because of some of the obvious observed differences between the two groups for particular error types on the two category types. Table 5 displays the mean number of errors for each error type for the goal-derived and common categories on both groups. Figure 2 displays the data representing the significant group × error type interaction. Data representing the significant category type × error type interaction are presented in Figure 3.

Several significant results were observed. The RBD group produced significantly more out-of-set unrelated responses than did the NBD group overall; it also produced significantly more of these responses on the goal-derived categories in particular. The NBD group produced significantly more hierarchically off responses than the RBD subjects did overall and also produced significantly more of these responses on the goal-derived categories. Overall, more out-of-set related, out-of-set unrelated, and hierarchically off errors were produced on the goal-derived than on the common categories ($p < .01$).

Subject responses were evaluated in regard to the number of exemplars produced during each minute of the experimental task in a repeated measures 2 Arcsin ($\sqrt{p}$) ANOVA. Significant findings included category type, $F(1,18) = 26.20, p < .0001$; time in minutes, $F(4,72) = 292.67, p < .0001$; and category type x time, $F(4,72) = 14.99, p < .0001$. There were no significant group differences. Figure 4 displays the mean proportion of responses for both category types based on time per minute across groups. Both groups produced significantly more responses for the common than for the goal-derived categories during the first minute of exemplar generation. During all other minutes, both groups produced significantly more responses for the goal-derived categories than for the common categories ($p < .05$).

Table 4. Error Types

Name	Description
Out-of-set unrelated	Responses that are outside the category boundary and have no relationship to a given category (e.g., "table" for the category "clothes")
Out-of-set related	Responses that are not category members of a given category but are members of a related category (e.g., "sunglasses" for the category "clothes")
Repetitions	Exact productions of previously produced responses for the same category
Hierarchically off	Responses that are not directly subordinate to the category label (e.g., producing "kitchen chair," "dinette chair," or "vinyl chair" for the category "furniture")
Functionally off	Responses that describe action or function of an object but are not specific referents of the category (e.g., for category, "clothes," producing "something you wear on your head")
Jargon	Nonmeaningful word or unintelligible response

Table 5. Mean Number of Responses per Error Type for the Goal-Derived and Common Categories

	Group			
Error Type	RBD[a]		NBD[b]	
	Common	Goal-derived	Common	Goal-derived
OSU	1.03 (.70)	3.42(2.32)	.65(1.04)	.95 (.75)
OSR	3.46(2.29)	5.36(2.61)	1.72(1.08)	4.39(2.99)
REP	8.69(5.61)	9.62(6.35)	8.88(5.35)	9.14(6.04)
HO	1.25(1.04)	3.87(3.94)	4.53(2.60)	14.95(9.06)

Note: Standard deviations are in parentheses. OSU = out-of-set unrelated; OSR = out-of-set related; REP = repetition; HO = Hierarchically off.
[a]Right hemisphere brain-damaged.
[b]Non-brain-damaged.

Pearson product-moment correlations were conducted between accuracy performance on the *Boston Naming Test* (BNT), standard scores on the *Test of Adolescent/Adult Word Finding* (TAWF), and the proportion of accurate responses and mean typicality ratings on the common and goal-derived categories for both groups. Table 6 presents the correlation matrices. For both groups, significant correlations of interest were found only between

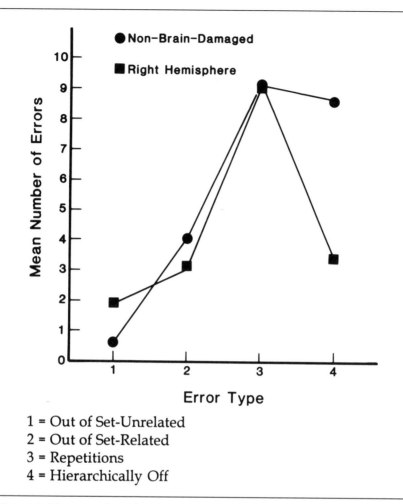

1 = Out of Set-Unrelated
2 = Out of Set-Related
3 = Repetitions
4 = Hierarchically Off

Figure 2. Mean number of errors per error type for the non-brain-damaged and the right hemisphere groups across category type.

the TAWF and BNT. For the NBD group only, a significant correlation was observed between the proportion of accuracy for both category types. For the RBD group only, a significant correlation was found between the proportion of accuracy for common categories and both the TAWF and the BNT. Overall, the results suggest that accuracy for goal-derived categories was related to accuracy for common categories only for the NBD group. Accuracy for the two category types was not related for the RBD group. Not surprisingly, significant correlational findings were not observed between the standardized tests and accuracy for either category type for

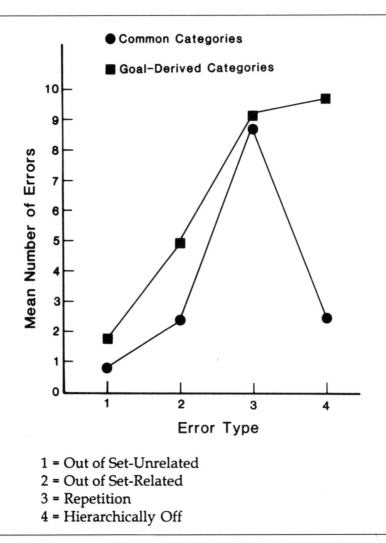

Figure 3. Mean number of errors per error type for the common and goal-derived categories across groups.

the NBD group. Interestingly, however, significant correlations were found between accuracy and standardized test results, for the RBD group, but only for the common categories. These results may suggest that exemplar generation for common categories is an appropriate measure of word retrieval skills, at least for adults with right hemisphere brain damage.

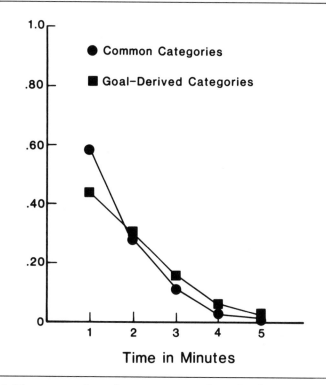

Figure 4. Mean proportion of responses per minute for the common and goal-derived categories across group.

DISCUSSION

In general, although the adults with right hemisphere brain damage produced fewer total and accurate responses for the common categories than the NBD subjects did, the two groups showed a similar overall pattern of performance for this category type. This finding is in agreement with Grossman (1981) and overall may be related to the construction of common categories. These categories appear to consist of actual structures for which an individual has a relatively defined representation in memory. Frequent processing of category information gives rise to the structures for these categories. Thus, the construction process for common categories may involve *automatic* access to the lexicon because of this familiarity with the category information. It is possible, therefore, that generation of category exemplars for common categories is not highly dependent on completely intact directed attentional or organizational skills. These skills

Table 6. Correlation Matrices: Task Performance and Standardized Naming Tests

	MT-C	MT-GD	BNT	TAWF	PRO-C	PRO-GD
			Right Hemisphere			
MT-C		.260	.152	.022	.316	.178
MT-GD			.141	.078	.165	.276
BNT				.591*	.927+	.237
TAWF					.559*	.433
PRO-C						.297
PRO-GD						

	MT-C	MT-GD	BNT	TAWF	PRO-C	PRO-GD
			Non-Brain-Damaged			
MT-C		.021	.173	.028	.357	.192
MT-GD			.153	.056	.142	.293
BNT				.881+	.372	.432
TAWF					.255	.458
PRO-C						.751+
PRO-GD						

MT-C: Mean typicality-common
MT-GD: Mean typicality-goal-derived
BNT: Boston Naming Test
TAWF: Test of Adolescent/Adult Word Finding
PRO-C: Proportion of accurate responses-common
PRO-GD: Proportion of accurate responses-goal-derived

+ = Highly significant (p < .01)
** = Moderately significant (.01 < p < .05)
* = Mildly significant (.05 < p < .10)

have been frequently cited as deficient areas for the RBD population (Hough, 1990; Joanette, Goulet, & Hannequin, 1990; Joanette, Goulet, Ska, & Nespoulous, 1986; Myers, 1986). Consequently, damage to the right hemisphere does not appear to affect the construction of common categories.

For the goal-derived categories, the RBD adults produced significantly fewer total and accurate responses than the NBD subjects did. More importantly, however, they showed a pattern of performance qualitatively different from that of the NBD subjects for the goal-derived categories. Other investigations have shown that normal aging adults produce more exemplars for goal-derived than for common categories (Hough & Snow, 1989) and produce more hierarchically off responses for goal-derived than for common categories (Hough, in press). Aphasic adults also have shown this pattern and have been observed to perform similarly to NBD adults on exemplar generation for goal-derived categories (Hough, in press; Hough & Pierce, 1988). In the current study, the RBD group showed no difference between category types in regard to the number of either total or accurate responses. Furthermore, although this group showed increased production of out-of-set unrelated errors and reduced production of hierarchically off errors for both category types compared to the NBD subjects, this pattern was significantly more apparent for the goal-derived categories. It is possible that right hemisphere brain damage inhibits the production of hierarchically off responses, particularly for goal-derived categories. The production of these responses by NBD adults may be an actual strategy used to produce more exemplars or to prime memory for production of other in-set responses.

The nature of goal-derived categories may have influenced the RBD subjects' performance. Whereas common categories may consist of defined entities represented in memory, goal-derived category construction appears to involve an actual creation process based on an individual's needs. This category development rests on an organized series of steps that a person must undertake to achieve the goal. Specifically, goal-derived category construction involves a generate-test process in which individuals rely on their previous knowledge and experience to produce dimensions relevant to the goal of a particular category. Persons use the associative structure of related well-established categories, such as common categories, to compare and then generate possible instances of a less established category. Normally aged as well as aphasic adults appear able to use their previous knowledge and experience and apply this information to current situations to achieve goal-derived category goals.

Goal-derived category construction may depend on the ability to make inferences. That is, to develop a goal-derived category, an individual must recognize the primary dimensions of the category and recognize their relationship to one another and to the category context or goal. It has been suggested that individuals with right hemisphere brain damage possess deficient inferential skills (Brownell, Potter, Bihrle, & Gardner, 1986; Joanette, Goulet, Ska, & Nespoulous, 1986; Mackisack, Myers, & Duffy, 1987; McDonald & Wales, 1986; Myers, 1986, 1990). Recently, it has been hypothesized that an inference failure may underlie most of the communication disorders associated with right hemisphere brain damage (Myers, 1990). This impairment may at times disrupt the necessary sequence of events involved in achieving goal-derived category objectives. That is, RBD individuals may not be able consistently to determine the relationship between key elements of a goal-derived category. Furthermore, they may have difficulty relating their previous knowledge and experience to achieve the goal of the goal-derived category in the current context. Consequently, they (a) produce more out-of-set responses that are unrelated to reaching the category objective; (b) produce a small number of hierarchically off responses, which may inhibit additional production of in-set goal-derived category responses; and (c) produce a greater proportion of atypical responses than NBD subjects do, although they produce fewer responses overall. Thus, it is possible that difficulties with inferential relationships may disrupt RBD adults' ability to generate exemplars consistently throughout the typicality spectrum for goal-derived categories. Their exemplar production patterns across the referential fields of goal-derived categories differ from the patterns of NBD adults. Inferencing ability may be less relevant to the construction of common categories because they are defined constructs in memory involving more automatic access to the lexicon.

Alternative explanations for the underlying bases of deficits observed after right hemisphere brain damage may be applicable to interpreting the current findings. As was previously mentioned, one of the hallmark behavioral characteristics of adults with right hemisphere brain damage is impaired organizational skills. Because these individuals may lack an organizing principle or have poor organizational strategies, they may fail to organize goal-derived category information in a logical pattern, thereby producing many tangential responses. They may verbalize relevant, less relevant, and irrelevant details in trying to achieve the goal of the goal-derived category. Consequently, they produce more atypical and out-of-set exemplars in attempting to organize dimensions relevant to the goal-derived category.

Another possible explanation for the present results relates to a generalized impairment in semantic processing. Although research findings have been unclear as to whether RBD adults display a true lexico-semantic processing deficit (Brownell, 1988; Joanette & Goulet, 1988; Joanette, Goulet, & Hannequin, 1990), this population has been observed to exhibit decreased performance on a variety of lexical and semantic tasks. Adults with right hemisphere brain damage have been observed to identify or produce literal rather than figurative or metaphoric interpretations for contexts or situations (Myers & Linebaugh, 1981; Winner & Gardner, 1977) and choose denotative rather than connotative meanings of words (Brownell, Potter, Michelow, & Gardner, 1984; Brownell, Simpson, Bihrle, Potter, & Gardner, 1990; Gardner & Denes, 1973). In conjunction with the present findings, these results suggest that RBD adults may have difficulty interpreting information beyond the perceptual level. This may occur because of problems integrating or combining semantic cues or associations, which appear to be necessary for the adequate construction of a goal-derived category.

Another possible underlying basis for the current observations may be a deficit in directed attention. RBD adults may be able to focus their attention to perceive or name exemplars but have difficulty combining or relating exemplars to one another to achieve the goal of a goal-derived category. It's possible that these individuals do not attend to the context or cues of the category label, particularly when it is not a defined representation in memory, as is the case for goal-derived categories.

Finally, the underlying basis for the present findings may be related to the *controlled* or *conscious* activation or access of the semantic component of the lexicon in constructing goal-derived categories. As was stated previously, common category construction may involve only *automatic* activation of the lexicon. Either hemisphere appears to be capable of this type of activation (Chiarello, 1985, 1988b; Joanette & Goulet, 1988); hence, RBD adults displayed minimal deficits in generating exemplars for common categories as they relied on their intact left hemisphere in undertaking this task. Controlled activation of the lexicon may be required for the appropriate generation of goal-derived category exemplars. This type of activation sometimes may involve the integration or semantic facilitation of both hemispheres to varying degrees. However, each hemisphere is unique in its semantic system, with the left hemisphere having a more focal, selective semantic system and the right hemisphere having a diffuse, nonselective system (Chiarello, 1985, 1988a). In the construction of goal-derived categories, there frequently is revision of the initial interpretation of the category goal or supplementation of this interpretation throughout the exemplar generation process. Right hemisphere brain damage may result in overreliance on the left hemisphere's selective semantic system, thus yielding limited interpretations of goal-derived category labels.

REFERENCES

Barsalou, L. (1983). Ad hoc categories. *Memory and Cognition, 8,* 211–227.
Barsalou, L. (1987). The instability of graded structure: Implications for the nature of concepts. In U. Neisser (Ed.), *Concepts and conceptual development* (pp. 101–140). New York: Cambridge University Press.
Brownell, H. H. (1988). Appreciation of metaphoric and connotative word meaning by brain-damaged patients. In C. Chiarello (Ed.), *Right hemisphere contributions to lexical semantics* (pp. 19–32). New York: Springer-Verlag.
Brownell, H. H., Potter, H., Bihrle, A., & Gardner, H. (1986). Inference deficits in right brain-damaged patients. *Brain and Language, 27,* 310–321.
Brownell, H. H., Potter, H., Michelow, D., & Gardner, H. (1984). Sensitivity to lexical denotation and connotation in brain-damaged patients: A double dissociation? *Brain and Language, 22,* 253–265.
Brownell, H. H., Simpson, T. L., Bihrle, A., Potter, H., & Gardner, H. (1990). Appreciation of metaphoric alternative word meanings by left and right brain-damaged patients. *Neuropsychologia, 28,* 375–383.
Chiarello, C. (1985). Hemispheric dynamics in lexical access: Automatic and controlled priming. *Brain and Language, 26,* 146–172.

Chiarello, C. (1988a). Lateralization of lexical processes in the normal brain: A review of visual half-field research. In H. Whitaker (Ed.), *Contemporary reviews in neuropsychology* (pp. 36–76). New York: Springer-Verlag.

Chiarello, C. (1988b). Semantic priming in the intact brain: Separate roles for the right and left hemispheres? In C. Chiarello (Ed.), *Right hemisphere contributions to lexical semantics* (pp. 59–70). New York: Springer-Verlag.

Daniel, W. W. (1987). *Biostatistics: A foundation for analysis in the health sciences* (4th ed.). New York: Wiley.

Gardner, H., & Denes, G. (1973). Connotative judgments by aphasic patients on a pictorial adaptation of the semantic differential. *Cortex, 9,* 183–196.

German, D. (1990). *Test of Adolescent/Adult Word Finding.* Allen, TX: DLM Teaching Resources.

Grossman, M. (1981). A bird is a bird is a bird: Making reference within and without superordinate categories. *Brain and Language, 12,* 313–331.

Hough, M. S. (1988). *Categorization in aphasia: Access and organization of ad hoc and common categories.* Unpublished doctoral dissertation, Kent State University, Kent, Ohio.

Hough, M. S. (1990). Narrative comprehension in adults with right and left hemisphere brain-damage: Theme organization. *Brain and Language, 38,* 253–277.

Hough, M. S. (in press). Categorization in aphasia: Access and organization of goal-derived and common categories. *Aphasiology.*

Hough, M. S., & Pierce, R. S. (1988). Word fluency revisited: Common and functional category structure in aphasic adults. Paper presented at the annual American Speech-Language-Hearing Association convention, Boston.

Hough, M. S., & Pierce, R. S. (in press). Contextual and thematic influences on narrative comprehension of left and right hemisphere brain-damaged adults. In H. Brownell & Y. Joanette (Eds.), *Narrative discourse in normal aging and neurologically-impaired adults.* San Diego: Singular.

Hough, M. S., & Snow, M. A. (1989). Category structure for goal-derived and common categories in aging. Paper presented at the annual American Speech-Language-Hearing Association convention, St. Louis.

Joanette, Y., & Goulet, P. (1986). Criterion-specific reduction of verbal fluency in right brain-damaged right-handers. *Neuropsychologia, 24,* 875–879.

Joanette, Y., & Goulet, P. (1988). Word-naming in right-brain-damaged subjects. In C. Chiarello (Ed.), *Right hemisphere contributions to lexical semantics* (pp. 1–18). New York: Springer-Verlag.

Joanette, Y., Goulet, P., & Hannequin, D. (1990). *Right hemisphere and verbal communication.* New York: Springer-Verlag.

Joanette, Y., Goulet, P., & LeDorze, G. (1988). Impaired word naming in right-brain-damaged right-handers: Error types and time-course analysis. *Brain and Language, 34,* 54–64.

Joanette, Y., Goulet, P., Ska, B., & Nespoulous, J. (1986). Informative content of narrative discourse in right-brain-damaged right-handers. *Brain and Language, 29,* 81–105.

Kaplan, E., Goodglass, H., & Weintraub, S. (1983). *Boston Naming Test.* Philadelphia: Lea & Febiger.

Kertesz, A. (1982). *Western Aphasia Battery.* New York: Grune & Stratton.

Kirk, R. E. (1982). *Experimental design: Procedures for the behavioral sciences* (2nd ed.). Belmont, CA: Brookes/Cole.

Mackisack, E., Myers, P., & Duffy, J. (1987). Verbosity and labeling behavior: The performance of right hemisphere and non-brain-damaged adults on an inferential picture description task. In R. Brookshire (Ed.), *Clinical aphasiology conference proceedings* (pp. 143–151). Minneapolis: BRK.

McDonald, S., & Wales, R. (1986). An investigation of the ability to process inferences in language following right hemisphere brain-damage. *Brain and Language, 29,* 68–80.

Myers, P. (1986). Right hemisphere communication impairment. In R. Chapey (Ed.), *Language intervention strategies in adult aphasia* (pp. 444–461). Baltimore: Williams & Wilkins.

Myers, P. (1990). Inference failure: The underlying impairment in right-hemisphere communication disorders. In T. Prescott (Ed.), *Clinical aphasiology,* Vol. 20 (pp. 167–180). Austin, TX: PRO-ED.

Myers, P., & Linebaugh, C. (1981). Comprehension of idiomatic expressions by right-hemisphere-damaged adults. In R. Brookshire (Ed.), *Clinical aphasiology conference proceedings* (pp. 254–261). Minneapolis: BRK.

Rosch, E. (1975). Cognitive representation of semantic categories. *Journal of Experimental Psychology: General, 104,* 192–233.

Rosch, E., & Mervis, C. (1975). Family resemblances: Studies in the internal structure of categories. *Cognitive Psychology, 7,* 573–605.

Winner, E., & Gardner, H. (1977). The comprehension of metaphor in brain-damaged patients. *Brain, 100,* 719–727.

Clinical Aphasiology, Vol. 22, 1994, pp. 53–65

Verbal Learning with the Right Hemisphere

Pelagie M. Beeson, Steven Z. Rapcsak,
Alan B. Rubens, and Kathryn A. Bayles

It is well documented that individuals with aphasia frequently exhibit verbal memory impairment (Albert, 1976; Butters, Samuels, Goodglass, & Brody, 1970; Goodglass, Gleason, & Hyde, 1970; Heilman, Scholes, & Watson, 1976). Short-term memory impairment, or reduced immediate serial recall, has been associated with all aphasia types (except the transcortical aphasias) and with lesions throughout the distribution of the left middle cerebral artery (DeRenzi & Nichelli, 1975; Gordon, 1983). A selective impairment of short-term verbal memory has been associated with lesions localized to the posterior parietal region (Shallice & Warrington, 1970; Warrington, Logue, & Pratt, 1971). Alternatively, deficits in verbal learning and long-term verbal recall have been associated with anterior lesions, particularly in the dorsolateral region of the left frontal lobe (Beeson, Bayles, Rubens, & Kaszniak, in press; Risse, Rubens, & Jordan, 1984). In the case of left hemisphere lesions that significantly damage the anterior *and* posterior regions served by the middle cerebral artery, impairment of both span memory and verbal learning would be expected.

In the process of testing 46 individuals with chronic aphasia as part of a larger study on memory impairment after stroke (Beeson, 1991), it was noted that two individuals with massive left hemisphere lesions performed surprisingly well on tests of verbal learning and long-term verbal memory. We report here on those two cases in relation to group data from Beeson (1991) and Beeson et al. (in press) that included normal control subjects and individuals with aphasia due to lesions confined to anterior or posterior brain regions.

METHODS

Subjects

Case 1. Subject GK was a 60-year-old male, 12.5 years post stroke at the time of testing. This previously right-handed man had undergone eleven years of formal education, had received a high school graduate equivalency diploma (GED), and had worked as a machinist and truck driver. Prior to his stroke, GK had no significant neurological history. His intelligence quotient estimated from demographic variables was 101.4 (Barona, Reynolds, & Chastain, 1984). There was no history of familial left-handedness.

Following a massive left hemisphere stroke at age 47, GK exhibited right hemiparesis, right hemisensory loss, right hemianopia, and global aphasia. His aphasia evolved to a Broca's type, and administration of the *Western Aphasia Battery* (WAB) (Kertesz, 1982; Shewan & Kertesz, 1980) yielded an Aphasia Quotient (AQ) of 69.5. GK's nonfluent, agrammatic speech consisted primarily of single words and short phrases of high communicative value.

Postacute CT and MRI scans revealed virtually complete destruction of GK's left hemisphere, including all regions served by the anterior, middle, and posterior cerebral arteries. A T_2-weighted MRI scan obtained close to the time of testing is displayed in Figure 1. The small islands of cortical tissue in the left hemisphere that are evident on the scan appear to be completely undercut and isolated and are of questionable viability.[1]

Case 2. Subject VH was a 73-year-old male, 5.5 years post stroke at the time of testing. He was previously right-handed, had 18 years of education, and was a retired U.S. Air Force colonel. He experienced a massive left hemisphere stroke at age 68 resulting in right hemiparesis, right visual field defect, and severe aphasia. During the 10 months preceding the stroke, VH had experienced intermittent right paresthesia without concomitant language difficulty. He has no known familial history of left-handedness other than one of his children, whose left-handedness was considered to be of maternal origin because of a documented history of left-handedness in his wife's family.

Administration of the WAB yielded an AQ of 60.7, with a profile of Broca's aphasia. VH's spontaneous speech was similar to GK in that it was nonfluent and agrammatic, but it yielded fairly successful communication with an active listener.

---

1. The extent of left hemisphere damage experienced by GK aroused our interest with regard to many aspects of performance, and accounts of GK's reading, writing, and praxis appear elsewhere (Rapcsak, Beeson, & Rubens, 1991a, 1991b; Rapcsak, Ochipa, Beeson, & Rubens, in press).

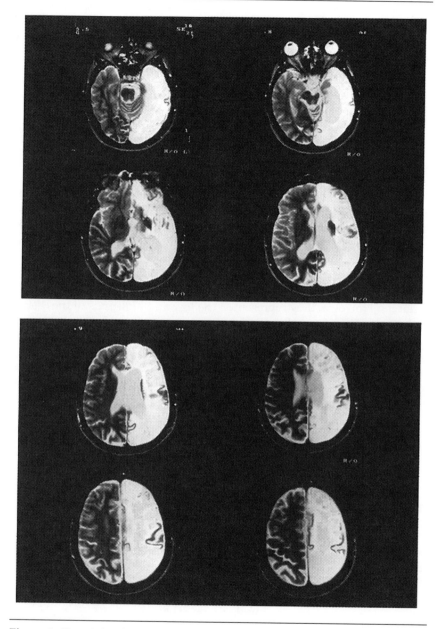

Figure 1. T_2-weighted MRI head scan of Subject GK demonstrating virtually complete destruction of the left hemisphere.

A recent CT head scan revealed an extensive left hemisphere lesion embracing essentially the entire distribution of the left middle cerebral artery, including the lenticulostriate branches, and most of the distribution of the anterior cerebral artery (Figure 2). Other than the left thalamus, the regions served by the left posterior cerebral artery were spared.

Group Data. The verbal memory performances of GK and VH were compared with group data from Beeson (1991) and Beeson et al. (1993). The subject groups comprised fourteen individuals who had experienced a single left hemisphere stroke resulting in persistent aphasia and fourteen demographically matched control subjects. Of the stroke patients, seven individuals had lesions of the frontal lobe (referred to as the anterior group) and seven individuals had lesions of the temporoparietal region (referred to as the posterior group). All subjects were native speakers of English and passed screening tests for vision and speech discrimination. The stroke patients were right-handed individuals who were neurologically normal prior to a single clinically documented stroke. All were at least six months post stroke at the time of testing.

GK and VH fell within the range of the group data for the demographic variables. However, they represented the low and high ends of the distribution, respectively, with regard to age, education, and estimated premorbid intelligence (Table 1). Whereas VH fell within the range of time post stroke for the group data, GK was tested at a later postonset time than any other subject. Both GK and VH obtained WAB AQ that were lower than the group means but still within one standard deviation from the mean of the anterior group.

Table 1. Subject Characteristics

Group	Age (years)	Education (years)	IQ (est.)	AQ (WAB)	Post CVA (years)
Subject GK	60	11	101.4	69.5	12.5
Subject VH	73	18	122.4	60.7	5.5
Anterior CVA (N = 7)[a]	63.5(7.0)	11.6(1.8)	105.1(6.7)	74.8(16.7)	4.8(5.9)
Posterior CVA (N = 7)[a]	67.0(7.2)	13.5(4.5)	108.6(11.8)	80.1(12.9)	2.5(2.7)
M	67.0	13.5	108.6	80.1	2.5
(SD)	(7.2)	(4.5)	(11.8)	(12.9)	(2.7)
Control (N = 14)[a]	68.7(8.6)	15.3(3.1)	113.4(5.9)	N/A	N/A

Note: AQ = Aphasia Quotient; WAB = Western Aphasia Battery.
[a]Data for anterior CVA, posterior CVA, and control groups are given as mean (standard deviation).

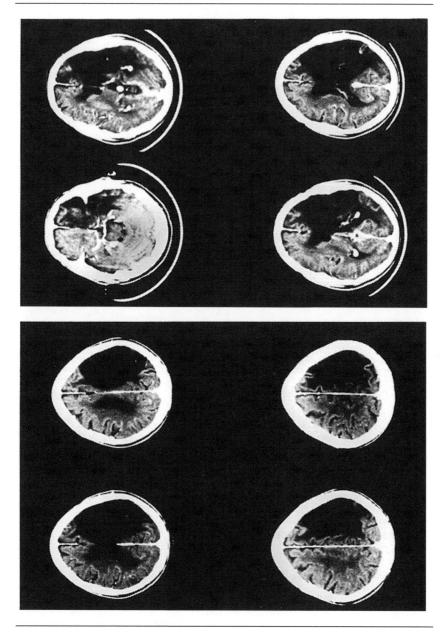

Figure 2. CT head scan of Subject VH demonstrating massive left hemisphere lesion affecting the entire distribution of the left middle cerebral artery and most of the distribution of the left anterior cerebral artery.

PROCEDURE AND RESULTS

Two verbal memory tests were administered to examine multitrial verbal learning and recall. One test was a replication of the selective reminding test (SRT) used by Risse, Rubens, and Jordan (1984) (after Buschke, 1973), which consisted of free recall of a nine-word list. High-frequency, concrete nouns selected from three semantic categories were presented orally. Immediately following list presentation, subjects were asked to recall as many words as possible, in any order. Subjects were selectively reminded of omitted words on 10 recall trials. GK was given a delayed recall trial (Trial 11) following a filled 15-minute delay.

The total number of words recalled on each trial included some words that were recalled immediately following list presentation or selective reminding (i.e., short-term memory) and some words that were recalled without reminding. According to the convention established by Buschke (1973), words that were recalled on two successive trials (i.e., recalled once without reminding) were thereafter considered recall from long-term memory.

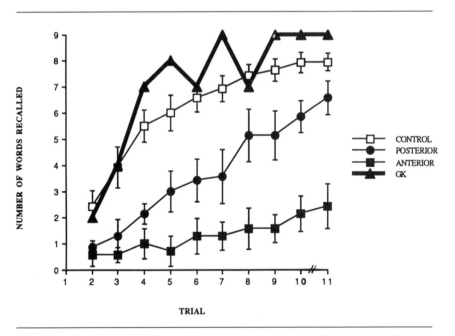

Figure 3. Recall from long-term memory on nine-word selective reminding test. (Subject GK's performance is shown along with the mean performance of control group and individuals with aphasia grouped by lesion location. Note that a 15-min delay was imposed between Trials 10 and 11. Anterior = frontal lesions; posterior = temporoparietal lesions. Vertical bars represent the standard error of the group mean.)

Long-term memory recall is depicted in Figures 3 and 4 for GK and VH, respectively, in relation to the anterior, posterior, and control groups. Both GK and VH exhibited verbal learning that most closely approximated the performance of the monaphasic control subjects.

The second verbal memory test required free recall and cued recall of an 18-word list presented using a guided semantic encoding task modeled after Grober and Buschke (1987). Labeled pictures were initially presented in groups of three for an auditory comprehension task that associated each item with its semantic category. For example, when presented with labeled pictures of a *trumpet,* a *foot,* and a *horse,* subjects had to point and say *"trumpet"* when asked *"Which one is the musical instrument?"* The stimuli were removed after all three items were identified, and an immediate cued recall trial was given wherein subjects were asked to recall the items in response to their semantic category (e.g., *"Which one was the musical instrument?").* All subjects successfully performed the comprehension task, and the immediate recall task was accomplished with no more than three opportunities given. Thus, it was documented that all subjects comprehended the list items, were capable of producing the item names, and had associated each item with its semantic category.

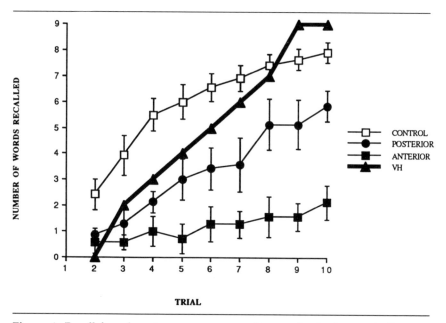

Figure 4. Recall from long-term memory on nine-word selective reminding test. (Subject VH's performance is shown along with the mean performance of control group and individuals with aphasia grouped by lesion location. Anterior = frontal lesions; posterior = temporoparietal lesions. Vertical bars represent the standard error of the group mean.)

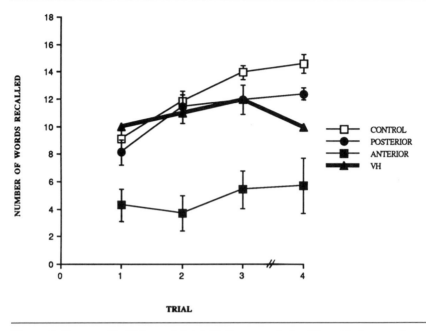

Figure 5. Free recall of 18-word list initially presented with guided semantic encoding procedure. (Subject GK's performance is shown along with the mean performance of control group and individuals with aphasia grouped by lesion location. Note that a 15-min delay was imposed between Trials 3 and 4. Anterior = frontal lesions; posterior = temporoparietal lesions. Vertical bars represent the standard error of the group mean.)

After all 18 list items were presented and a 30-second distraction task was performed, three free recall trials were presented. Each free recall trial was followed by semantically cued recall for unrecalled items and another 30-second distraction task to eliminate sustained subvocal rehearsal of list items. A delayed recall trial was administered following a 15-minute filled interval.

Figures 5 and 6 display free recall on the verbal-learning test with guided semantic encoding for GK and VH, respectively, in relation to the mean group performance. Their performance approximated the posterior and control groups on the initial recall trials and continued to approximate the performance of the posterior group over the repeated recall trials. Free recall by GK and VH was notably superior to the anterior aphasia group. Cued recall performance was high for all groups. The total number of words recalled by free recall plus cued recall was essentially undifferentiated for GK, VH, the posterior group, and the control group.

Short-term verbal memory was tested using the Digits Forward subtest from the *Wechsler Memory Scale–Revised* (WMS–R) (Wechsler, 1988). GK

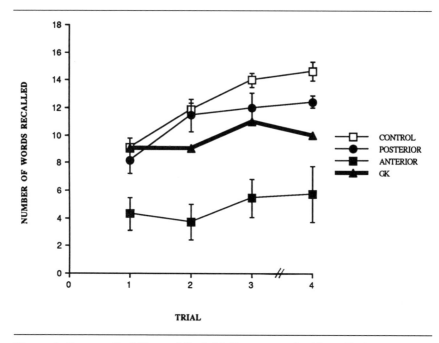

Figure 6. Free recall of 18-word list initially presented with guided semantic encoding procedure. (Subject VH's performance is shown along with the mean performance of control group and individuals with aphasia grouped by lesion location. Note that a 15-min delay was imposed between Trials 3 and 4. Anterior = frontal lesions; posterior = temporoparietal lesions. Vertical bars represent the standard error of the group mean.)

and VH each received raw scores of 3 for digit span, indicating spans of about three digits. The mean raw scores for the anterior ($M = 4.7$, $SD = 2.4$), posterior ($M = 2.3$, $SD = 1.4$), and control groups ($M = 7.9$, $SD = 1.4$) represented digit spans of approximately four to five digits, three digits, and six digits, respectively (Figure 7).

Visual memory span was assessed using the Tapping Forward subtest from the WMS–R (Figure 7). GK and VH exhibited visual memory spans of approximately 4–5 (raw scores = 6 and 7, respectively); the anterior, posterior, and control groups exhibited visual memory spans of 5–6 (raw score Ms = 8.3, 7.7, 8.5, respectively).

DISCUSSION

The relatively unimpaired, or mildly impaired, performance of GK and VH on tests of verbal learning and recall was quite surprising, consider-

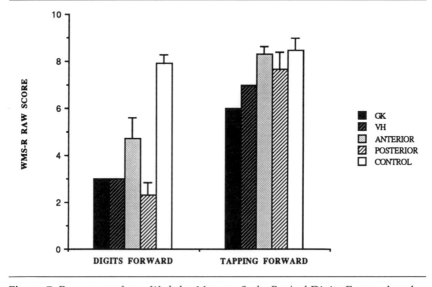

Figure 7. Raw scores from *Wechsler Memory Scale–Revised* Digits Forward and Tapping Forward subtests for Subjects GK and VH along with the mean performance of control group and individuals with aphasia grouped by lesion location. (Anterior = frontal lesions; posterior = temporoparietal lesions. Vertical bars represent the standard error of the group mean.)

ing the massive left hemisphere damage each had experienced. GK and VH consistently performed in a superior fashion when compared to the verbal learning of aphasic individuals with smaller lesions confined to the left frontal region. Their performance was either better than or similar to the mean performance of individuals with temporoparietal lesions. The findings could not be accounted for by aphasia severity because the AQs for GK and VH were lower than the mean AQs for the comparison groups. Furthermore, verbal-learning performance was independent of digit span, which was significantly limited for GK and VH, illustrating the dissociation of short- and long-term verbal memory noted by others (Risse, Rubens, & Jordan, 1984; Shallice & Warrington, 1970).

In view of the extent of the left hemisphere lesions in GK and VH, it is reasonable to conclude that their right hemispheres were responsible for accomplishing the verbal memory tasks. In the case of GK, the virtually complete destruction of his left hemisphere scarcely leaves an alternative explanation. A right hemisphere explanation is also favored for VH, rather than attributing his language and verbal memory abilities to the remaining tissue of the left frontal and occipital poles.

The linguistic demands of the verbal-learning tasks used in this study were relatively well suited to right hemisphere processing. The stimuli were highly imageable concrete nouns that are optimal for the lexical-semantic system of the right hemisphere, as revealed in studies of split-brain and left hemispherectomized patients (Joanette, Goulet, & Hannequin, 1990; Zaidel, 1985). A digit span of about 3 ± 1 is also consistent with previously reported right hemisphere capacity (Zaidel, 1985).

We hypothesize a shift to right hemisphere processing may be explained as a release of the right hemisphere from left hemisphere inhibition, thus allowing it to manifest its competence for verbal learning. Landis and colleagues similarly reported evidence of a release of right hemisphere linguistic processing with large left hemisphere lesions (Landis, Regard, & Serrat, 1980; Landis, Regard, Graves, & Goodglass, 1983). They claimed a correlation between left hemisphere lesion size and the release of the right hemisphere for verbal processing. We infer from our findings that the tenacity of the partially damaged left hemisphere in maintaining its role as the verbal processor may impede the right hemisphere's assumption of certain language-related functions.

It is important to acknowledge that large individual differences have been noted in the literature with regard to the verbal capacity of the right hemisphere (Gazzaniga, 1983; Sidtis, Volpe, Wilson, Rayport, & Gazzaniga, 1981; Zaidel, 1985). Clearly, GK and VH represent particularly well developed right hemisphere verbal ability, and all individuals with extensive left hemisphere lesions may not benefit from the shift of verbal processing to the right hemisphere to the extent that GK and VH did. Nevertheless, these two subjects demonstrate that in some cases, the right hemisphere is capable of accomplishing verbal learning with considerable competence.

ACKNOWLEDGMENTS

Preparation of this paper was supported in part by the National Institute of Deafness and Other Communication Disorders grant DC-01409 to the Institute for Neurogenic Communication Disorders at the University of Arizona.

The authors would like to acknowledge the cooperation of the Tucson Veteran's Administration Medical Center, Dr. Enrique Labadie of the Department of Neurology, in particular, and the Rehab Institute of Tucson. We also express our thanks to GK, VH, and Mrs. H for their cheerful participation in this research effort.

REFERENCES

Albert, M. L. (1976). Short-term memory and aphasia. *Brain and Language, 3,* 28–33.
Barona, A., Reynolds, C., & Chastain, R. (1984). A demographically based index of premorbid intelligence for the WAIS–R. *Journal of Clinical and Consulting Psychology, 52,* 885–887.

Beeson, P. M. (1991). Memory impairment associated with stroke and aphasia (Doctoral dissertation, University of Arizona, 1990). *Dissertation Abstracts International, 51,* 10-B, 4807.

Beeson, P. M., Bayles, K. A., Rubens, A. B., & Kaszniak, A. W. (in press). Memory impairment and executive control in individuals with stroke-induced aphasia. *Brain and Language, 45.*

Buschke, H. (1973). Selective reminding for analysis of memory and learning. *Journal of Verbal Learning and Verbal Behavior, 12,* 543–550.

Butters, N., Samuels, I., Goodglass, H., & Brody, B. (1970). Short-term visual and auditory memory disorders after parietal and frontal lobe damage. *Cortex, 6,* 440–459.

DeRenzi, E., & Nichelli, P. (1975). Verbal and non-verbal short-term memory impairment following hemispheric damage. *Cortex, 11,* 341–354.

Gazzaniga, M. S. (1983). Right hemisphere language following brain bisection: A 20-year perspective. *American Psychologist, 38,* 525–537.

Goodglass, H., Gleason, J. B., & Hyde, M. (1970). Some dimensions of auditory language comprehension in aphasia. *Journal of Speech and Hearing Research, 13,* 595–606.

Gordon, W. P. (1983). Memory disorders in aphasia: I. Auditory immediate recall. *Neuropsychologia, 21,* 325–339.

Grober, E., & Buschke, H. (1987). Genuine memory deficits in dementia. *Developmental Neuropsychology, 3,* 13–36.

Heilman, K. M., Scholes, R., & Watson, R. T. (1976). Defects of immediate memory in Broca's and Conduction aphasia. *Brain and Language, 3,* 201–208.

Joanette, Y., Goulet, P., & Hannequin, D. (1990). *Right hemisphere and verbal communication.* New York: Springer-Verlag.

Kertesz, A. (1982). *Western Aphasia Battery.* New York: Grune & Stratton.

Landis, T., Regard, M., Graves, R., & Goodglass, H. (1983). Semantic paralexia: A release of right hemispheric function from left hemispheric control. *Neuropsychologia, 21,* 359–364.

Landis, T., Regard, M., & Serrat, A. (1980). Iconic reading in a case of alexia without agraphia caused by a brain tumor: A tachistoscopic study. *Brain and Language, 11,* 45–53.

Rapcsak, S. Z., Beeson, P. M., and Rubens, A. B. (1991a). "Reading with the right hemisphere." Poster Session, 19th Annual Meeting of the International Neuropsychological Society, San Antonio, Texas, February, 1993. *Journal of Clinical and Experimental Neuropsychology, 14,* 39 (Abstract).

Rapcsak, S. Z., Beeson, P. M., and Rubens, A. B. (1991b). Writing with the right hemisphere. *Brain and Language, 41,* 510–530.

Rapcsak, S. Z., Ochipa, C., Beeson, P. M., & Rubens, A. B. (in press). Praxis and the right hemisphere. *Brain and Cognition.*

Risse, G. L., Rubens, A. B., & Jordan, L. S. (1984). Disturbances of long-term memory in aphasic patients. *Brain, 107,* 605–617.

Shallice, T., & Warrington, E. K. (1970). Independent functioning of verbal memory stores: A neuropsychological study. *Quarterly Journal of Experimental Psychology, 22,* 261–273.

Shewan, C. M., & Kertesz, A. (1980). Reliability and validity characteristics of the *Western Aphasia Battery* (WAB). *Journal of Speech and Hearing Disorders, 45,* 308–324.

Sidtis, J. J., Volpe, B. T., Wilson, D. H., Rayport, M., & Gazzaniga, M. S. (1981). Variability in right hemisphere language function after callosal section: Evidence for a continuum of generative capacity. *Journal of Neuroscience, 1,* 323–331.

Warrington, E. K., Logue, V., & Pratt, R. T. C. (1971). The anatomical localization of auditory-verbal short-term memory. *Neuropsychologia, 9,* 377–387.

Wechsler, D. A. (1988). *Wechsler memory scale–revised manual.* New York: Psychological.

Zaidel, E. (1985). Right hemisphere language. In D. F. Benson and E. Zaidel (Eds.), *The dual brain.* New York: Guilford Press.

Clinical Aphasiology, Vol. 22, 1994, pp. 67–80

Analysis of First-Encounter Conversations of Right-Hemisphere-Damaged Adults

Mary R. T. Kennedy, Edythe A. Strand, Wendy Burton, and Connie Peterson

The study of discourse has a long history in the field of speech-language pathology (Ervin-Tripp, 1979; Prutting & Kirchner, 1987; Sarno, 1969; Taylor, 1965; Ulatowska, North, & Macaluso-Haynes, 1981; Yorkston & Beukelman, 1980). Research in narrative and procedural discourse focuses on the examination of coherence and content in monologues, whereas conversational discourse emphasizes the dyadic interaction in turns (Duncan & Fiske, 1985; Searle, 1976). Conversational analysis provides an important vehicle through which to examine functional communication. Unfortunately, although narrative and procedural discourse have received much attention, there is little applied research on conversation (Stover & Haynes, 1989).

A limited number of studies have employed conversational analysis methods with brain-injured populations. Wambaugh, Thompson, Doyle, and Camarata (1991) compared conversations of six aphasic individuals to those of a control group (60 adults) and found that aphasic individuals displayed a variety of conversational skills, many of which differed considerably from the control groups. Conversational studies of cognitively impaired adult populations have employed a variety of elicitation procedures, measurements, and both familiar and unfamiliar partners, making comparisons of results difficult (Coelho, Liles, & Duffy, 1991; Mentis & Prutting, 1991; Penn & Cleary, 1988; Ripich & Terrell, 1988). However, the results of these studies generally seem to indicate that individuals with traumatic brain injury (TBI) and dementia produce more turns and words in their conversations. TBI individuals appear to be more passive participants, allowing the partners to direct the conversation, whereas individuals with dementia are frequently judged as being incoherent (Coelho et al., 1991; Ripich & Terrell, 1988).

Research on conversational characteristics of individuals with right hemisphere damage (RHD) is extremely limited. Descriptions of conversational management skills of the RHD group have been anectodal and include poor topic maintenance and termination, cohesion deficits, tangentiality, verbosity, poor eye contact, and inadequate prosody (Gianotti, Caltagirone, Miceli, & Masullo, 1981; Myers, 1986; Ross, 1981). Although these descriptive terms are useful clinically, they do not lend themselves to quantitative investigation. No studies have quantified the topic skills and turn-taking skills observed in this population's dyadic interactions.

PURPOSE

The purposes of this study were: (1) to identify and compare the dyadic interaction in turns between RHD and non-brain-damaged (NBD) groups; (2) to investigate the degree to which RHD and NBD individuals' conversation exhibits specific topic manipulation and turn-taking skills during first encounters; and (3) to examine the individual RHD subjects' patterns of performance in conversation.

METHOD

Subjects

Twelve RHD adults and 11 NBD adults served as the experimental and control groups. The RHD subjects were acute rehabilitation inpatients whose speech intelligibility was adequate for conversational discourse. Many of the RHD subjects demonstrated mild to moderate speech deficits, such as inadequate prosody and reduced vocal quality. All RHD subjects had been screened by a speech-language pathologist and had been referred for a complete communication evaluation and treatment program. Their mean time post onset was 3 months, and all had experienced a single cerebrovascular accident (CVA) in the right hemisphere resulting in a left-sided hemiparesis or hemiplegia. Subjects who had experienced hemorraghic and subcortical CVAs were included in the study, because the behavioral information from the communication screening did not indicate that their deficits were uniquely different from those who had experienced cortical thromboembolic CVAs. At the time of data collection, none of the RHD subjects had received discourse therapy. The NBD group matched the RHD group in age and years of education. No

Table 1. Characteristics of (RHD) Subjects

Subj.	Age (years)	Education (years)	Months post onset	Gender	Left neglect	Initial communication screening language/ cognition deficits
1	50	12	3	M	mild	mild/mod.–mild
2	45	14	1	F	min/mild	mod.–mild/mod.–mild
3	51	08	2	F	moderate	mild/mod.–mild
4	42	13	1	F	none	mod.–mild/mod
5	52	12	2	M	mod./sev.	mod/severe
6	33	14	2	M	moderate	mod.–mild/mod
7	61	12	3	F	severe	mod.–mild/mod
8	46	12	3	M	none	mod.–mild/ mod. sev.–mod
9	57	10	1	F	moderate	mod.–mild/mod.–sev.
10	39	14	12	M	mild	minimal/mild
11	38	14	2	M	moderate	mild/mod.–sev.
12	48	12	2	M	moderate	mild/mod.
Mean	46.8	12.25	3			
SD	7.9	1.7				

subjects in the study had a history of drug or alcohol abuse, seizures, or periods of unconsciousness. All subjects' primary language was English, and all had visual and hearing acuity adequate for speech communication purposes. Descriptive data are presented in Tables 1 and 2.

Procedure

The experimental protocol consisted of a first-encounter conversation between each subject and one of four certified speech-language pathologists or one trained graduate student in speech pathology who served as conversational patterns. Standardized instructions were given to the subjects and guidelines given to the therapists prior to their meeting:

> **Instructions to subjects:** I would like you to meet someone that you have not met before. She's a therapist here and I would like you to get to know her. This is not an interview, so she doesn't have a list of questions to ask you. She'll just talk with you to try to get to know you, too. A tape recorder will be used.
> **Guidelines to therapists:**
> 1. This is not an interview. Converse as you would with anyone you have met for the first time. Allow the partner to initiate topics.

Table 2. Characteristics of Non-Brain-Damaged (NBD) Subjects: Age in Years, Years of Education, and Gender

Subject	Age	Education	Gender
1	30	14	F
2	38	14	F
3	48	13	F
4	31	12	F
5	47	12	F
6	25	14	F
7	41	14	M
8	36	14	M
9	39	12	F
10	60	14	M
11	49	11	M
Mean	40.3	13.0	
SD	9.9	1.0	

2. Converse freely, giving your opinion and personal experiences so that the subject can get to know you.
3. Do not take notes during the conversation, but be a full participant.

Each subject was taken into a quiet room that contained a sofa, coffee table, and chair and was introduced to the clinician, whom the subject had not met before. The two were left alone to converse. A tape recorder was placed in an inconspicuous location. The clinician introduced a familiar topic typical of first encounters, such as "Do you live around here?" or "What do you do for a living?" (Kellermann, Broetzmann, Tae-Seop, & Kenji, 1989). After 12–15 minutes of audiotaped conversation, the clinician brought the conversation to a close.

Method of Analysis

Conversational parameters selected as dependent variables were organized into two broad categories: topic skills and conversational turn-taking skills. These dependent variables are part of a larger analysis called the *Adult Conversational Analysis Tool* (ACAT) and are summarized here (Kennedy, Burton, & Peterson, 1990):

Topic skills
Introduce: to bring up a topic in the conversation for the first time
Maintain: to continue with the same topic identified in the previous utterance without adding any additional information; to restate

Expand: to maintain the topic while incorporating additional information or details

Shade: to subtly shift the topic by adding new or detailed information

Reintroduce: to bring up a topic that has already been introduced

Terminate: to end a topic in conversation by explicitly bringing it to a close

Turn-taking skills

Represent: to make a statement as an assertion or conclusion of fact or opinion

Direct: to express an indirect or direct request for information or for action

Express: to make a statement that communicates a psychological state or emotion

Acknowledge: to produce an utterance that communicates that the listener heard or understood the speaker

Commit: to make a statement that indicates that the speaker will do something in the future

Each subject's conversation was transcribed using a turn-by-turn approach. The following characteristics were used to identify turns and are based on sequential-production (Sacks, Schegloff, & Jefferson, 1974) and signaling models (Duncan & Fiske, 1985). Turns were identified by

1. a period of silence by the speaker signaling the relinquishment of the turn;

2. an intonational change by the speaker signaling the relinquishment of the turn;

3. the taking of a turn, or interruption, in the absence of a signal by the speaker;

4. the grammatical completion of an ideational unit or strings of ideational units; or

5. one-word utterances such as "yes," "oh," "uh-huh," if occurring with characteristics 1 or 2 (see Stover and Haynes, 1989, for rationale).

The middle eight minutes of the conversation were extracted from the tape recording to avoid the highly ruled-governed introductory and closing phases of the first encounter. This portion of the recording was transcribed by three of the four authors. Individual turns were counted, and each turn was coded by type of topic skill (introduce, maintain, expand, etc.) and type of turn-taking skill (represent, direct, express, etc.). Results were then converted to percentages of total turns, to eliminate the variability of the number of turns in each conversation.

Reliability

To ensure interjudge coding agreement, 21% of the original transcripts were selected randomly. Two investigators, other than the original coder, coded the transcript, resulting in three analyses per transcript. Using turn-by-turn agreement in coding, judges reached 88% agreement for topic skills and 95% agreement for turn-taking skills.

RESULTS

The results of between-group comparisons are reported first, followed by individual profile data for the RHD group. To compare group data, a Mann-Whitney U test (Bruning & Kintz, 1977) was used to determine the presence of statistical differences. Table 3 provides the group mean percentages for the total number of turns and for each topic and turn-taking skill, as well as standard deviations and the U values for each.

The RHD group's conversations contained significantly more turns than the conversations of the NBD group. To determine whether an inverse

Table 3. Parameter Occurrence as Percentage of Total Turns

Parameters	NBD[a] mean	sd	RHD[a] mean	sd	U value*
Topic skills					
Introduce	.8	.4	.81	.7	59.5
Maintain	35	9.5	41	10.8	45
Expand	51	7.8	46	10	46.5
Shade	13	5.7	10.6	7.6	40
Reintroduce	0	0	1.7	2.6	48
Terminate	0	0	0	0	0
Turn-taking skills					
Represent**	81	5.3	86	10.5	32
Direct**	9	4.7	3.5	.8	21
Express	2.7	2.8	4.6	5.1	55
Acknowledge	7	3.9	5.5	.4	48.5
Commit	.27	.8	.5	1.4	49
Total turns**	31	6.2	45	8.9	12

[a]NBD = non-brain-damaged; RHD = right hemisphere damaged.
*Using a two-tailed test, the critical value of U at alpha > .05 was 33 or less for the difference to be significant (N_1 = 12; N_2 = 11).
**Significant differences present between groups on Mann-Whitney U test ($p < .05$).

relation existed between the number of turns in the conversation and the number of words per turn, a post-hoc analysis was performed. The number of words per turn was counted, averages were obtained for each subject, and using a Mann-Whitney U test, the number of words per turn for the two groups was found to be significantly different (U value = 23). In the RHD conversations, the subjects' mean words per turn was 15.8, whereas the therapists' mean words per turn was 9.9. However, in the NBD conversations, turns were longer, as is demonstrated by the subjects' mean words per turn of 25.8 and the therapists' mean words per turn of 13.7.

None of the topic skill parameters statistically differentiated the groups. In turn-taking skills the RHD group produced significantly more representative statements than the NBD group. The parameter of direct statements (requests for information) also statistically differentiated the two groups. The RHD group made significantly fewer requests for information (direct statements) than did the NBD group (see Table 3).

Figure 1 displays a comparison of the topic skills of the two groups using group mean percentages. Overall, the patterns of topic skills were

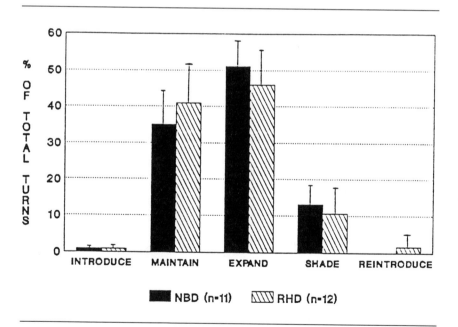

Figure 1. Group mean percentages of the total number of turns for each topic skill parameter for the non-brain-damaged (NBD) and right-hemisphere-damaged groups. (The bars indicate standard deviations. Terminating the topic was not displayed as neither group used this strategy.)

similar, although the standard deviations of the RHD group were larger than those of the NBD group (Table 3). It is interesting to note the frequency with which particular parameters occurred in both groups. Topics were expanded most frequently by both groups, although the NBD group used this strategy more than the RHD group did. Maintaining topics, which is a simpler strategy, was used more frequently by the RHD group than by the NBD group. Topics were changed in these first encounters by shading, which the RHD group used less than the NBD group. Topics were never reintroduced by the NBD group, whereas a third of the RHD group (4 out of 12) used this strategy.

Figure 2 displays a comparison of the turn-taking skills of the groups using group mean percentages. Representative statements (facts, opinions, etc.) dominated this category as subjects shared information about themselves. However, the RHD group produced significantly more representative statements than did their NBD counterparts. In requesting information demonstrated by direct statements, the RHD group used this strategy significantly less than the NBD group did. The other statement categories occurred infrequently and did not statistically differentiate the groups.

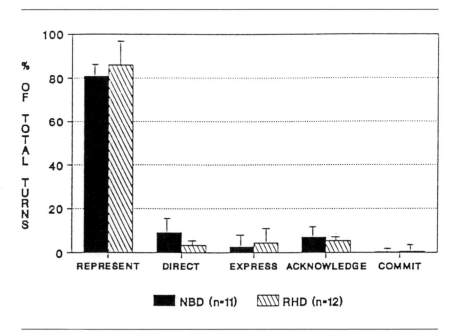

Figure 2. Group mean percentages of the total number of turns for each turn-taking skill parameter for the non-brain-damaged (NBD) and right-hemisphere-damaged groups. (The line bars indicate standard deviations.)

Table 4. Total Turns and Percentage of Total Turns for Each Topic and Turn-Taking Skill Parameter for Every RHD Subject

Parameters	1	2	3	4	5	6	7	8	9	10	11	12
					Subjects							
Topic skills												
Introduce	0	0	0	0	0	2[a]	2[a]	6[a]	0	0	0	0
Maintain	56[a]	32	57[a]	60[a]	37	40	30	45	44	24	33	37
Expand	36[a]	39	35[a]	40	58	50	50	40	45	65[a]	37[a]	5
Shade	8	22	6	0[a]	5	8	18	7	11	11	27[a]	5
Reintroduce	0	7[a]	2[a]	0	0	0	0	2[a]	0	0	3[a]	0
Terminate	0	0	0	0	0	0	0	0	0	0	0	0
Turn-taking skills												
Represent	88	92[a]	66[a]	96[a]	98[a]	75	91[a]	62	91[a]	91[a]	88	93[a]
Direct	0[a]	0[a]	6	2	2	9	5	6	2	4	6	0[a]
Express	5	4	14[a]	2	0	2	2	16[a]	5	0	6	0
Acknowledge	7	4	14	0[a]	0[a]	10	2	16[a]	0[a]	5	0[a]	7
Commit	0	0	0	0	0	4[a]	0	0	2[a]	0	0	0
Total turns	59[a]	28	49[a]	42[a]	40	52[a]	44[a]	55[a]	45[a]	55[a]	33	43[a]

[a]Values ≥ 2 standard deviations above or below the non-brain-damaged group's mean.

Because of the variable performance across parameters in the RHD group, it is perhaps more useful clinically to examine individual profile data demonstrating strengths and weaknesses in conversational skills. Tables 4 and 5 provide individual data in percentages of the total turns for each of the topic skills and turn-taking skills. Each RHD subject's profile is different from the others'. Figure 3 exemplifies this by comparing profiles of three RHD subjects. The NBD group mean is shown as 0 on the y-axis. The standard deviation from the normal group mean is represented by the bars. Each subject will be described individually.

CR (Subject 11) manipulated topics by shading while not expanding enough. He switched topics frequently without elaborating on them. The acknowledgments category was the only potentially problematic area in turn-taking skills. EC (Subject 4), however, used a more limited repertoire of parameters. Topic manipulation was characterized by redundant and repetitive maintenance and little topic shading. Turn-taking skills were limited to an overabundance of representative statements and infrequent acknowledgments. Likewise, there were many turns in her conversation as she relied on the partner to carry the conversation while she remained a passive participant. RG (Subject 3) excessively maintained topics while not expanding on them. In her turn-taking skills, she made emotional statements in the form of expressives, which inversely affected the frequency of representative statements. RG's conversation contained many turns.

Table 5. Total Turns and Percentage of Total Turns for Each Topic and Turn-Taking Skill Parameter for Every NBD Subject

	Subjects										
Parameters	*1*	*2*	*3*	*4*	*5*	*6*	*7*	*8*	*9*	*10*	*11*
Topic skills											
Introduce	0	0	0	0	0	0	0	4	3	0	0
Maintain	36	27	32	28	18	44	52	46	27	39	36
Expand	50	55	49	63	55	44	35[a]	43	62	53	52
Shade	14	18	19	9	27[a]	10	10	7	8	8	12
Reintroduce	0	0	0	0	0	0	0	0	0	0	0
Terminate	0	0	0	0	0	0	0	0	0	0	0
Turn-taking skills											
Represent	79	82	83	72	82	73	78	86	81	83	88
Direct	18	9	11	9	9	15	13	4	8	6	0[a]
Express	3	0	3	6	0	0	0	7	3	0	8
Acknowledge	0[a]	9	3	13	9	12	6	3	8	11	4
Commit	0	0	0	0	0	0	3[a]	0	0	0	0
Total turns	28	22	37	32	22	41	31	28	37	36	25

[a]Values ≥ 2 standard deviations above or below the non-brain-damaged group's mean.

DISCUSSION

The finding that the RHD subjects took significantly more turns than the NBD group is consistent with the findings of other conversational studies on individuals with TBI and dementia (Coehlo et al., 1991; Ripich & Terrell, 1989). One explanation for this finding is the inverse relationship between the number of words per turn and the total number of turns in the conversation. The RHD subjects produced far fewer words per turn than the NBD subjects. The therapists allowed the subjects in both groups to set the pace, as indicated by the relative adjustment in the length of their turns (shorter turns with the RHD subjects and longer turns with the NBD subjects). Therefore, it appears that although some RHD subjects' conversations contained proportions of topic skills and turn-taking skills similar to the NBD subjects', this was accomplished with less elaboration.

During these first-encounter conversations, some RHD individuals were likely to ask fewer questions of their partners and talk more about themselves than their NBD counterparts. For these individuals, the more they talked about themselves, the less they requested information from their partners. Additionally, some of the RHD subjects used the simpler topic skills of maintaining and reintroducing the topic. Instead of asking a

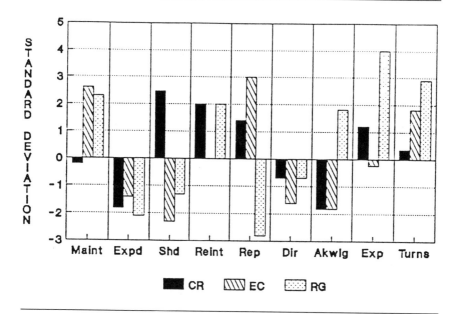

Figure 3. Conversational profiles for three right-hemisphere-damaged subjects. (CR = Subject 11; EC = Subject 4; RG = Subject 3. The non-brain-damaged [NBD] group mean is shown as 0 on the y-axis. The standard deviation from the NBD group mean is represented by the shaded bars. Bars with values below 0 indicate the number of standard deviations below the NBD group mean. Bars with values above 0 indicate the number of standard deviations above the NBD group mean.)

question of their partner, they relied on these two simpler strategies. For these subjects, perhaps there were more turns because their strategies had become simplified and thus required fewer words.

The fact that the various topic skill parameters did not differentiate the NBD and RHD groups is intriguing, given the anecdotal descriptions of topic skills in the literature. One explanation may be related to the use of the turn as the unit of analysis regardless of its length. The turn is sensitive to various turn-taking skills, but topic manipulation may require a smaller unit of analysis, such as the propositional unit recommended by narrative researchers (Joanette & Goulet, 1990). Conversely, however, the coherence skills of cognitively impaired individuals may provide more information regarding overall topic organization than a finer level of analysis would allow (Glosser & Deser, 1990). These two types of analyses warrant further investigation.

The group data from this study should be interpreted with caution. First, as indicated by the large standard deviations within the RHD group, some RHD individuals are severely limited in their conversational skills, whereas others are close to the norm. Second, the small size of both groups in this study makes it difficult to draw conclusions about the populations in general. Third, the groups may have differed in their perceived social relationship to the communication partner. Although both subject groups were aware that the partners were speech-language pathologists, the RHD subjects may have assumed a more passive role in the conversation because they might not have perceived the partner as being on equal ground. Nevertheless, though this perceived inequity might have been a factor, it should have applied across the board. The NBD subjects were all individuals who were employed at the hospital in clerical, maintenance, or therapy assistant positions. Thus, there was also an unequal social relationship between the NBD subjects and the speech pathologist partners. An additional control group of non-brain-damaged patients would be needed to resolve this issue. Finally, the gender proportion in the RHD and NBD groups was slightly unequal. Tannen (1990) indicates that men and women differ in their conversational styles, particularly in the use and comprehension of indirect requests. To determine whether there were conversational differences between men and women in this study, a post hoc analysis was performed on all the dependent measures using the Mann-Whitney U test ($p > .05$). No significant differences were found.

The above discussion highlights the point that studies using small groups to investigate conversational skills are difficult to interpret. Future research should focus on large group studies of normal and neurologically impaired populations to document various conversational patterns. Longitudinal studies should also be implemented to investigate communicative skill in conversation. Examination of dyadic discourse during disease progression (e.g., for Alzheimer's patients) and during periods of spontaneous recovery of cognitively impaired patients will lead to a better understanding of how these conversational deficits affect communication efficiency and the ability to complete communicative intent.

This study illustrates the clinical importance of examining individual profile data in planning treatment. Although these profiles identify specific communication patterns, they do not indicate *how* conversational skills have changed as a result of a CVA. Interviews with family members and the use of a communication inventory to determine the individual's premorbid conversational style could provide clinicians with useful information from which to make comparisons. Perhaps instead of identifying a conversational impairment based on group normative data, it would be more clinically useful to identify a conversational impairment based on premorbid conversational style.

Continued research in dyadic conversational discourse in neurologically impaired individuals is clearly warranted. Through such work, clinical researchers will be better able to identify communicative impairment and plan appropriate treatment. Further, this research will facilitate continued refinement of models of pragmatic/language performance.

REFERENCES

Bruning, J. L., & Kintz, B. L. (1977). *Computational handbook of statistics* (pp. 224–227). Glenview, IL: Scott, Foresman.

Coelho, C., Liles, B., & Duffy, R. (1991). Analysis of conversational discourse in head-injured adults. *Journal of Head Injury Rehabilitation, 6* (2), 92–99.

Duncan, F., & Fiske, D. (1985). *Interaction structure & strategy.* New York: Cambridge University Press.

Ervin-Tripp, S. (1979). Children's verbal turn taking. In E. Ochs & B. Schieffelin (Eds.), *Developmental pragmatics* (pp. 391–429). New York: Academic Press.

Gianotti, G., Caltagirone, C., Miceli, G., & Masullo, C. (1981). Selective semantic-lexical impairment of language comprehension in right-brain-damaged patients. *Brain and Language, 13,* 201–211.

Glosser, G., & Deser, T. (1990). Patterns of discourse production among neurological patients with fluent language disorders. *Brain and Language, 40,* 67–88.

Joanette, Y., & Goulet, P. (1990). Narrative discourse in right-brain-damaged right-handers. In Y. Joanette & H. H. Brownell (Eds.), *Discourse ability and brain damage: Theoretical and empirical perspectives* (pp. 131–153). New York: Springer-Verlag.

Kellermann, K., Broetzmann, S., Tae-Seop, L., & Kenji, K. (1989). The conversation mop: Scenes in the stream of discourse. *Discourse Processes, 12,* 27–61.

Kennedy, M., Burton, W., & Peterson, C. (1990). *Adult conversational analysis tool.* Unpublished manuscript, Rancho Los Amigos Medical Center, Downey, CA.

Mentis, M., & Prutting, C. (1991). Analysis of topic as illustrated in a head-injured and a normal adult. *Journal of Speech and Hearing Research, 34* (3), 583–595.

Myers, P. (1986) Right hemisphere communication impairment. In R. Chapey (Ed.), *Language intervention strategies in adult aphasia* (pp. 444–461). Baltimore: Williams & Wilkins.

Penn, C., & Cleary, J. (1988). Compensatory strategies in the language of closed head injured patients. *Brain Injury, 2,* 3–17.

Prutting, C., & Kirchner, D. (1987). A clinical appraisal of the pragmatic aspects of language. *Journal of Speech and Hearing Disorders, 52,* 105–119.

Ripich, D., & Terrell, B. (1988). Patterns of discourse cohesion and coherence in Alzheimer's disease. *Journal of Speech and Hearing Disorders, 53,* 8–15.

Ross, E. (1981). The aprosodias. *Archives of Neurology, 38,* 561–569.

Sacks, H., Schegloff, E., & Jefferson, G. (1974). A simplest systematics for the organization of turn-taking for conversation. *Language, 50,* 696–735.

Sarno, M. (1969). *The Functional Communication Profile.* New York: NYU Medical Center, Institute of Rehabilitation Medicine.

Searle, J. (1976). A classification of illocutionary acts. *Language in Society, 5,* 1–23.

Stover, S., & Haynes, W. (1989). Topic manipulation and cohesive adequacy in conversations of normal adults between the ages of 30 and 90. *Clinical Linguistics & Phonetics, 3* (2) 137–149.

Tannen, D. (1990). *You just don't understand: Women & men in conversation.* New York: William Morrow.

Taylor, M. (1965, Jan.). A measurement of functional communication in aphasia. *Archives of Physical Medicine and Rehabilitation*, 101–107.

Ulatowska, H., North, A., & Macaluso-Haynes, S. (1981). Production of narrative and procedural discourse in aphasia. *Brain and Language, 13*, 345–371.

Wambaugh, J. L., Thompson, C. K., Doyle, P. J., & Camarata, S. (1991). Conversational discourse of aphasic and normal adults: An analysis of communicative functions. In T. E. Prescott (Ed.), *Clinical aphasiology*, Vol. 20 (pp. 343–353). Austin, TX: PRO-ED.

Yorkston, K., & Beukelman, D. (1980). An analysis of connected speech samples of aphasic and normal speakers. *Journal of Speech and Hearing Disorders, 45*, 27–36.

Clinical Aphasiology, Vol. 22, 1994, pp. 81–96

A Topographic Event-Related Potential Analysis of the Attention Deficit for Auditory Processing in Aphasia

Richard K. Peach, Scott S. Rubin, and
Marilyn Newhoff

McNeil (1982, 1988) and McNeil, Odell, and Tseng (1991) have hypothesized that the variability seen in aphasia may be due, at least in part, to a disorder in attention, effort allocation, or both. In a recent study, Peach, Newhoff, and Rubin (1993) employed electrophysiological testing procedures described by Naatanen (1990) to identify attentional deficits in auditory information processing following aphasia.

According to Naatanen (1990), a component referred to as the mismatch negativity (MMN) is elicited in event-related potentials (ERPs) when subjects are instructed to ignore auditory input consisting of standard and deviant tones (oddball paradigm) and attend to some distracting task such as reading or watching a video. The MMN component is extracted from a difference waveform produced by subtracting the standard stimulus ERP from the rare stimulus ERP (see Figure 1). This MMN component is said to reflect the subjects' automatic, preconscious attention to unattended auditory stimuli (Naatanen, 1990; Nyman et al., 1990).

In the study performed by Peach et al. (1993), aphasic subjects were tested under two conditions: ignoring and attending to auditory stimuli. The stimuli were composed of standard (frequent) and deviant (rare) tone bursts at 1000 and 2000 Hz, respectively. The MMN peaks for each subject were identified from the difference waveforms, and the peak latencies were then computed. Based on the pattern of latencies observed in the ignore condition, aphasic subjects were said to have demonstrated automatic attentional abilities similar to those of normal control subjects. The authors suggested, therefore, that aphasic subjects engage attention

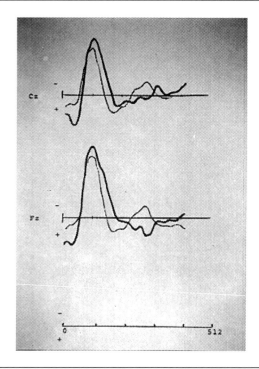

Figure 1. Normal ERP waveforms in elderly control subject to standard 1000 Hz tones (thin line) and rare 2000 Hz tones (heavy line).

for auditory stimuli as normal listeners do. Performance in the attend condition, however, indicated that the aphasic subjects' attention for completing discriminative tasks was deficient.

Recent investigations of the MMN have further defined this component in normals, in terms of its morphologic and topographic characteristics, and have provided some neurophysiological implications for these findings. Looking at the ignore conditions, Giard, Perrin, Pernier, and Bouchet (1990) identified a positive-going polarity in temporal regions below the Sylvian fissure accompanying the frontocentral negativity. Giard et al. (1990) and Paavilainen, Alho, Reinikainen, Sams, and Naatanen (1991) have suggested that these two components reflect a temporal generator located in the auditory cortex and a frontal generator that preferentially involves the right hemisphere. Giard et al. (1990) also suggested that the temporal component arising in the auditory cortex may be associated with a sensory memory trace and that the frontal component may represent an attention-switching process caused by the detection of a change at the sensory memory system.

These findings also have influenced the way in which MMN has been identified. Previously, the MMN has been measured at the peak of the negativity in the difference waveform corresponding to this component. Recognizing the contributions of the temporal cortex to the spatial characteristics of the MMN, Novak, Ritter, Vaughan, and Wiznitzer (1990) have reported an alternative approach that measures this component at the peak of its positive polarity in the temporolateral regions.

These findings led us to investigate more extensively the attentional mechanisms underlying auditory information processing in aphasia. To do this, we analyzed the morphologic and topographic characteristics of the MMN waveform elicited from aphasic subjects using the more recent methods of waveform identification described by Novak et al. (1990). The results were then compared to the findings obtained by Peach et al. (1993) when analyzing waveform latencies based on frontocentral negativities only. The following questions were addressed:

1. Are the morphologic characteristics (relative component amplitudes, onsets/offsets, time course) of the MMN waveforms found in the event-related potentials of aphasic subjects similar to those obtained in normal subjects?

2. What topographic patterns are associated with the MMN waveform in aphasic patients, and how are they related to those identified in normal subjects?

METHOD

Subjects

Seven subjects (five aphasic subjects and two controls) participated in this study (see Table 1). All subjects were native speakers of English and demonstrated normal hearing acuity for both ears in the frequency range between 500 and 2000 Hz. The aphasic group consisted of four males and one female ranging in age from 39 to 72 years. Aphasia was due to a single left hemisphere cerebrovascular accident for all subjects. Each aphasic subject was administered the *Western Aphasia Battery* (Kertesz, 1982) to obtain a measure of general language ability; the Aphasia Quotients for the group ranged from 88.9 to 14.4. The results were also used to determine the pattern of aphasia for each subject. Four patterns of aphasia were observed in this group, including anomic, Broca's, Wernicke's, and global aphasia. The time since onset of the aphasia ranged from 12 to 31 months.

Table 1. Subject Characteristics

Group	Age	Sex	WAB AQ[a]	Aphasia Type	Time Post Onset[b]
Control					
MN	47	F	—	—	—
IG	71	F	—	—	—
Aphasia					
EH	72	F	88.9	Anomia	24
PA	72	M	77.2	Broca	19
CS	72	M	49.8	Broca	15
AH	69	M	17.3	Wernicke	12
TL	39	M	14.4	Global	31

[a]WAB AQ = *Western Aphasia Battery* Aphasia Quotient. [b]Time post onset reported in months.

Instrumentation

Evoked potential testing and brain mapping was performed using the Biologic Brain Atlas Electrodiagnostic Testing System. Electrodes were placed using an ECI electro-cap electrode system. Twenty electrodes with impedances of less than 3 kΩ were placed according to the International 10–20 system. All electrodes were referenced to linked ears. The low- and high-frequency filters were set at 0.3 Hz and 100 Hz, respectively, and gain was 30,000 μV.

Data Collection

Auditory stimuli consisting of tone bursts were presented to each subject over Telephonics TDH-39P headphones at a rate of 0.8 per second. Each tone was characterized by a 20-ms plateau and a 20-ms rise/fall time. Standard and deviant stimuli consisting of 1000- and 2000-Hz tones, respectively, were presented randomly at a ratio of 5:1. Stimulus presentation continued until 50 samples were obtained to deviant tones. All samples were obtained using automatic artifact rejection.

The auditory stimuli were presented under a condition of passive attending. In this condition, subjects watched an inaudible segment from a familiar movie while the tone bursts were presented over headphones. Subjects were instructed to ignore the tones and to attend only to the movie. To increase attention to the movie and decrease attention to the tones, subjects were also told to be prepared to answer questions about the video.

Data Analysis

The morphologic characteristics of the MMN event were examined in this study by analyzing difference waveforms as suggested by Naatanen (1990). The difference waveforms were derived by subtracting the standard stimulus ERPs from the deviant stimulus ERPs. Two components of the MMN event were investigated: the temporal positivity arising from the auditory cortex and the frontal negativity arising from the right frontal cortex. To achieve this, the waveforms arising from two electrode sites, T5 and F4, were selected for analysis. These sites correspond to the left temporolateral region and to the right frontal convexity, respectively.

The following guidelines were used to analyze the waveforms obtained from each of these sites. To identify the temporolateral positivity associated with the MMN event, the waveform at T5 was first examined in the region between 70 and 250 ms, that is, in the area where the positive polarity is expected to occur (Giard et al., 1990; Nyman et al., 1990). The peak with the highest positive amplitude in this region that was also associated with frontal negativity at F4 was then selected and analyzed (Novak et al., 1990). MMN frontal negativity was identified subsequently by locating the greatest pattern of right frontal asymmetry at F4 following the temporolateral positivity at T5 and selecting the peak with the highest amplitude in this region of the waveform. Latencies and amplitudes for each of these peaks were then computed.

The topographic patterns associated with the MMN waveform were demonstrated in the brain maps constructed from the waveform amplitudes at each electrode site. The patterns observed in the aphasic subjects were compared with those of the control subjects, as well as with the expected patterns reported for normal subjects in the literature. Similarities and differences were noted and summarized descriptively.

RESULTS

Waveform Morphology

The morphological characteristics of the MMN difference waveforms at T5 and F4 are summarized in Table 2. All aphasic subjects demonstrated peak positive temporolateral latencies that were within the range both of the control subjects and also of normal subjects reported in the literature (70–250 ms). In fact, the latencies for the aphasic subjects were actually shorter in each case than those observed for either of the control subjects. The frontal latencies for the aphasic group were also similar to those of

Table 2. Peak Latencies and Amplitudes Associated With Temporal (T5) and Frontal (F4) Components of Mismatch Negativity Event

	Electrode Site				
	T5[a]		F4[b]		Latency
Group	ms	μV	ms	μV	Difference
Control					
MN	128	0.65	132	−4.73	4
IG	126	1.87	148	−3.02	24
Aphasia					
EH	84	4.00	132	−1.55	48
PA	108	4.41	162	−1.63	54
CS	106	0.65	140	−0.89	34
AH	78	2.00	166	−1.75	88
TL	102	0.85	150	−0.61	48

[a]Left, posterior temporal region. [b]Right, frontal convexity.

the control subjects and within the reported ranges. These latencies either overlapped with or were slightly longer than the latencies observed in the control subjects. Large differences were observed, however, between the aphasic subjects and the control subjects in the amount of time between the onset of the peak positive temporolateral and peak negative frontal polarities. The younger control subject exhibited the expected pattern, consisting of a peak temporolateral positivity at T5 followed by a peak frontal negativity in close proximity at F4. The difference between the onset of these two events in this subject was 4 ms. In the older control subject, this difference increased to 24 ms, an effect that may be consistent with aging. For the aphasic subjects, though, the latency differences more than doubled to an average of 54.4 ms (SD = 20.2). These findings suggest that the aphasic subjects established a sensory trace of the deviant stimuli within normal limits but experienced abnormally long delays in switching their attention to these changes once they detected them.

Inspection of the amplitude data for these groups revealed a wide range of peak amplitudes for the temporolateral positivity at T5 in both the control and aphasic subjects. The amplitude for the F4 frontal negativity in the older normal (−3.02 μV) was less than that observed for the younger normal (−4.73 μV). This pattern is consistent with the age-related decreases in evoked potential amplitudes that have been reported consistently in the literature (Bashore, 1990). The F4 amplitudes for the aphasic subjects, however, were substantially below those observed in either of the control subjects. This decrease in amplitude suggests a reduction in the attentional resources allocated to the changes detected in the trace in sensory memory. These findings also support the increased latencies observed between the previously described peak temporolateral positivity and frontal negativity. It appears that aphasic subjects required more time and allocated fewer attentional resources to the stimulus changes in this study than did either control subject.

Topographic Patterns

The topographic patterns of the aphasic subjects also showed distinct differences from the normal expected patterns. In normal subjects, the two components of the MMN event are associated with functional processes arising from two generators, one in the supratemporal plane of the auditory cortex and the other preferentially involving the right frontal region (Giard et al., 1990). The temporal generator underlies a neuronal mismatch process created by the deviant stimulus, whereas the frontal generator gives rise to an orientation to that mismatch. Our younger control subject exhibited the expected pattern of left temporal activity concurrent with bilateral frontal activity having right hemisphere preference. Temporal activity subsequently dissipated, leaving a strongly lateralized state in the frontal regions (see Figures 2 and 3). The older control subject initially displayed temporal activity with only minimal right frontal activity. This pattern did give way, however, to the bilateral frontal activity with right-sided preference that was observed in the younger control subject (see Figures 4–5).

The aphasic subjects produced several unexpected patterns. Two patients, EH and PA, demonstrated no frontal activity accompanying early left temporal activity. In addition, although right frontal asymmetry was observed subsequently, the amplitudes for these patients were significantly reduced in this region, as well as in all other cortical regions, relative to those of the control subjects (see Figures 6–9). Two other aphasic subjects, CS and AH, demonstrated a preference for left hemisphere frontal activity in conjunction with the activity of the temporal generator. For CS, the pattern associated with the frontal generator changed only with regard to the intensity of the associated amplitudes (see Figures 10 and 11). For AH, right frontal preference was established, but with persistent activity in the temporal region (see Figures 12 and 13). Finally, TL showed only right frontal activity in conjunction with the temporal activity corresponding to the mismatch process. This, of course, deviates from the expected pattern of bilateral frontal activity with a right hemisphere preference. As peak right frontal activity was established, temporal activity diminished as expected, but the amplitudes over the entire region were significantly reduced (see Figures 14 and 15). In fact, right frontal activity never exceeded that associated with the temporal mismatch process observed in the older control subject.

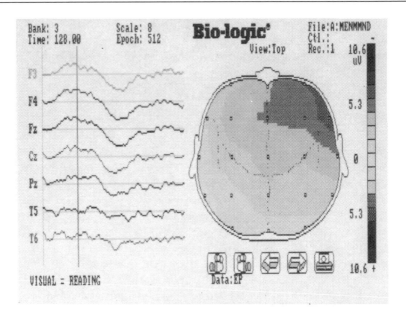

Figure 2. Difference waveforms and topographic pattern in younger control subject demonstrating left temporal activity with bilateral frontal activity having right hemisphere preference.

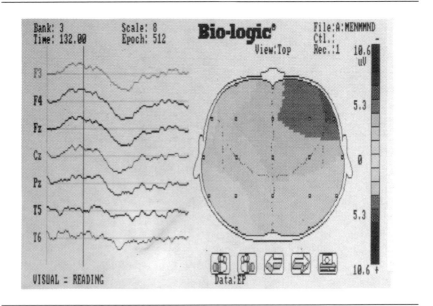

Figure 3. Strongly lateralized right frontal activity in younger control subject.

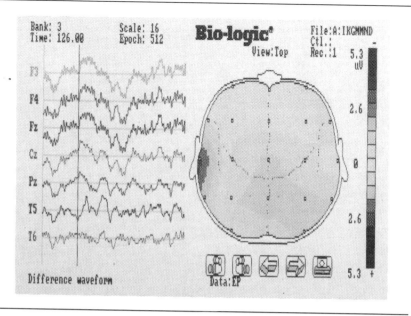

Figure 4. Temporal activity in elderly control subject with minimal right frontal activity.

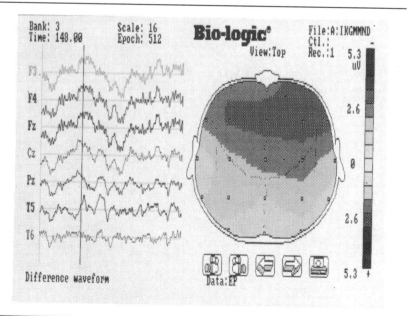

Figure 5. Late bilateral frontal activity with right-sided preference in elderly control subject.

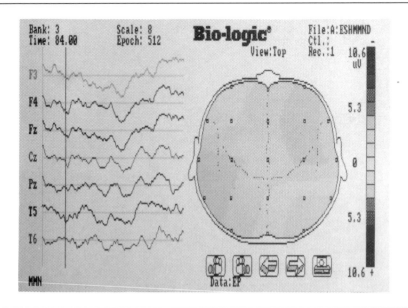

Figure 6. Early left temporal activity without accompanying frontal activity in aphasic subject EH.

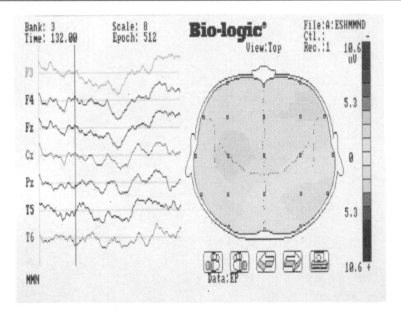

Figure 7. Late right frontal activity with reduced amplitude in aphasic subject EH.

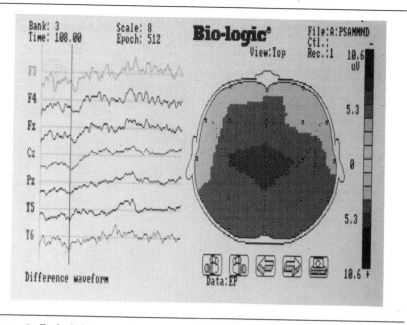

Figure 8. Early left temporal activity without accompanying frontal activity in aphasic subject PA.

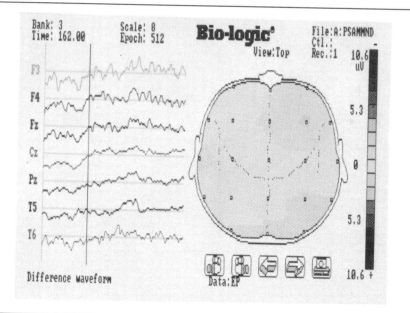

Figure 9. Late right frontal activity with reduced amplitude in aphasic subject PA.

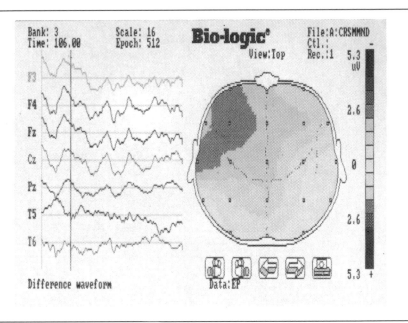

Figure 10. Left frontal preference in conjunction with activity of the temporal generator in aphasic subject CS.

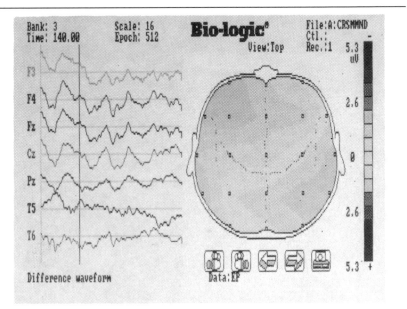

Figure 11. Late maintenance of left frontal preference with reduced amplitudes in aphasic subject CS.

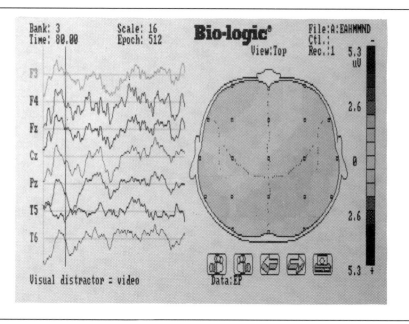

Figure 12. Left frontal preference in conjunction with activity of the temporal generator in aphasic subject AH.

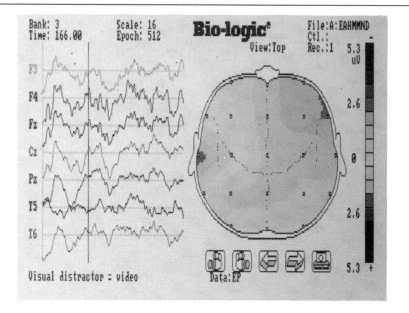

Figure 13. Late right frontal preference with persistent temporal activity in aphasic subject AH.

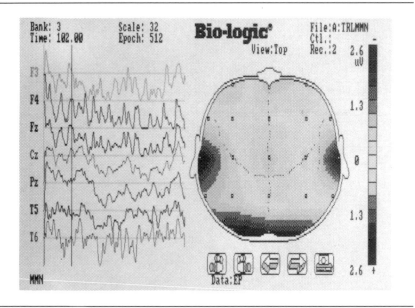

Figure 14. Right frontal activity only in conjunction with temporal activity in aphasic subject TL.

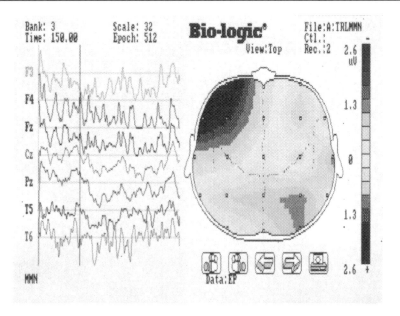

Figure 15. Peak right frontal activity with reduced amplitudes in aphasic subject TL.

DISCUSSION

In this study, aphasic subjects demonstrated increased latencies between waveform peaks reflecting the temporal and frontal components of the mismatch negativity event. In addition, the peak waveform amplitudes associated with the cognitive processes underlying the MMN event were significantly reduced from those observed in control subjects. Together, these data indicate that these aphasic subjects required more time to allocate fewer attentional resources to the detection of changes in an auditory signal; as McNeil et al. (1991) would put it, the aphasic subjects expended less attentional effort per unit of time. In addition, the topographic patterns of the event-related potentials in these subjects demonstrate abberations in the neural generators underlying these attentional processes. In sum, these findings are consistent with attentional deficits at the earliest, preconscious levels of attention.

McNeil et al. (1991) have suggested that some attentional deficits may result from an arousal impairment. According to these authors, "arousal subserves the ability of the organism to generate and allocate mental attention" (p. 32). Our current findings provide evidence that the attentional deficit in these aphasic subjects does not result simply from reduced arousal. The peak temporal latencies indicate the height of the timeframe within which our subjects detected and registered the change in the sensory stimulus. These latencies were well within the normal range; in fact, they preceded even those demonstrated by our control subjects. Had an arousal deficit been present, the aphasic subjects would have been expected to present longer temporal latencies than those of the control subjects, thereby indicating a difficulty in physiologically activating sensory systems to respond to the stimulus changes. Instead, the increased latency between detecting the stimulus changes and orienting to these changes, as indicated by the frontal latencies, is more consistent with a difficulty in effectively allocating attention to these changes.

The methodologic changes incorporated in this study produced results that contrast with those reported by Peach et al. (1993). Whereas those authors reported the attentional deficit following aphasia to be restricted to the completion of discriminative tasks, the present findings demonstrate that aphasic subjects do not engage attention for auditory stimuli as do normal listeners, even at the earliest, preconscious phases of orientation.

These findings do not provide a direct link between the attentional deficits observed in these aphasic subjects and their linguistic deficits, yet they do provide compelling evidence for an impairment in resource allocation that produced online processing deficits for auditory information. These deficits may, in turn, underlie some of the computational deficits associated with the language problems in aphasia. To address this issue, we are using evoked potentials to assess linguistic discriminations as a means of further exploring the link between these attentional deficits and aphasic language. Perhaps the findings from work of this kind will provide the additional evidence needed to help determine how variations in attentional resources relate to the linguistic deficits observed in aphasia.

REFERENCES

Bashore, T. R. (1990). Age-related changes in mental processing revealed by analyses of event-related brain potentials. In J. W. Rohrbaugh, R. Parasuraman, & R. Johnson (Eds.), *Event-related brain potentials: Basic issues and applications.* New York: Oxford University Press.

Giard, M. H., Perrin, F., Pernier, J., & Bouchet, P. (1990). Brain generators implicated in the processing of auditory stimulus deviance: A topographic event-related potential study. *Psychophysiology, 27* (6), 627–640.

Kertesz, A. (1982). *The Western Aphasia Battery.* New York: Grune & Stratton.

McNeil, M. R. (1982). The nature of aphasia in adults. In N. J. Lass, L. V. McReynolds, J. L. Northern, & D. E. Yoder (Eds.), *Speech, language, and hearing: Volume II, Pathologies of speech and language* (pp. 692–740). Philadelphia: W. B. Saunders.

McNeil, M. R. (1988). Aphasia in the adult. In N. J. Lass, L. V. McReynolds, J. L. Northern, & D. E. Yoder (Eds.), *Handbook of speech-language pathology and audiology* (pp. 738–786). Toronto: B. C. Decker.

McNeil, M. R., Odell, K., & Tseng, C. H. (1991). Toward the integration of resource allocation into a general theory of aphasia. *Clinical aphasiology, 20,* 21–39.

Naatanen, R. (1990). The role of attention in auditory information processing as revealed by event-related potentials and other brain measures of cognitive function. *Behavioral and Brain Sciences, 13,* 201–288.

Novak, G. P., Ritter, W., Vaughan, H. G., & Wiznitzer, M. L. (1990). Differentiation of negative event-related potentials in an auditory discrimination task. *Electroencephalography and Clinical Neurophysiology, 75,* 255–275.

Nyman, G., Alho, K., Laurinen, P., Paavilainen, P., Radil, T., Reinikainen, K., Sams, M., & Naatanen, R. (1990). Mismatch negativity (MMN) for sequences of auditory and visual stimuli: Evidence for a mechanism specific to the auditory modality. *Electroencephalography and Clinical Neurophysiology, 77,* 436–444.

Paavilainen, P., Alho, K., Reinikainen, K., Sams, M., & Naatanen, R. (1991). Right hemisphere dominance of different mismatch negativities. *Electroencephalography and Clinical Neurophysiology, 78,* 466–479.

Peach, R. K., Newhoff, M., & Rubin, S. S. (1993). Attention in aphasia as revealed by event-related potentials: A preliminary investigation. *Clinical aphasiology, 21,* 323–334.

Clinical Aphasiology, Vol. 22, 1994, pp. 97–106

Preliminary Investigations Into the Effects of Changing the Attentional Target on Left Hemisphere Function in Aphasic Patients

Marilyn Selinger and Thomas E. Prescott

The relationship between attention and aphasia has enjoyed increased discussion in the past decade (McNeil, Odell, & Tseng, 1991; Peach, Rubin, & Newhoff, 1994). Although attention is believed to be involved in multiple processes in the central nervous system, it is generally accepted as a process of selection. Attention can be defined as the selection of a specific type of sensory information on which to focus, with a concomitant reduction or elimination of concentration on other impinging sensory information (Robinson & Petersen, 1986).

In an elegant discussion calling for the integration of attention and resource allocation theory with concepts of aphasia, McNeil et al. (1991) suggest that aphasia is more than a disruption in specific attributes of language. They propose that aphasia might result from decreased abilities in arousing and directing processing energy to the task at hand. The notion that aphasia may be a deficit in attention and resource allocation should provoke further research.

Attention can be examined by presenting a test manipulation and observing either overt behaviors or changes in brain activity that result from it. The evoked potential paradigm presented in this chapter attempts to answer questions concerning aphasic patients' changes in brain activity resulting from differences in instructional set.

For the most part, evoked potential studies designed to test hemispheric changes in brain activity have used tasks defined as consistent with the processing styles of each hemisphere. The left hemisphere has been found to process information in a sequential or analytical manner

(e.g., language). The right hemisphere has been found to process information in a holistic manner (e.g., music). Consequently, music and language
are presented to the subjects and resulting asymmetries are measured
(Brown, Marsh, & Smith, 1976; Friedman, Simpson, Ritter, & Rapin, 1975;
Shucard, Shucard, & Thomas, 1977).

The evoked potential technique reported here, known as a probe paradigm, involves imposing a task-irrelevant sensory stimulus on an ongoing complex task. Conclusions are subsequently drawn about the hemisphere most involved in the complex task based on each hemisphere's
response to the irrelevant probe. Assumptions of this paradigm are based
on the notion that the brain is a limited capacity system; that is, the brain
is limited by more than structure in the number of things it can do at one
time, and increasing the demand of a task causes some performance
deterioration. Such degradation of performance may result from the brain's
reduced attentional allocation for the task.

Task demand has been compared to the attentional allocating abilities
for the individual (Allen, 1983; Crossley & Hiscock, 1987). A task that
requires a great deal of effort also requires the allocation of increasing
amounts of processing resources. A task that is simpler or more familiar
requires less attention (Crossley & Hiscock, 1987) and decreased resources.
Laterality differences using evoked potentials may be related to the effort
required to complete the task. A severely impaired aphasic patient may
need increased effort for language processing, whereas a less impaired
patient may use less effort to perform language tasks. It is suggested that
when the amount of attention needed for the task surpasses the capacity
of the specialized hemisphere, additional processing is shifted to the
other hemisphere.

Using a directed attention task, Thomas, Shucard, and Selinger (1980)
and Thomas and Shucard (1983) tested the hypothesis that interhemispheric asymmetries change as a function of the instructional set given to
the subject, even though the physical properties of the stimuli are held
constant. They hypothesized that holding the stimuli constant and varying the instructions to the subject may result in cerebral asymmetries
based on the subjects' attention to the stimuli and the resulting specialized processing style they apply to the task. In the Music condition of
these studies, subjects received ongoing classical musical passages with
irrelevant superimposed tone pairs. The subjects were instructed to ignore
the tones, listen to the music, and identify recurring melodies within the
music. In the Tones condition (where the stimuli were identical to the
music condition), the subjects were instructed to ignore the music and to
count various sequences of pairs of tones; the tones thus were no longer
irrelevant to the task.

Using this paradigm, the results with normal subjects indicated that
the pattern of interhemispheric activation when the subjects ignored the

tones differed from when they counted the tones. In the Tones condition, the evoked potential amplitude response was larger over the left hemisphere. In the Music condition, either there was no hemisphere differentiation, or the amplitude response was larger over the right hemisphere.

The purpose of the present study was to determine whether left-hemisphere-damaged patients exhibit hemispheric asymmetries when the relevant targets in a task are changed through instructional set while the stimuli themselves remain constant.

The study addressed the following specific questions:

1. Is there an interhemispheric amplitude asymmetry change between conditions as subjects change their problem-solving strategies for each task?

2. Is there an intrahemispheric amplitude asymmetry change between conditions as subjects change their problem-solving strategies for each task?

3. Are there hemispheric or task differences in the latencies of the evoked potential responses?

METHOD

Subjects

The aphasic patients studied were 5 premorbidly right-handed males (as measured by the Handedness Questionnaire [Raczkowski, Kalat, & Nebes, 1974]) between the ages of 60 and 64 ($x = 61.7$; $SD = 1.67$) whose only episode of hemisphere damage was on the left side. Table 1 shows results for *Boston Severity (Boston Diagnostic Aphasia Examination)* (Goodglass & Kaplan, 1972) and the *Porch Index of Communicative Ability* (PICA) (Porch, 1967).

Procedure

To examine effects of changing instructional set on hemispheric response to the same stimuli, two conditions were given to each aphasic subject. The stimuli consisted of five classical music pieces with simple recurring melodies. In the Music condition, subjects were instructed to listen to the music and identify the presence of a recurring melody while ignoring the tones. In the Tones condition, subjects were instructed to ignore the music and count the tone pairs in the recurring sequence of two pairs, three pairs, then four pairs.

Table 1. Subjects' Age and Test Result Data

Subject	Age (years)	PICA[a] Overall	PICA[a] VI	PICA[a] X	Boston Severity
1	60	89	74	73	4
2	64	88	99	99	4
3	62	97	99	99	4
4	60	92	99	99	5
5	62	65	99	99	2

Note: PICA scores are reported as percentiles.
[a]*Porch Index of Communicative Ability.*
Boston Severity from *Boston Diagnostic Aphasia Examination (BDAE).*

A third condition was added as a comparative measurement of hemispheric response to language. The Verbal condition consisted of several short stories with irrelevant tone pairs superimposed on the passage. Subjects were instructed to identify a recurring word within a story.

During each task the subject was seated in a sound-attenuated, electrically shielded room. The subjects kept their eyes closed during each 3-min segment. The subjects were instructed to listen to each stimulus and to respond by exhaling through their nostrils each time a recurring word occurred in the verbal task or a recurring melody occurred in the music task and at the correct series of tone pairs in the tones task. A specified key word, melody, or tone sequence was presented to the subjects prior to the onset of the appropriate segment. In addition, two multiple-choice questions were asked following each verbal segment. These behavioral tasks were used as indicators of the subjects' alertness and their understanding of and ability to perform the task. Each target item occurred 6 to 14 times within each segment.

Approximately 20 pairs of 600-Hz, 100-msec tones with an interstimulus interval of 2 sec and an interpair interval of 4 to 6 sec were superimposed on each musical selection. The AEPs were recorded from T4-to-Cz and T3-to-Cz electrode placements (Jasper, 1958) during all three conditions. Grass gold-plated disk electrodes were affixed to the scalp sites. Impedances from each electrode were measured at the beginning and end of each session; none was greater than 5 kΩ.

Auditory AEPs were averaged online and separately for Tone 2 of each pair as the subjects performed the tasks. The number of measurements of evoked potentials to the second tone of the pair ranged from 55 to 80 across subjects.

A Modular Instruments Signal Averaging system, interfaced with an AMDEC computer, generated the tones and averaged and scored the data. Microvolt amplitude and msec latency scores were obtained for each subject on the AEP component known as N2, a negative-going peak with a mean latency of 294 msec. This peak tends to represent processing of information in more associative stages. N2 has previously been found to be most sensitive to hemisphere asymmetries reflecting higher or later cortical processing (Shucard et al., 1977; Shucard, Cummins, Thomas, & Shucard, 1981).

RESULTS

Our first two questions referred to inter- and intrahemispheric amplitude differences in the three conditions. Because of the preliminary nature of this investigation and its application to only five subjects, we used descriptive statistics to examine differences in mean latencies and mean amplitudes between tasks and hemispheres.

We compared the latencies (time of occurrence) between the tasks and the hemispheres for N2. The mean latency across tasks for N2 in the right hemisphere was 297 milliseconds; for the left hemisphere it was 292 milliseconds. Mean latencies for the tasks described by hemisphere are shown in Table 2.

Amplitudes in microvolts for each hemisphere and each task were also examined; these measurements are believed to represent the amount of activation or involvement in each task. Figure 1 represents the differences between the hemispheres on the verbal task. The right hemisphere exhibits a larger response to the task than does the left hemisphere. Figure 2 illustrates the differences between the hemispheres on the tones task. In this task, the left hemisphere is characterized by a larger response than the right hemisphere's. Figure 3 represents the differences between the two hemispheres for the music task. There were no hemispheric differences in responses to this task.

Table 2. Millisecond Results for Peak 3

Task	Right Hemisphere	Left Hemisphere
Verbal	287 msec	293 msec
Tones	301 msec	294 msec
Music	304 msec	288 msec

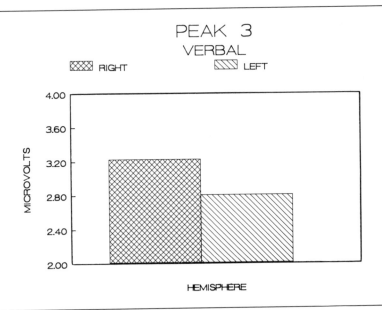

Figure 1. Differences in microvolt amplitudes between the right and left cerebral hemispheres as measured from bipolar temporal to Cz leads on the Verbal task.

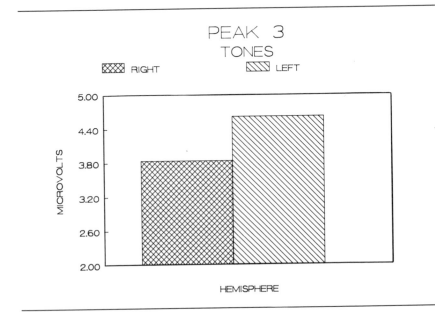

Figure 2. Differences in microvolt amplitudes between the right and left cerebral hemispheres as measured from bipolar temporal to Cz leads on the Tones task.

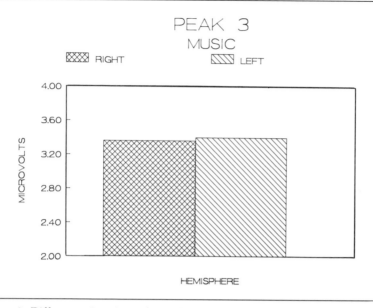

Figure 3. Differences in microvolt amplitudes between the right and left cerebral hemispheres as measured from bipolar temporal to Cz leads on the Music task.

DISCUSSION

The purpose of this study was to establish some preliminary data about the effects of varying instructional set on differential hemispheric involvement as measured by auditory evoked potentials between right and left hemisphere temporal sites. We attempted to measure a change in hemispheric involvement by presenting the same ongoing stimuli to the aphasic patients but directing their attention to different aspects of those stimuli.

When the aphasic patients were instructed to attend to classical music and ignore the superimposed tones, there was no differential hemisphere activation to the task in N2 data. This finding is consistent with previous findings on the music task, with both aphasic and normal subjects exhibiting no strong hemispheric differentiation for this task.

When the aphasic patients were attending to and counting sequences of tone pairs and ignoring the ongoing music, N2 indicated a difference in hemispheric response. That is, aphasic patients showed a higher left hemisphere response during the tones task. The results from the tones task are consistent with previously reported results using this paradigm with normal adults. To obtain a comparative measurement of left hemisphere function during verbal tasks, a language task was also presented to each subject. This task did not use the same stimuli as those reported in the music and tones tasks. The findings indicated that, when our aphasic patients were attending to verbal material and ignoring superimposed tones the right hemisphere showed a higher amplitude response than did the left hemisphere. The findings for the verbal task reflect the results previously reported by Selinger, Shucard, and Prescott (1980) and by Selinger, Prescott, and Shucard (1989). Of particular significance was the relatively larger right hemisphere response that occurred during the processing of verbal information in the aphasic group.

The aphasic patients in this preliminary investigation exhibited changes in the amount of hemispheric activity based on directing attention toward different facets of the same stimuli. Therefore, the required strategy and level of difficulty for accomplishing the task at hand seem to have affected which hemisphere's resources were allocated toward the solution.

Intrahemispheric activity in these aphasic patients was characterized by more variability of responses in the left hemisphere. This is consistent with behavioral observations concerning the variability in aphasia. The left hemisphere exhibited differential specialization of function on the two left-hemisphere-style tasks. This differential function suggests the left hemisphere to have a greater involvement than the right during the counting task and the right to have a greater involvement than the left during the verbal task. Counting is often classified as an overlearned function or more automatic task; thus, it should be easier than processing connected language. This finding suggests that the damaged left hemisphere in aphasic patients is able to respond within normal limits to tasks that are sequential or analytical but do not necessarily place a high task demand on processing complex language. It appears that, when task demand is reduced, attentional allocation of resources does not reach its limit and performance deterioration or shift to other resources is unnecessary.

Our previous findings using the stimuli of language and music had led us to the conclusion that the right hemisphere in aphasic patients had a larger response to language than the left. This conclusion raised the following question: Is the right hemisphere showing increased activation to language, or are we actually seeing that the left hemisphere is unable to respond to the stimuli because of the damage in the left hemisphere?

These data suggest that our aphasic patients exhibited increased activation in the left hemisphere when processing information in a predominately sequential or analytic task (e.g., counting in sequence). The left hemisphere, therefore, was not unable to respond, but it might have been limited in its response according to the increasing complexity or difficulty of the language material. When the task demand fell heavily into verbal processing, the left hemisphere exhibited reduced processing of the information. It appears that our earlier conclusions concerning reduced performance abilities in the left hemisphere may be supported by these data, in that they indicate that the left hemisphere does process left-hemisphere-style tasks that are not heavily loaded toward language. These results imply that directing attention toward tasks at appropriate levels of difficulty may bias the left hemisphere, thereby allowing for practice and use of the left hemisphere's abilities.

Finally, these findings also suggest that our aphasic patients were able to attend appropriately to the directed task in a manner similar to normal subjects. However, it should be remembered that this was a directed attention task and not a dual-task paradigm; that is, it involved attending to one type of target without a concurrent task requirement. It is possible that had we increased the difficulty or complexity of an attention task, our aphasic patients would have exhibited a deficit response pattern. However, this possibility simply reiterates the necessity of attending to the level of task demand when drawing conclusions about behavioral and neurophysiological deficits in aphasic patients.

ACKNOWLEDGMENT

This research was funded in part by Department of Veterans Affairs Rehabilitation Research and Development Grant C-493.

REFERENCES

Allen, M. (1983). Models of hemispheric specialization. *Psychological Bulletin, 93,* (1), 73–104.

Brown, W. S., Marsh, J. T., & Smith, J. C. (1976). Evoked potential waveform differences produced by the perception of different meanings of an ambiguous word. *Electroencephalography and Clinical Neurophysiology, 41,* 113–123.

Crossley, M., & Hiscock, M. (1987). Concurrent-Task Interference indicates asymmetric resource allocation in children's reading. *Developmental Neuropsychology 3* (3&4), 207–225.

Friedman, D., Simpson, R., Ritter, W., & Rapin, I. (1975). Cortical evoked potentials elicited by real speech words and human sounds. *Electroencephalography and Clinical Neurophysiology, 38,* 13–19.

Goodglass, H., & Kaplan, E. (1972). *The assessment of aphasia and related disorders.* Philadelphia: Lea & Febiger.

Jasper, H. H. (1958). The ten-twenty electrode system of the international federation of societies for electroencephalography: Appendix to the report of the committee of methods of clinical examination in electroencephalography. *Electroencephalography and Clinical Neurophysiology, 10,* 371.

McNeil, M. R., Odell, K., & Tseng, C. H. (1991). Toward the integration of resource allocation into a general theory of aphasia. In T. E. Prescott (Ed.), *Clinical aphasiology,* Vol. 20 (pp. 21–40). Austin, TX: PRO-ED.

Peach, R. K., Rubin, S. R., & Newhoff, M. (1994). A topographic event-related potential analysis of the attention deficit for auditory processing in aphasia. In M. L. Lemme (Ed.), *Clinical aphasiology*, Vol. 22 (pp. 81–96). Austin, TX: PRO-ED.

Porch, B. (1967). *The Porch Index of Communicative Abilities*. Palo Alto: Consulting Psychologists Press.

Raczkowski, D., Kalat, J. W., & Nebes, R. (1974). Reliability and validity of some handedness questionnaire items. *Neuropsychologia, 12*, 43–47.

Robinson, D. L., & Petersen, S. E. (1986). The neurobiology of attention. In J. E. LeDoux & W. Hirst (Eds.), *Mind and brain: Dialogues in cognitive neuroscience.* New York: Cambridge University Press.

Selinger, M., Schucard, D., & Prescott, T. E. (1980). Relationships between behavioral and electrophysiological measures of auditory comprehension. In R. H. Brookshire (Ed.), *Clinical Aphasiology Conference Proceedings* (pp. 217–225). Minneapolis: BRK Publishers.

Selinger, M., Prescott, T. E., & Shucard, D. W. (1989). Auditory event-related potential probes and behavioral measures of aphasia. *Brain and Language, 36*, 3.

Shucard, D. W., Shucard, J. L., & Thomas, D. G. (1977). Auditory evoked potentials as probes of hemispheric differences in cognitive processing. *Science, 197*, 1295–1298.

Shucard, D. W., Cummins, K. R., Thomas, D. G., & Shucard, J. L. (1981). Evoked potentials to auditory probes as indices of cerebral specialization of function— replication and extension. *Electroencephalography and Clinical Neurophysiology, 52*, 389–393.

Thomas, D. G., & Shucard, D. W. (1983). Changes in patterns of hemispheric electrophysiological activity as a function of instructional set. *International Journal of Neuroscience, 18*, 11–20.

Thomas, D. G., Shucard, D. W., & Selinger, M. (1980). Auditory event-related potentials as measures of differential hemispheric processing: Stimulus and cognitive factors. *Psychophysiology, 17*, 289–290.

Clinical Aphasiology, Vol. 22, 1994, pp. 107–118

Duke *Prognosis Profile Worksheet:* Inter- and Intraobserver Reliability

Jennifer Horner, Mary Ann Eller,
Deborah V. Dawson, and
Frances G. Buoyer

In clinical aphasiology, prognostication is a process by which clinicians assess a range of biographic, neurologic, linguistic, and behavioral data for the purpose of predicting a patient's future communication performance. Prognostication may pertain to the anticipated benefits of spontaneous recovery, the anticipated benefits of treatment, or both (Darley, 1982; Marquardt, 1982). According to Wertz (1978), "The task . . . is to make a prospective statement for each patient individually" (p. 26). Both Wertz (1978) and Darley (1982) advised clinicians to ask, *prognosis . . . for what, for whom,* and *at what point in time?* Horner and Rothi (1984) stated, "Because no single factor is sufficient for estimating prognosis, and because variables interact in complex and individual ways, we recommend rating as many variables as possible" (p. 24). One goal of a comprehensive approach is to avoid "test-driven" prognostication in favor of patient- and clinician-driven prognostication. A final introductory point is that—at least in the acute phase of recovery—prognosis for communication recovery is a dynamic phenomenon, not a static one. In Marquardt's (1982) words, "The clinician's responsibility is not always to be right; rather it is to make the best judgment possible and to be willing to change an opinion if the patient's situation warrants it" (p. 104).

The literature pertaining to prognosis is too extensive to review here, but the foundation for our worksheet can be found in Darley (1982); Hier, Mondlock, and Caplan (1983); Holland, Greenhouse, Fromm, and Swindell (1989); Horner and Rothi (1984); Kertesz (1979); Levin, Benton, and Grossman (1982); Marquardt (1982); and Rosenbek, LaPointe, and Wertz (1989). One recent study (Holland et al., 1989) reported the acute language recovery of left and right hemisphere stroke patients. Using the *Western Aphasia Battery* (Kertesz, 1979, 1982), they defined language recovery as an aphasia quotient of 93.8 or better. They submitted select variables to a multiple logistic regression analysis and found that language recovery favored younger patients, shorter hospital stays, males, hemorrhagic strokes, and right hemisphere strokes.

The purpose of this study was to assess the inter- and intraobserver reliability of a prognosis worksheet designed to help us prognosticate recovery from communication disability in adults sustaining brain damage. The prognosis worksheet was adapted from Horner and Rothi (1979, 1984). In the context of current clinical practice, the original prognosis worksheet had several shortcomings. First, the worksheet helped the clinician describe but not quantify relevant parameters. Second, there were no data on inter- or intraobserver reliability. Third, several developments in the clinic mandated a change in our perspective on the question of prognosis. The first of these developments was increased diversity in our patient caseload, from narrowly defined "aphasic" syndromes to a host of poststroke, postsurgical, posttraumatic, and post-"other" etiologies. The second development was the introduction of the concept of "cognitive-communication" disorders. Despite the 1991 position statement of the American Speech-Language-Hearing Association (ASHA), clinicians lack consensus regarding the definition or measurement of cognitive-communication disorders. The third development was the gradual accumulation of research concerning prognosis for recovery. The fourth development—a result of the increasing cost of health care—was the shorter duration of hospital stays for the purpose of rehabilitation.

All of these developments provoked questions relevant to our clinical practice and research design. First, should we use one test battery for all patients? Second, should we use one set of prognostic indicators for all patients? Third, what is the reliability of the prognostic estimate that we generate? And fourth, what is the predictive validity of the prognostic estimate?

Clinicians treating adult neurogenic communication disorders are faced with an ever-increasing diversity of theory, clinical perspectives, and caseload composition (Duffy & Myers, 1991), yet we do not yet have a consistent or satisfactory approach or nomenclature. Therefore, we decided to use a standard admission battery for all patients. Further, we decided to use a common prognosis worksheet for all patients, regardless of etiology, side of brain damage, or severity of brain damage. We deferred the question of predictive validity to a later time. In this study we addressed the clinicians' lack of a systematic, reliable approach to estimating prognosis for recovery from communication disorders during acute rehabilitation. The specific question of this study was: what is the reliability of the *Duke Prognosis Profile Worksheet*?

METHOD

Subjects

During the 12-month study period, 128 patients admitted to Duke Rehabilitation Center received evaluations by speech-language pathologists. Excluded from this study were 70 patients with isolated dysarthria or dysphagia, as well as patients who were too severely impaired to tolerate standardized language testing. Of the remaining 58 patients (Table 1), 37 were men, 21 were women, and all but one were right-handed. Stroke—left, right, or bilateral—was the most frequent etiology; the nonstroke patients were mostly neurosurgical and head trauma patients.

Table 1. Characteristics of Patients for Whom Prognostic Estimates Were Derived

	Diagnostic Category			
Patient Characteristic	LHS[a] (N = 18)	RHS[b] (N = 14)	BHS[c] (N = 10)	Nonstroke (N = 16)
Gender				
Male	14	9	6	8
Female	4	5	4	8
Handedness				
Right	17	14	10	16
Left	1	0	0	0
Education (years)				
< 6–8	5	2	3	3
9–12	7	5	2	8
13–16, college	5	6	5	4
> 16, college	1	1	0	1
Age (years)	61.8	62.4	65.6	57.5
SD	[12.9]	[13.0]	[13.2]	[16.6]
Days post onset				
Mean	39.4	52.9	18.8	40.1
Median	29.5	26.5	14.5	30.0
Range	5–190	10–335	9–40	18–138
Western Aphasia Battery				
Aphasia Quotient				
Mean	40.2	92.0	76.8	87.1
SD	[3.0]	[7.3]	[23.6]	[19.8]
Range	1.0–94.0	70.8–99.6	9.9–94.2	14.2–100.0
Cortical Quotient				
Mean	40.2	83.7	69.6	81.2
SD	[28.6]	[11.6]	[21.3]	[18.9]
Range	3.1–87.7	59.4–94.8	10.6–91.9	52.5–96.5

[a]LHS = left hemisphere stroke. [b]RHS = right hemisphere stroke. [c]BHS = bilateral hemisphere stroke.

Materials

The *Prognosis Profile Worksheet* (Appendix A) consists of two pages. The front page allows a summary of etiologic and neurodiagnostic data and notes aphasia type (if applicable), number of hospital days, former occupation, and so on. The second page, the worksheet per se, comprises 24 variables yielding four subscores. The first set of data (the top half of the form) pertains to demographic and neurologic information, each assigned a relative weight of 1, 2, or 3 points. The remaining subscores (on the bottom half) pertain to language performance, other higher cortical functions, and visuomotor functions—each assigned a relative severity rating of 1 to 5 points. By tallying these subscores, the clinician derives the total prognosis score (maximum 100 points) and then assigns an overall qualitative estimate for extent of improvement in communication.

Procedure

The standard admission battery for the *Speech and Language Pathology Program* at Duke Rehabilitation Center included the *Neurobehavioral Cognitive Status Examination* (1983) and the *Western Aphasia Battery* (Kertesz, 1979; 1982). Both tests have proven reliability and validity (Kiernan, Mueller, Langston, & Van Dyke, 1987; Shewan & Kertesz, 1980), and they allow evaluation of both language and nonlanguage abilities. A variety of clinician-selected supplementary tests and informal observations supplemented standardized testing. At the completion of the evaluation, the patient's primary clinician completed a *Prognosis Profile Worksheet.*

For the interobserver reliability question, five clinicians—*in pairs*—participated in this study of 58 patients. Each had a master's degree, a Certificate of Clinical Competence, (CCC), and a state license. The range of experience was from 1 to 9 years; the average was 4.6 years. The primary clinician (the primary observer) evaluated the patient, completed test forms in a routine manner, wrote a comprehensive diagnostic report including an addendum summarizing test scores, and then completed the two-page *Prognosis Profile Worksheet.* Subsequently, a randomly assigned independent observer who had never met or had no more than incidental knowledge of the patient reviewed background information, test data (including test record forms), and the diagnostic report. From this review, the independent observer completed a *Prognosis Profile Worksheet.*

For the intraobserver reliability question, one observer completed prognosis worksheets on 27 patients. She had appropriate qualifications and 4 years of experience. She was blinded to her original, baseline worksheet, and she was blinded to the actual treatment outcome.

RESULTS

Tables 2, 3, and 6 summarize statistical analyses for interobserver reliability; Tables 4, 5, and 7 do the same for intraobserver analyses. First, we calculated Spearman Rank Correlation Coefficients for all 58 pairs of observations for the four category subscores and the total score (see Table 2). We also looked at *intraclass* coefficients, which treated the interobserver observations as replicates and ignored the specific roles of primary and independent observers. (These were calculated using ranks for comparability with the Spearman coefficients.) All correlations were significant at $p < .0001$.

Next, we investigated possible systematic differences between observers (see Table 3). These comparisons were made by examining the differences between the scores of the primary and independent observers and testing whether the median difference was zero using the nonparametric Wilcoxon signed rank procedure. Again, this was done for the subscores and the total scores. In no instance was the result significant at the 5% level. In fact, the only result that could even be termed suggestive was for language performance ($p = .06$). However, even here the median difference was zero. The observers agreed exactly in 20 of 58 cases and within one point in 45 of 58 cases.

We then conducted parallel analyses for intraobserver reliability. In Table 4 we report Spearman and intraclass coefficients for initial and repeat scores. As in the case of interobserver reliability, we found all intraobserver correlations to be statistically significant. Table 5 presents comparisons between subscores and total scores using the Wilcoxon procedure. In only one instance—that for the Demographic/Neurologic category—was the

Table 2. Correlation Coefficients Between Primary Clinician and Independent Observer Using the *Prognosis Profile Worksheet* Contrasted With Intraclass Correlation Coefficients Based on Ranks

Category	Spearman Correlation Coefficients*	Intraclass Correlation Coefficients*
Demographic/lesion	.857	.857
Language performance	.909	.906
Other higher cortical	.896	.900
Visuomotor	.890	.891
Total	.968	.965

Note: $N = 58$.

*All correlations were significant at $p < .0001$. The p-values are those associated with the test of the null hypothesis of zero correlation.

Table 3. Comparisons Between Primary and Independent Observers on *Prognosis Profile Worksheet* Scores Using the Nonparametric Wilcoxon Signed Rank Procedure

Worksheet Component	p*	Mean	S.E.	Median
Subscore Category				
Demographic/lesion	.60	−.07	.15	0
Language performance	.06	.34	.22	0
Other higher cortical	.88	0.33	.29	0
Visuomotor	.91	−.19	.24	0
Total	.79	.09	.38	0

*p-values are those associated with the test of the null hypothesis that the median difference is zero.

Table 4. Correlation Coefficients Between Initial and Repeat Scores Using the *Prognosis Profile Worksheet* Contrasted With Intraclass Correlation Coefficients Based on Ranks

Category	Spearman Correlation Coefficients*	Intraclass Correlation Coefficients*
Demographic/lesion	.940	.915
Language performance	.756	.767
Other higher cortical	.812	.782
Visuomotor	.901	.901
Total	.902	.895

Note: N = 27.
*All correlations were significant at $p < .0001$. The p-values are those associated with the test of the null hypothesis of zero correlation.

result significant at the 5% level, though even here the median difference score was zero. Scoring agreed perfectly in this category for 10 of 27 records. Disparities suggested that the p-value actually reflected *skewness* in disagreement: that is, the initial score was less than the repeat score in 4 cases and greater than the repeat score in 13 cases.

The prognosis worksheet allows the clinician to generate a prognosis score and a prognosis estimate. The score is based on 24 categorical variables yielding 100 possible points. The qualitative prognostic estimate is based on the clinician's overall appraisal of the individual's potential for improvement, that is, as excellent, good, fair, guarded, or poor. Using these data, the kappa statistic is a measure of agreement, corrected for the agreement one would expect by chance: A kappa of 0 indicates a level of

Table 5. Comparisons Between the Initial and Repeat Scoring by One Observer on *Prognosis Profile Worksheet* Using the Nonparametric Wilcoxon Signed Rank Procedure

Worksheet Component	p*	Mean	S.E.	Median
Subscore Category				
Demographic/neurologic	.013	−.52	.19	0
Language performance	.480	−.07	.29	0
Other higher cortical	.139	1.04	.61	0
Visuomotor	.688	.04	.17	0
Total	.128	1.52	.87	1

*p-values are those associated with the test of the null hypothesis that the median difference is zero.

Table 6. Assessment of Interobserver Agreement for the Overall Prognostic Estimate of Improvement After Completion of the *Prognosis Profile Worksheet*

Observed Agreement	Unweighted Kappa	S.E.	p*
44.8%	.231	.075	.002

Observed Agreement	Weighted Kappa	S.E.	p*
93.1%	.735	.128	.001

Note: Acceptable agreement is defined as either precise agreement or disparity of only one *prognosis estimate* category. The *prognosis estimate* categories are excellent, good, fair, guarded, and poor. N = 58.
*p-values are associated with the test of the null hypothesis that the level of agreement observed does not differ from that expected by chance alone.

agreement no different from that expected by chance alone; a kappa of 1 indicates perfect agreement.

As shown in Table 6, the first and second observer agreed on the prognostic estimate precisely 44.8% of the time (this represents 26 of 58 cases). The weighted kappa showed that the two observers agreed in 54 of 58 cases, or 93.1%. (The first observer rated "lower" in 16 instances; the second observer rated "lower" in 12.) For interobserver comparisons, both unweighted and weighted kappas were statistically significant.

As shown in Table 7, intraobserver agreement using the kappa statistic was based on 40.7% observed agreement; the weighted kappa, on 96.3% observed agreement. The weighted kappa achieved statistical significance; the unweighted did not.

Table 7. Assessment of Intraobserver Agreement for the Overall Prognostic Estimate of Improvement After Completion of the *Prognosis Profile Worksheet*

Observed Agreement	Unweighted Kappa	S.E.	p*
40.7%	.196	.105	.062

Observed Agreement	Weighted Kappa	S.E.	p*
96.3%	.860	.137	.0001

Note: Acceptable agreement is defined as either precise agreement or disparity of only one *prognosis estimate* category. The *prognosis estimate* categories are excellent, good, fair, guarded, and poor. N = 27.
*p-values are associated with the test of the null hypothesis that the level of agreement observed does not differ from that expected by chance alone.

DISCUSSION

After having observer pairs formed from a group of five speech-language pathologists with an average of about 5 years experience evaluate 58 acute rehabilitation patients, we compared both scores and estimates derived from the *Prognosis Profile Worksheet*. In addition, we compared both scores and estimates made by a single observer for 27 patients.

We conclude from our data that the *Prognosis Profile Worksheet* has acceptable inter- and intraobserver reliability.

We offer several caveats for this research study. First and foremost, we recognize that some of the variables comprising the Demographic/Neurologic subscore of the *Prognosis Profile Worksheet* have controversial prognostic significance—handedness, sex, age, education, and hemiplegia, to name a few. In turn, our assignment of 3-point ratings to these and other variables may be blatantly premature. Isolating these controversial variables in a logistic regression model will help us rectify this. Second, the *Prognosis Profile Worksheet,* although comprehensive, is not exhaustive. For example, we excluded from the worksheet *per se* information on lesion *site* and ratings of patient motivation because of the difficulty of fitting these complex variables into a quantitative approach. Third, we are aware of Marquardt's (1982) warning that "a determination of which patient has the best prognosis is not possible by mathematic computation" (p. 104). If this statement is true, we may be at fault for fitting our prognostic indicators into an all-too-neat 100-point package.

In closing, we suggest that research using a quantified approach to prognostication (such as the *Prognosis Profile Worksheet*) might proceed as follows. First, subjects should be stratified prospectively, by etiology, using large numbers of patients in each group. Or, as Rosenbek et al. (1989) suggested, one might "establish and study cohorts who differ only on a single variable" (p. 94). Second, rather than using a common battery (in this instance, the *Neurobehavioral Cognitive Status Examination* and the *Western Aphasia Battery*), we should explore prognosis based on "etiology-specific" batteries. Third, as Holland and colleagues did in 1989, we can subject select items catalogued on the *Prognosis Profile Worksheet* to logistic regression once sufficient subject numbers are available in each diagnostic group. (Other statistical methods are described by Rosenbek et al., 1989, p. 97.) Fourth, we envision a study that might assess cross-disciplinary prognostic estimates (e.g., asking whether neurologists' prognostic estimates agree with speech-language pathologists' prognostic estimates). Fifth, we think it would be valuable to explore the reliability of prognostication at different points in time. Rather than making estimations at roughly 1 month post onset, as we did, one might examine prognosis at 1 week, or 3 months, or 6 months post onset. Ideally, such a study would use the same group of patients. Finally, we plan to test the prognostic validity of the *Prognosis Profile Worksheet* by comparing prognostic scores and estimates with actual improvement in communication ability.

ACKNOWLEDGMENTS

Lisa A. Carr, M. H. S., Barbara K. Dodson, M. S., and Mary S. Brennan, M. S.

REFERENCES

American Speech-Language-Hearing Association (1991). Guidelines for speech-language pathologists serving persons with language, socio-communicative, and/or cognitive-communicative impairments. *Asha, 33* (Supplement 5), 21–28.

Darley, F. L. (1982). *Aphasia* (pp. 110–143). Philadelphia: W. B. Saunders.

Duffy, J. R., & Myers, P. S. (1991). Group comparisons across neurologic communication disorders: Some methodological issues. In T. E. Prescott (Ed.), *Clinical aphasiology*, Vol. 19 (pp. 1–14). Austin: PRO-ED.

Hier, D. B., Mondlock, J., & Caplan, L. R. (1983). Recovery of behavioral abnormalities after right hemisphere stroke. *Neurology, 33*, 337–343.

Holland, A. L., Greenhouse J. B., Fromm, D., & Swindell, C. S. (1989). Predictors of language restitution following stroke: A multivariate analysis. *Journal of Speech and Hearing Research, 32*, 232–238.

Horner, J., & Rothi, L. J. (1979). Aphasia recovery: Theory and treatment. *Asha, 21,* 604–605. (Abstract.)

Horner, J., & Rothi, L. J. (1984). Prognosis for recovery from aphasia: Estimating extent of improvement. *Communique* (North Carolina Speech-Language-Hearing Association Journal) (Research Edition: 20–29).

Kertesz, A. (1979). *Aphasia and related disorders.* New York: Grune & Stratton.

Kertesz, A. (1982). *Western Aphasia Battery.* New York: Grune & Stratton.

Kiernan, R. J., Mueller, J., Langston, J. W., & Van Dyke, C. (1987). The neuro-behavioral cognitive status examination: A brief but differentiated approach to cognitive assessment. *Annals of Internal Medicine, 107,* 481–485.

Levin, H. S., Benton, A. L., & Grossman, R. G. (1982). *Neurobehavioral consequences of closed head injury.* New York: Oxford University Press.

Marquardt, T. P. (1982). *Acquired neurogenic disorders* (pp. 67–104). Englewood Cliffs, NJ: Prentice-Hall.

Neurobehavioral Cognitive Status Examination Manual (1983). Fairfax, CA: Northern California Neurobehavioral Group.

Rosenbek, J. C., LaPointe, L. L., & Wertz, R. T. (1989). *Aphasia: A clinical approach* (pp. 55–103). Austin, TX: PRO-ED.

Shewan, C. M., & Kertesz, A. (1980). Reliability and validity characteristics of the *Western Aphasia Battery* (WAB). *Journal of Speech and Hearing Disorders, 45,* 308–324.

Wertz, R. T., (1978). Neuropathologies of Speech and Language: An introduction to patient management. In D. F. Johns (Ed.), *Clinical management of neurogenic communicative disorders* (pp. 1–101). Boston: Little, Brown.

APPENDIX A:
DUKE PROGNOSIS PROFILE WORKSHEET

ESTIMATING POTENTIAL FOR EXTENT OF IMPROVEMENT
(Horner et al., Experimental Version, 1989)
(Adapted from Horner & Rothi, 1984)

Patient: Date of Evaluation:
Date of Onset: Clinician:

ETIOLOGY

STROKE
..... Ischemic
..... Embolic
..... Thrombotic
..... Hemorrhagic
..... Intracerebral (ICH)
..... Subarachnoid (SAH)
..... Aneurysm
..... Arteriovenous
      malformation (AVM)

TRAUMA
..... Closed head injury (CHI)
..... Concussion
..... Contusion
..... Subdural hematoma (SDH)
..... Intracerebral hemorrhage (ICH)
..... Coup ..... Contre coup
..... Open head injury (OHI)/with skull fracture
..... Concussion
..... Contusion
..... SDH
..... ICH
..... Coup ..... Contre-coup

TUMOR
..... Glioblastoma Multiforme
..... Astrocytoma
..... Meningioma
..... Metastatic
..... Other:

..... Loss of consciousness—or coma RLA I, II, III—and duration:

Neuroradiology:

..... Head CT Scan   ..... Head MRI   ..... Angiography   ..... PET or SPECT   ..... Other

Aphasia Profile (W.A.B.-A.Q.) [if applicable]

..... Anomic
..... Conduction
..... Wernicke
..... Transcortical Sensory

..... Broca
..... Transcortical motor
..... Global
..... Mixed transcortical

..... Unclassifiable; NOT aphasic; normal
..... Unclassifiable; NOT aphasic; ABnormal

ADDITIONAL VARIABLES:

Race: Caucasian   Black   Hispanic   Other:

Occupation (now or in past):

Number of TOTAL hospital days (i.e., from acute hospital admission through discharge from rehabilitation):

Appendix A. (continued)

RATING:	3	2	1
HANDEDNESS:	..... Left	..... Right	..... Ambidextrous
SEX:	..... Male	..... Female	
AGE:	..... ≤ 40	 41–69	..... ≥ 70
EDUCATION:	..... > 12	 9–12	..... < 9
LESION TYPE: Stroke	..... Hemmorhagic	..... Ischemic	..... Hemorrhagic infarct
Trauma	..... Focal	..... Diffuse	..... Focal and diffuse
Tumor	..... Slow growing	..... Rapid growing	
LESION NUMBER:	.... Single	..... Multiple	..... Multiple with atrophy
LESION SIDE:	..... Right	..... Left	..... Bilateral
NEUROLOGIC SIGNS:	..... No weakness	..... L or R arm/leg	..... Bilateral arm/leg
VISUAL FIELD DEFECT:	..... No	..... Yes	..... (Neglect precludes unequivocal test)
MONTHS POST ONSET:	 0–1	 1–6	..... > 6
			{ /30}

RATING:	5	4	3	2	1	0 = Not testable
LANGUAGE PERFORMANCE:	Normal	Mild	Moderate	Severe	Profound	
Auditory	.....	.....	.....	.....	.....	{ /5}
Oral-verbal	.....	.....	.....	.....	.....	{ /5}
Reading	.....	.....	.....	.....	.....	{ /5}
Writing	.....	.....	.....	.....	.....	{ /5}
						{ /20}
OTHER HIGHER CORTICAL FUNCTIONS:						
Construction (Copying, Drawing, Blocks)	.....	.....	.....	.....	.....	{ /5}
Calculations	.....	.....	.....	.....	.....	{ /5}
Abstract reasoning	.....	.....	.....	.....	.....	{ /5}
Verbal memory	.....	.....	.....	.....	.....	{ /5}
Visual memory	.....	.....	.....	.....	.....	{ /5}
						{ /25}
VISUAL-MOTOR FUNCTIONS:						
Praxis: Buccofacial	.....	.....	.....	.....	.....	{ /5}
Praxis: Limb	.....	.....	.....	.....	.....	{ /5}
Praxis: Verbal	.....	.....	.....	.....	.....	{ /5}
Dysarthria	.....	.....	.....	.....	.....	{ /5}
Visual neglect	.....	.....	.....	.....	.....	{ /5}
						{ /25}
TOTAL:						{ /100}

OVERALL PROGNOSTIC ESTIMATE FOR EXTENT OF IMPROVEMENT
IN APHASIA/COGNITION/COMMUNICATION

..... Excellent   ..... Good   ..... Fair   ..... Guarded   ..... Poor

Clinical Aphasiology, Vol. 22, 1994, pp. 119–133

Test-Retest Stability of Measures of Connected Speech in Aphasia

Robert H. Brookshire and Linda E. Nicholas

Almost all aphasic adults have impairments in connected speech. Clinicians often are called on to describe, measure, and treat connected speech impairments in adults with aphasia, and they may categorize persons in terms of the severity and type of their aphasia based in large part on their connected speech. Clinicians may also use samples of connected speech to establish baselines against which to assess the effects of neurologic recovery or treatment. Such uses of connected speech require two assumptions: (a) that the speech samples are representative of the speaker's general connected speech abilities and (b) that differences in connected speech among patients, or differences in a given patient's connected speech on different test occasions, are reliable differences. Although these assumptions are crucial, their legitimacy has not been established, in large part because we know little about the test-retest stability of measures typically used to assess connected speech in adults with aphasia.

Numerous studies in the area of child language have shown that the size of a speech sample often has potent effects on the stability of the measures used to quantify it (Hess, Haug, & Landry, 1989; Hess, Sefton, & Landry, 1986). Consequently, it is generally recognized that children's speech samples should meet certain minimum length requirements, although no generally accepted minimum length exists (Miller, 1981).

We know very little, however, about the effects of sample size on measures of connected speech for adults with aphasia. The issue of speech sample size seems particularly germane to aphasiology, because speech samples collected in clinical and research activities with aphasic adults tend to be quite short—often fewer than 100 words. Such samples often come from an aphasic person's description of a single picture, which is frequently the so-called Cookie Theft picture from the *Boston Diagnostic Aphasia Examination* (BDAE) (Goodglass & Kaplan, 1983).

We became concerned with the issue of sample size as we were working to validate measures of connected speech of adults with aphasia and to measure how different elicitation stimuli affected the speech samples obtained. On the average, our stimuli each elicited fewer than 100 words from aphasic speakers, and it seemed to us that basing our measures on such short speech samples might compromise their stability. Consequently, we decided to evaluate whether measures based on short speech samples are unstable and, if so, whether combining short speech samples to make longer ones increases test-retest stability.

METHOD

Subjects

Subjects were 20 non-brain-damaged (NBD) adults and 20 aphasic (APH) adults. All were native speakers of English who had hearing and vision adequate for the tasks. Aphasic subjects were at least 3 months post onset of a single left-hemisphere cerebrovascular brain injury. Six exhibited nonfluent (essentially Broca's) aphasia and 14 exhibited fluent aphasia (fluent speech with literal paraphasias and word retrieval difficulty). Their aphasia severity, as estimated by their overall percentile on a four-subtest shortened version (SPICA) (Disimoni, Keith, & Darley, 1980) of the *Porch Index of Communicative Ability* (PICA) (Porch, 1971), ranged from the 40th to the 85th percentile. Aphasic subjects ranged in age from 51 to 77 years ($M = 64.9$, $SD = 6.8$) and in education from 10 to 16 years ($M = 13.1$, $SD = 1.7$). Non-brain-damaged subjects were nonhospitalized and noninstitutionalized adults who were similar to the aphasic adults in age ($M = 64.2$ years, $SD = 7.0$; range = 50–73) and education ($M = 12.8$; $SD = 2.2$; range = 8–16).

Stimuli

Connected speech was elicited from aphasic and non-brain-damaged speakers with a set of 10 stimuli. The stimuli included two aphasia test pictures, the Cookie Theft picture from the BDAE and the Picnic picture from the *Western Aphasia Battery* (WAB) (Kertesz, 1982). The stimuli also included the following:

- two single pictures drawn for the study (*Cat in Tree* and *Birthday Party*, see Figure 1);

- two picture sequences drawn for the study (*The Argument* and *Directions*, see Figure 2);

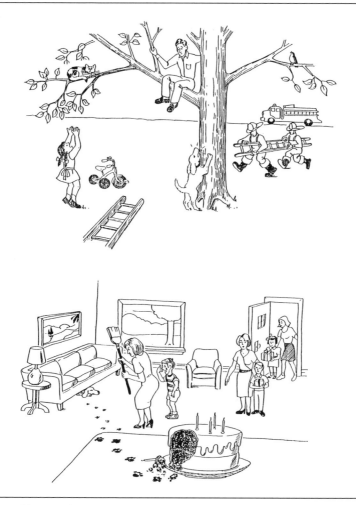

Figure 1. Two single-picture elicitation stimuli drawn for the study. (Copyright 1992, Robert H. Brookshire and Linda E. Nicholas. Reproduced with permission.)

- two requests for personal information:
  "Tell me what you usually do on Sundays," and
  "Tell me where you live and describe it to me"; and

- two requests for procedural information:
  "Tell me how you would go about doing dishes by hand," and
  "Tell me how you would go about writing and sending a letter."

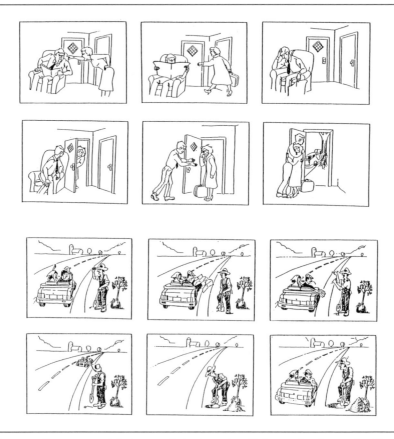

Figure 2. Two sequential picture elicitation stimuli drawn for the study. (Copyright 1992, Robert H. Brookshire and Linda E. Nicholas. Reproduced with permission.)

Measures of Connected Speech

This study evaluated the test-retest stability of three measures of connected speech, *words per minute, correct information units per minute,* and *percent correct information units.*[1] Speech samples were elicited from the non-brain-damaged and the aphasic subjects with the 10 elicitation stimuli

---

1. We developed correct information unit (CIU) analysis to quantify the *informativeness* of connected speech (Nicholas & Brookshire, 1993). Correct information units are words that are intelligible in context and accurately convey information relevant to the eliciting stimulus. Percent correct information units is calculated by dividing the number of CIUs in a speech sample by the number of words in the sample.

on two occasions. The second session followed the first after 7 to 10 days. A different random order of stimuli was established for each subject, and each subject responded to the 10 stimuli in the same random order in both sessions. Each subject's responses to the stimuli were recorded on audiotape and orthographically transcribed. Two judges independently verified the accuracy of the transcripts and made corrections as needed. The corrected transcripts were then timed and scored for words and correct information units (CIUs).

To assess scoring reliability, two scorers independently scored the transcripts of six non-brain-damaged and six aphasic subjects. Point-to-point percentage agreement on words ranged from 97 to 100 percent; on CIUs, it ranged from 90 to 99 percent.

Procedures

To evaluate the effects of sample size on the stability of the measures, we divided the 10 elicitation stimuli into two sets of 5 stimuli each, which we labeled Sets A and B; Table 1 shows their contents. We then evaluated the test-retest stability of the three measures for all 10 stimuli combined (hereafter called Set AB), for Sets A and B (which contained 5 stimuli each), and for one single stimulus—the *Cookie Theft* picture from the BDAE. We chose the *Cookie Theft* picture as the single stimulus because it has been a popular vehicle for eliciting connected speech from aphasic adults, not because we believed that it would yield samples with either greater or less stability than any other single elicitation stimulus.

RESULTS

To determine an overall measure of test-retest stability, we first calculated correlation coefficients between subjects' Session 1 and Session 2 scores

Table 1: Elicitation Stimuli Contained in Set A and Set B

Category of Stimulus	Set A	Set B
Aphasia test picture	BDAE Cookie Theft	WAB Picnic
Single picture	Birthday Party	Cat in Tree
Picture sequence	Argument	Directions
Personal information	Sunday	Live
Procedures	Dishes	Letter

Note: BDAE = *Boston Diagnostic Aphasia Examination;* WAB = *Western Aphasia Battery.*

for Sets AB, A, and B and for the "Cookie Theft" picture. The results are shown in Table 2. The correlations were always higher for scores based on sets of stimuli than for scores based on the single stimulus, suggesting greater test-retest stability for scores based on larger speech samples.

To determine the magnitude of changes in scores from Session 1 to Session 2, we calculated the absolute difference between the scores from both sessions for each subject on each measure and averaged them for each of the two groups. We ignored the sign of the differences so that negative differences would not cancel out positive differences when we calculated group statistics. Also, we were interested in *how much* scores changed, not the direction in which they changed.

Figure 3 shows the average absolute change in words per minute from Session 1 (T_1) to Session 2 (T_2) for the set of 10 stimuli, for the two 5-stimulus subsets, and for each stimulus. Change scores for both groups were considerably smaller when they were based on sets of either 5 or 10 stimuli than when they were based on single stimuli. Aphasic subjects' average change scores for sets of stimuli ranged from about six to eight words per minute. When the scores were based on individual stimuli, change scores often doubled or tripled. A similar pattern can be seen for the non-brain-damaged subjects, although their scores were more unstable overall.

Figure 4 shows test-retest stability for correct information units per minute. The pattern is similar to that for words per minute. Both groups' change scores for sets of stimuli generally were considerably smaller than those for individual stimuli. Once again, non-brain-damaged subjects' scores were somewhat more unstable overall than aphasic subjects' scores.

Table 2: Correlations Between Session 1 and Session 2 Scores of Non-Brain-Damaged and Aphasic Subjects

Measure	Set AB[a]	Set A[a]	Set B[a]	BDAE[b]
Non-Brain-Damaged Subjects				
Words per minute	.90	.90	.82	.79
CIUs[c] per minute	.90	.89	.83	.77
% CIUs	.96	.84	.92	.62
Aphasic Subjects				
Words per minute	.98	.98	.97	.86
CIUs[c] per minute	.97	.94	.97	.75
% CIUs	.98	.93	.94	.71

[a]Set AB contained 10 stimuli; Set A and B contained 5 each. [b]*Boston Diagnostic Aphasia Examination* (Goodglass & Kaplan, 1983) Cookie Theft picture. [c]CIU = correct information unit.

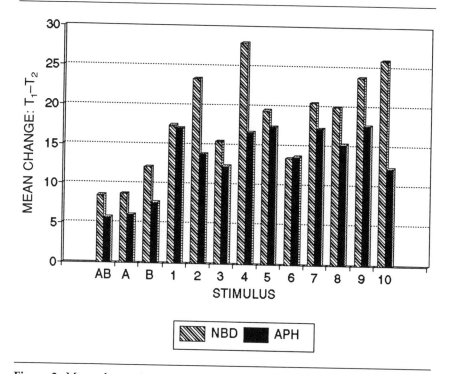

Figure 3. Mean change in words per minute from Test 1 (T_1) to Test 2 (T_2) for non-brain-damaged (NBD) and aphasic (APH) subjects when speech was elicited with Set AB (10 stimuli), Sets A or B (5 stimuli each), or each of 10 single elicitation stimuli (numbers 1–10). (1 = BDAE Cookie Theft picture; 2 = WAB picnic picture; 3, 4 = single pictures; 5, 6 = sequence pictures; 7, 8 = personal information; 9, 10 = procedures.)

Figure 5 shows the results for percent correct information units. The percent CIUs measure was more stable overall than the other two measures. However, as was true for the other measures, the average change from Session 1 to Session 2 generally was greater for individual stimuli than for sets of either 5 or 10 stimuli, especially for aphasic subjects. Their average change scores usually more than doubled when scores were based on individual stimuli rather than a 5- or 10-stimulus set. Non-brain-damaged subjects' scores show a similar relationship; however, their percent CIU scores tended to be more stable overall than the percent CIU scores for aphasic subjects.

To determine whether the five categories of elicitation stimuli differed in test-retest stability, we calculated an average change score for each category. (These average change scores represent change scores that could be expected from testing and retesting with a single stimulus in each

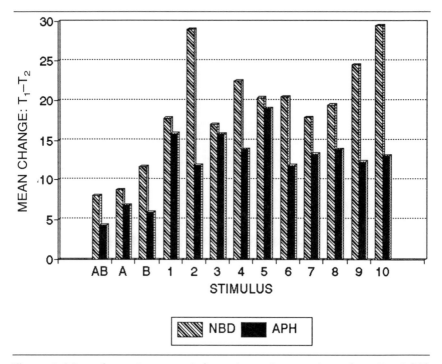

Figure 4. Mean change in correct information units per minute from Test 1 (T_1) to Test 2 (T_2) for non-brain-damaged (NBD) and aphasic (APH) subjects when speech was elicited with Set AB (10 stimuli), Sets A or B (5 stimuli each), or each of 10 single elicitation stimuli (numbers 1–10).

category. They do not represent what would be expected if the speech samples obtained for the two stimuli within each category were *combined*.) The results for words per minute are shown in Figure 6. For aphasic subjects, no category of elicitation stimuli was appreciably more or less stable than any other; they all averaged about a 15-words-per-minute change from Session 1 to Session 2. Non-brain-damaged subjects showed greater variability, with change scores ranging from 18 to 27 words per minute across categories.

Figure 7 shows the results for correct information units per minute. For aphasic subjects the differences among stimulus categories for CIUs per minute were somewhat greater than they had been for words per minute. However, the actual difference between procedures (which yielded the most stable scores) and sequence pictures (which yielded the least stable scores) was less than three CIUs per minute—probably not a clinically significant difference. Again, non-brain-damaged subjects showed greater variability in change scores across stimulus categories than aphasic subjects did.

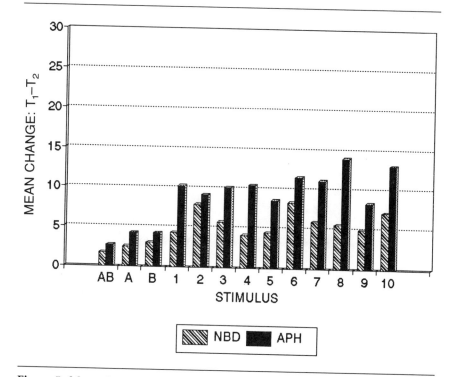

Figure 5. Mean change in percent correct information units from Test 1 (T$_1$) to Test 2 (T$_2$) for non-brain-damaged (NBD) and aphasic (APH) subjects when speech was elicited with Set AB (10 stimuli), Sets A or B (5 stimuli each), or each of 10 single elicitation stimuli (numbers 1–10).

Figure 8 shows the results for percent correct information units. Differences in the categories of elicitation stimuli had little effect on the stability of aphasic and non-brain-damaged subjects' percent CIU scores. The largest difference (between aphasia test pictures and requests for personal information for aphasic subjects) was less than 3%.

To go beyond group averages, and to assess the test-retest stability of the measures on an individual-subject basis, we compared each of the 20 aphasic subjects' change scores for samples elicited with the Cookie Theft picture with their change scores for samples elicited with Set A. Only the results for Set A are presented, because the results for Set B were similar, and although differences between Set AB (with 10 stimuli) and the Cookie Theft picture would be greater yet, a 5-stimulus set seemed clinically more practical.

Figure 9 shows the subject-by-subject results for words per minute. In most cases, scores for the *Cookie Theft* picture were more unstable than

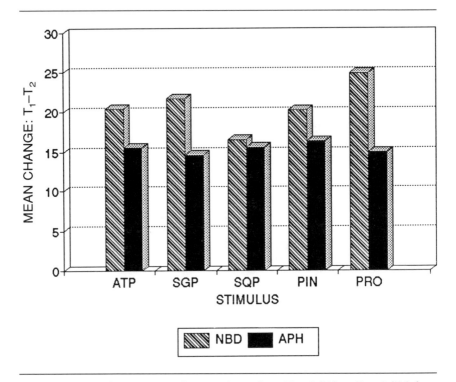

Figure 6. Mean change in words per minute from Test 1 (T_1) to Test 2 (T_2) for non-brain-damaged (NBD) and aphasic (APH) subjects when speech was elicited with aphasia test pictures (ATP), single pictures (SGP), sequence pictures (SQP), requests for personal information (PIN), or requests for descriptions of procedures (PRO).

scores for Set A, with some subjects exhibiting dramatic instability on the *Cookie Theft* picture. Only 3 of 20 aphasic subjects exceeded a 10-words-per-minute difference between Session 1 and Session 2 on Set A, whereas 12 of 20 exceeded this difference on the BDAE picture, including 4 whose change scores exceeded 30 words per minute.

The results were similar for correct information units per minute (Figure 10). Again, scores for the Cookie Theft picture were more unstable than scores for the five-stimulus set, with 4 subjects showing changes of more than 30 CIUs per minute.

Figure 11 shows the results for percent correct information units. Overall, percent CIU scores were more stable than either words per minute or CIUs per minute scores, but scores on the *Cookie Theft* picture again were less stable than scores on the five-stimulus set. Only 1 of the 20 aphasic subjects exhibited a greater than 10% change in percent CIUs on Set A, whereas 11 exhibited changes of this magnitude or more on the Cookie Theft picture.

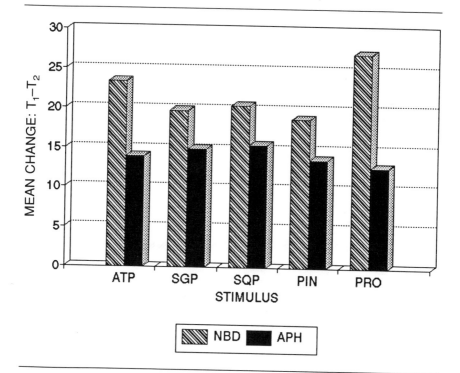

Figure 7. Mean change in correct information units per minute from Test 1 (T_1) to Test 2 (T_2) for non-brain-damaged (NBD) and aphasic (APH) subjects when speech was elicited with aphasia test pictures (ATP), single pictures (SGP), sequence pictures (SQP), requests for personal information (PIN), or requests for descriptions of procedures (PRO).

DISCUSSION

Our results clearly show that one should not make decisions about the connected speech of an adult with aphasia based on measures obtained from one short speech sample, because such measures can be highly unstable from test to test. Because of this instability, a patient's type or severity of aphasia might appear to have changed, even though no actual change has occurred. Likewise, if such short speech samples are used to establish baselines against which the effects of treatment or neurologic recovery are to be measured, actual differences may be obscured by test-retest instability, or spurious differences generated by test-retest instability may be misconstrued as the effects of treatment or neurologic recovery.

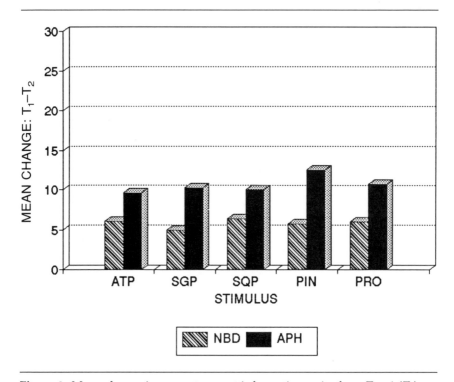

Figure 8. Mean change in percent correct information units from Test 1 (T_1) to Test 2 (T_2) for non-brain-damaged (NBD) and aphasic (APH) subjects when speech was elicited with aphasia test pictures (ATP), single pictures (SGP), sequence pictures (SQP), requests for personal information (PIN), or requests for descriptions of procedures (PRO).

On the other hand, our results show that when measures such as those described herein are based on longer speech samples, they are likely to have adequate test-retest stability. We do not know, at this time, how much one could reduce the number of elicitation stimuli below five and still maintain acceptable stability. Because transcribing and scoring connected speech samples can be time consuming, it seems clinically important to analyze only a large enough sample to ensure representativeness and stability. Our results suggest that there is substantial gain in stability by moving from 1 to 5 stimuli and that going from 5 to 10 stimuli yields substantially smaller gains. When the time needed to transcribe and score the extra 5 stimuli is considered, that small gain may not be worthwhile. At this time we do not know whether samples based on responses to 2, 3, or 4 stimuli would yield acceptably stable measures, but we plan to explore that possibility.

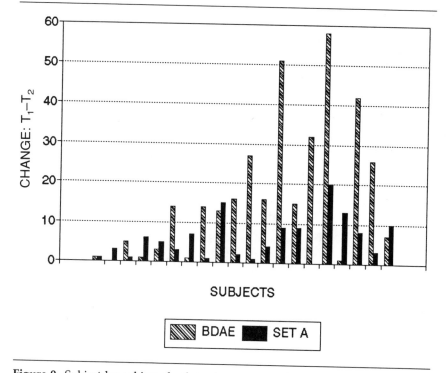

Figure 9. Subject-by-subject absolute change scores for words per minute when speech was elicited with the *Boston Diagnostic Aphasia Examination* Cookie Theft picture (BDAE) or with Set A (5 elicitation stimuli).

Although the results of this study do not speak directly to the issue of representativeness, we feel that speech samples composed of responses to a variety of elicitation stimuli are likely to be more representative of an individual's everyday connected speech than are samples based on a single type of stimulus. At this point, we believe that a combined sample representing an aphasic speaker's responses to the five types of elicitation stimuli described herein should, in most cases, satisfy the need for both stability and representativeness.

ACKNOWLEDGMENTS

This research was supported by the Department of Veterans' Affairs Medical Research Service and by the Medical Research Service of the Minneapolis VA Medical Center.

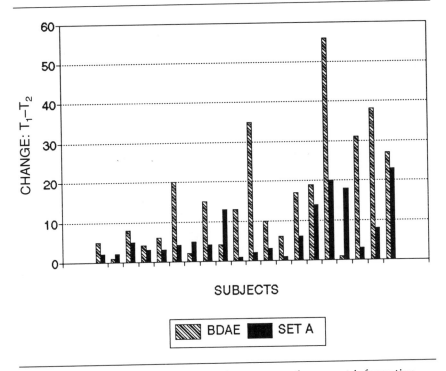

Figure 10. Subject-by-subject absolute change scores for correct information units per minute when speech was elicited with the *Boston Diagnostic Aphasia Examination* Cookie Theft picture (BDAE) or with Set A (5 elicitation stimuli).

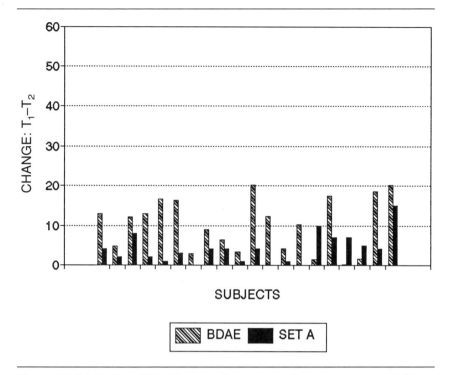

Figure 11. Subject-by-subject absolute change scores for precent correct information units when speech was elicited with the *Boston Diagnostic Aphasia Examination* Cookie Theft picture (BDAE) or with Set A (5 elicitation stimuli).

REFERENCES

Disimoni, F. G., Keith, R., & Darley, F. L. (1980). Prediction of PICA overall score by short versions of the test. *Journal of Speech and Hearing Research, 23,* 511–516.

Goodglass, H., & Kaplan, E. (1983). *The Boston Diagnostic Aphasia Examination.* Boston: Lea & Febiger.

Hess, C. W., Haug, H. T., & Landry, R. G. (1989). The reliability of type-token ratios for the oral language of school age children. *Journal of Speech and Hearing Research, 32,* 536–540.

Hess, C. W., Sefton, K. M., & Landry, R. G. (1986). Sample size and type-token ratios for oral language of preschool children. *Journal of Speech and Hearing Research, 29,* 129–134.

Kertesz, A. (1982). *The Western Aphasia Battery,* New York: Grune & Stratton.

Miller, J. F. (1981). *Assessing language production in children: Experimental procedures.* Baltimore: University Park.

Nicholas, L. E., & Brookshire, R. H. (1993). A system for quantifying the informativeness and efficiency of aphasic adults' connected speech. *Journal of Speech and Hearing Research, 36,* 338–350.

Porch, B. E. (1971). *The Porch Index of Communicative Ability,* Palo Alto, CA: Consulting Psychologists Press.

Clinical Aphasiology, Vol. 22, 1994, pp. 135–144

The Effects of Setting Variables on Conversational Discourse in Normal and Aphasic Adults

Patrick J. Doyle, Cynthia K. Thompson, Karen Oleyar, Julie Wambaugh, and Amy Jackson

Ecologically valid outcome measures are crucial to thoroughly assess the efficacy of language intervention in aphasic adults. In this regard, clinical researchers are, with increasing frequency, sampling conversational discourse as a means to evaluate generalization effects of treatment.

Collecting language samples under conversational discourse conditions has several advantages. First, the contextual elements that compose such conditions, and the functional purpose and structure of the samples obtained, more closely approximate typical sociocommunicative interactions than do narrative, procedural, or expository forms of discourse. Second, certain pragmatic aspects of communication, such as the appropriate and successful use of speaking turns, topic shifts, and various communicative functions, may be observed only under conversational discourse conditions.

Nevertheless, there are a number of problems inherent to conversational discourse sampling, especially as it relates to the measurement of communicative functions. These include a lack of quantitative data from normal adults regarding the range and proportionate use of various communicative functions and a lack of information regarding the effects of a number of setting variables, including the number and familiarity of conversational partners, the physical environment in which conversations occur, and the manner in which discourse samples are elicited.

Therefore, the purpose of this investigation was to describe the proportionate distribution of communicative functions in the conversations of aphasic and normal adults and to examine the effects of familiarity of conversational partner (i.e., familiar vs. unfamiliar), sampling procedure (i.e., topic-open vs. topic-constrained), number of conversational participants (i.e., dyad vs. triad), and physical environment (i.e., subjects' homes vs. simulated home environments) on the dependent variables. These dependent variables included the communicative function categories of statements, requests, answers, and ambiguous communicative attempts.

METHOD

Participants

Subjects. Two groups of subjects, 12 normal and 13 aphasic adults, participated in the study. The aphasic group consisted of 12 males and 1 female who ranged from 18 to 180 months post onset of a single left hemisphere cerebrovascular accident (CVA). They obtained *Porch Index of Communicative Ability* (PICA) (Porch, 1971) overall percentile scores between 54 and 87 and estimated premorbid IQs (Wilson, Rosenbaum, & Brown, 1979) between 90 and 138. The mean age of the group was 60.6 years (*SD* = 5.88). Individual subject data, including Western Aphasia Battery (WAB) type (Kertesz, 1982), are presented in Table 1. The normal subject group consisted of 11 males and 1 female with a mean age of 58.8 years

Table 1. Aphasic Subject Data

Subject	Age	Gender	Hand[a]	MPO[b]	EPIQ[c]	WAB Type[d]	PICA %ile[e]
S1	66	M	R	120	114	Broca's	57
S2	62	M	R	48	112	Broca's	63
S3	62	M	R	79	107	Broca's	70
S4	69	M	L	71	116	Conduction	78
S5	60	M	R	25	138	Broca's	87
S6	50	M	R	101	122	Broca's	54
S7	59	M	R	86	132	Broca's	84
S8	68	M	R	65	119	Broca's	57
S9	59	F	R	54	109	Broca's	79
S10	50	M	R	18	110	Broca's	87
S11	62	M	R	180	120	Broca's	81
S12	64	M	R	32	90	Broca's	–
S13	57	M	R	46	102	Broca's	62
M	60.6						
SD	5.88						

[a]Handedness, [b]Months post onset. [c]Estimated premorbid IQ. [d]*Western Aphasia Battery* type. [e]*Porch Index of Communicative Ability.*

(*SD* = 58.8) and estimated premorbid IQs between 109 and 130. The subject groups did not differ significantly with respect to age [*t* (23) = .69, *p* = .499], estimated premorbid IQ [*t* (23) = –.97, *p* = .342], or years of formal education [*t* (23) = –.99, *p* = .331]. All subjects lived at home and identified 2 individuals with whom they were closely acquainted to serve as their familiar partners.

Conversational Partners. Two groups of volunteers, 50 familiar (i.e., 2 acquaintances of each aphasic and normal subject) and 25 unfamiliar (i.e., 1 hospital voluntary service worker for each subject) served as conversational partners. The familiar group consisted of 16 males and 34 females with a mean age of 53.0 years (*SD* = 16.5). The unfamiliar group consisted of 13 males and 12 females with a mean age of 54.6 years (*SD* = 10.5). The volunteer groups did not differ significantly with respect to age [*t* (73) = –.45, *p* = .652] or years of formal education [*t* (73) = –.187, *p* = .065].

All study participants were monolingual English-speaking individuals who passed a pure tone audiometric screening at 30dB HL in the better ear.

Data Collection

Six-minute samples of conversational discourse were obtained in a counterbalanced order across subjects within each group by holding number of conversational participants (dyads) and physical environment (simulated) constant while manipulating familiarity of conversational partner and topic-open versus topic-constrained sampling procedures. In topic-constrained sampling conditions, subjects viewed and then discussed one of five 4-minute videotaped news segments that were presented in a counterbalanced order across conditions. The video recordings were selected from a pool of 12 *ABC News*, "American Agenda" segments that were equated on a number of interest and complexity parameters by a separate group of 19 age-matched volunteers prior to data collection. In topic-open conditions, subjects were instructed to talk about anything they chose.

Samples were also obtained under conditions in which familiarity of conversational partner (familiar) and sampling procedure (topic-constrained) were held constant while the number of conversational participants and physical environment (i.e., subjects' homes vs. simulated home environments) were manipulated. Simulated home environments were located in the speech clinics of two research sites. These rooms were carpeted and contained comfortable furniture, draperies, wall hangings, TV monitors, and VCRs. All recording equipment was unobtrusive.

Data Analysis

A total of 175 conversations were conducted. Two were lost because of recording equipment failure; the remaining 173 samples were orthographically transcribed from audio recordings, segmented into utterances, and entered into a microcomputer by a trained research assistant. Utterance segmentation was determined on the basis of prosodic, syntactic, and semantic criteria according to transcription conventions adapted from those described by Campbell and Dollaghan (1987). Each subject utterance was subsequently coded by two speech pathologists according to the dependent measures defined in Appendix A.

Frequency data for individual communicative functions were converted to proportions of the total number of subjects' communicative functions in each sample. Proportional data were subsequently subjected to ARCSIN transformations to stabilize the variances.

Repeated measures analyses of variance were performed on each dependent measure to examine the effects of (a) group, familiarity, sampling procedure, and their interactions, and (b) group, number of participants, physical environment, and their interactions.

Reliability

Tests of the reliability of transcription and utterance segmentation were performed on all samples. To determine reliability, a second rater was provided with the original transcripts and corresponding audio recordings and instructed to indicate any disagreements with respect to utterance content or utterance segmentation on the original transcript. Disagreements were reviewed by a third rater and either resolved by consensus or omitted from the data analysis. Less than 2% of the utterances sampled were omitted because of a lack of consensus among the raters. A test of the reliability of communicative function scoring was performed on one randomly selected conversation for each subject. For this dimension, two raters independently coded all subject utterances, and point-to-point reliability was calculated. The percentage of interobserver agreement was determined by dividing the number of agreements by the number of agreements plus disagreements and multiplying by 100. The mean percentage of agreement for the 25 transcripts sampled was 86%, with scores ranging from 79 to 100%.

RESULTS

Descriptive data are provided in the form of group means and standard deviations for the dependent measures within each setting condition

Table 2. Mean Values and Standard Deviations for Group, Familiarity, and Sampling Procedures

N = 13 N = 12	Aphasic Normal	Group	FAMILIARITY		SAMPLING PROCEDURE	
			Unfamiliar	Familiar	Topic-Open	Topic-Con.
		M (SD)	M (SD)	M (SD)	M (SD)	M (SD)
Statements	A	.1855(.1287)	.1751(.1195)	.1958(.1379)	.1805(.1058)	.1904(.1516)
	N	.5891(.1468)	.5438(.1520)	.6345(.1416)	.4971(.1400)	.6811(.1537)
Requests	A	.0275(.0283)	.0173(.0197)	.0377(.0368)	.0342(.0331)	.0208(.0234)
	N	.0728(.0588)	.0618(.0448)	.0838(.0726)	.0927(.0674)	.0530(.0502)
Answers	A	.1844(.1092)	.1823(.0859)	.1869(.1326)	.2202(.1154)	.1489(.1030)
	N	.0393(.0380)	.0386(.0249)	.0399(.0331)	.0628(.0876)	.0158(.0215)
ACA	A	.1357(.0869)	.1496(.1215)	.1219(.0852)	.1209(.0685)	.1505(.1054)
	N	.0562(.0401)	.0518(.0364)	.0607(.0483)	.0484(.0349)	.0641(.0453)

(Tables 2 and 3). Inferential analyses are provided in the form of F values obtained from repeated measures analysis of variance procedures. Because of the number of analyses conducted on the same data set, a conservative significance level of .01 was employed for each inferential comparison.

Group, Familiarity, and Sampling Procedure Effects

Under conditions in which the number of conversational participants and environment were held constant while familiarity and sampling procedure were manipulated, aphasic subjects' conversations contained significantly lower proportions of statements [$F (1, 22) = 92.33, p < .01$] and requests [$F (1, 22) = 14.88, p < .01$] and significantly higher proportions of answers [$F (1, 22) = 41.21, p < .01$] and ambiguous communicative attempts [$F (1, 22) = 12.74, p < .01$], relative to normals.

Familiarity of conversational partner was found not to influence significantly subjects' use of the dependent measures [All F values $(1, 22) < 6.75$, $p > .01$].

In contrast, sampling procedure was found to affect performance, with subjects producing significantly greater proportions of statements under topic-constrained sampling conditions [$F (1, 22) = 13.67, p < .01$] and significantly greater proportions of requests [$F (1, 22) = 10.26, p < .01$] and answers [$F (1, 22) = 19.19, p < .01$] under topic-open sampling conditions.

However, for the communicative function category of statements, group membership significantly interacted with sampling procedure. That is, normal subjects produced more statements in the topic-constrained as compared to topic-open sampling condition [$F (1, 22) = 11.00, p < .01$],

Table 3. Mean Values and Standard Deviations for Group, Number, and Setting

N = 13 N = 12	Aphasic Normal	Group	NUMBER		SETTING	
			Dyad	Triad	Home	Simulated
		M (SD)	M (SD)	M (SD)	M (SD)	M (SD)
Statements	A	.2068(.1705)	.2085(.2104)	.2051(.1305)	.2103(.1943)	.2075(.2069)
	N	.6974(.1358)	.7087(.1320)	.6861(.1398)	.7107(.1351)	.6841(.1365)
Requests	A	.0227(.0298)	.0265(.1320)	.0188(.0266)	.0163(.0274)	.0290(.0321)
	N	.0655(.0516)	.0787(.0609)	.0524(.0422)	.0666(.0433)	.0645(.0598)
Answers	A	.1653(.1269)	.1589(.1341)	.1715(.1197)	.1754(.1382)	.1551(.1156)
	N	.0230(.0275)	.0212(.0220)	.0258(.0330)	.0226(.0234)	.0234(.0316)
ACA	A	.1342(.1071)	.1412(.1064)	.1271(.1079)	.1417(.1132)	.1265(.1012)
	N	.0852(.0619)	.0759(.0549)	.0930(.0572)	.0929(.0572)	.0774(.0656)

whereas the proportionate use of statements by aphasic subjects was not affected by differences in sampling contexts.

Group, Number, and Setting Effects

Under conditions in which the familiarity of conversational partner and sampling procedure were held constant while the number of conversational participants and physical environments were manipulated, the main effects for group were essentially replicated. That is, aphasic subjects produced significantly smaller proportions of statements [F (1, 23) = 94.83, $p < .01$] and requests [F (1, 23) = 24.28, $p < .01$] and significantly greater proportions of answers [F (1, 23) = 23.89, $p < .01$] relative to normals.

However, neither number of conversational participants nor physical settings significantly influenced subjects' use of the dependent measures [All F values (1, 23) < 5.01, $p > .01$].

In summary, our findings revealed that aphasic subjects used significantly lower proportions of statements and requests and greater proportions of answers during their conversations than did normals across all setting conditions. These behaviors were particularly sensitive to the manner in which conversational discourse was elicited (i.e., topic-open versus topic-constrained sampling procedures) but were not significantly influenced by the familiarity or number of conversational partners, or by the physical environments in which the conversations occurred.

DISCUSSION

One of the purposes of this investigation was to describe the proportionate distribution of communicative functions in the conversational discourse of people with aphasia and of normal adults. The results indicated that aphasic and normal subject groups differed significantly in their proportionate use of the communicative functions measured. Normal subjects' conversations primarily comprised utterances that asserted information that was neither obligated nor requested (i.e., statements). In contrast, aphasic subjects provided information in the form of answers to direct requests as frequently as they provided unsolicited information. Clearly, aphasic subjects were asked many more direct questions about themselves and the topics of conversation by their conversational partners than were normal subjects. This pattern of interaction may be accounted for by a number of factors, including (a) differences in conversational participants' perceived roles when conversing with aphasic subjects as compared to normal language users, (b) the reduced efficiency with which aphasic subjects were able to initiate substantive turns, (c) aphasic subjects' use of conversational regulators as an active strategy to shift the communicative burden to their conversational partner, or (d) interactions of all these factors, as well as other uncontrolled variables. However, what is evident is that the aphasic subjects studied in this investigation demonstrated the full range of communicative functions in their conversations, although they assumed a primarily passive communicative role relative to normals.

Another aspect of this study concerned the influence of extralinguistic contextual variables on the subjects' use of communicative functions. The results revealed that only the manner in which conversational discourse was elicited (i.e., topic-open versus topic-constrained sampling procedures) significantly influenced subject performance. These conditions actually differed on three relevant stimulus parameters (i.e., mode of presentation, degree of topic constraint, and degree of shared knowledge or reference). Specifically, the topic-constrained condition employed a *videotaped mode* of stimulus presentation in which *topic selection was constrained* and the extent of *shared topic reference was maximized* (i.e., subjects and partners viewed the videotape together). In contrast, the topic-open condition employed a *verbal instruction mode* of stimulus presentation in which *topic selection was unconstrained* and the degree of *shared topic knowledge varied* depending on the familiarity and conceptual knowledge of the participants. It is difficult to explain why the aphasic subjects' use of statements (unlike the normals') was not affected by differences in these eliciting conditions. It is possible that the provision of topic structure and the shared knowledge base operating in the topic-constrained condition had a facilitative effect on the aphasic subjects' ability to assert information by minimizing the extent to which they were required to generate topics and by providing a mutually shared experience about which subjects could converse. This appears to be a plausible explanation for the significant differences observed in the normal subjects' use of statements across these conditions.

One possible explanation for the lack of observed differences in the aphasic group's use of statements across topic-open and -constrained sampling conditions may be related in part to the cognitive demands of the tasks. Topic-constrained conditions required subjects to retrieve auditory and visually presented information from short-term memory with essentially no opportunity for rehearsal. Although we attempted to control for task demands by selecting news segments that were rated low on complexity parameters and high on relevancy dimensions by age-matched volunteers, it may be that the memory demands of the task exceeded the potential facilitative properties of topic-structure and shared reference.

Both subject groups requested information and answered direct requests in greater proportions under topic-open conditions than in topic-constrained conditions, although careful examination of the group means for requests reveals that this communicative function category was used relatively infrequently by both aphasic and normal subjects. Given the limited frequency with which requests for information were observed regardless of subject group or elicitation condition, it is difficult to determine whether the differences observed under topic-open versus topic-constrained sampling conditions are clinically important. It may be that none of our sampling contexts provided sufficient obligatory contexts for requesting information.

Although the results of this investigation must be considered preliminary, there are several implications worth consideration with respect to the assessment and treatment of functional conversational skills in adults with aphasia. First, the lack of significant differences in subjects' performance across number and setting conditions suggests that all other factors being equal, one may observe a representative sample of conversational discourse in simulated natural environments that include one or two familiar conversational partners. Second, assessing requests for information under conversational discourse conditions may require specific instructions or the arrangement of obligatory contexts to provide sufficient opportunities to observe this particular communicative function. Third, although aphasic subjects' use of statements was not affected by the sampling procedures employed in this study, the facilitative effect observed in normal subjects under conditions in which topics were constrained and shared topic reference or knowledge was maximized should not be ignored. One may want to incorporate these contextual parameters into a sampling procedure that minimizes the cognitive demands placed on the subject, thus providing a more facilitative context for assessing aphasic subjects' ability to assert new information.

With respect to treatment, applied generalization theory advises that one way to enhance transfer of treatment effects to more natural performance environments is to incorporate salient dimensions of the generalization context into the training context. Given the facilitative effect of topic structure and shared reference observed in our normal subjects' use of statements, it may be useful to incorporate such stimulus parameters in the context of a conversation-based therapy program whose terminal goal would be the functional assertion of information with familiar partners in nontherapeutic contexts.

In conclusion, much work needs to be done to determine which extra-linguistic contextual variables do and do not affect the conversational discourse of aphasic individuals in important ways. The results of this investigation are a preliminary attempt to clarify the relationship between specific aspects of aphasic subjects' conversations and contextual variables that sample a range of natural contexts in which aphasic subjects need to communicate.

ACKNOWLEDGMENTS

This investigation was supported by the Department of Veterans Affairs Rehabilitation, Research, and Development Grant C330-3RA.

We gratefully acknowledge Tom Marshall, Linda McWilliams, Adele Pocavich, Brenda Peggs, and David DeAngelo for their assistance on various aspects of this project. Special thanks are extended to the Highland Drive VAMC volunteers who served as conversational participants in this study.

REFERENCES

Campbell, T. F., & Dollaghan, C. A. (1987). *Conventions for transcribing the spontaneous language samples of brain-injured children.* Unpublished manual. Language Analysis Laboratory, Department of Communication Disorders, Children's Hospital of Pittsburgh, Pittsburgh.

Kertesz, A. (1982). The Western Aphasia Battery. New York: Grune & Stratton.

Porch, B. E. (1971). The Porch Index of Communicative Ability, Vol. 1 (1st ed.). Palo Alto, CA: Consulting Psychologists Press.

Wilson, R. S., Rosenbaum, G., & Brown, G. (1979). The problem of premorbid intelligence in neuropsychological assessment. *Journal of Clinical Neuropsychology, 1,* 49–53.

APPENDIX A

Statements: utterances that were intelligible in context and communicated information relevant to the topic(s) of conversation that was not obligated or requested.

Requests: utterances that were intelligible in context and solicited information not previously provided and about the identity, location, or property of a person, object, or event.

Answers: utterances that were intelligible in context and provided information directly complementing a prior request.

Ambiguous Communicative Attempts: utterances containing intelligible words but whose meaning or intent was uninterpretable.

Clinical Aphasiology, Vol. 22, 1994, pp. 145–155

Longitudinal Assessment of Narrative Discourse in a Mildly Aphasic Adult

Carl A. Coelho, Betty Z. Liles, Robert J. Duffy, Janine V. Clarkson, and Deanne Elia

Traditionally, clinicians have been faced with the problem of identifying measures of communicative change for patients with mild aphasia. Such patients often present functional communication skills yet demonstrate subtle deficits that are difficult to quantify. Recent investigations of verbal communicative ability in adults with brain injuries have focused on the analysis of narrative discourse. Populations studied have included individuals with traumatic brain injury (e.g., Liles, Coelho, Duffy, & Zalagens, 1989; Mentis & Prutting, 1987), those with right hemisphere damage (e.g., Gardner, Brownell, Wapner, & Michellow, 1983; Joanette & Goulet, 1990), and aphasic individuals (e.g., Bottenberg, Lemme, & Hedberg, 1985; Ulatowska, North, & Macaluso-Haynes, 1981). Accurate narrative production and comprehension require a complex interaction of cognitive, linguistic, and social abilities and may be sensitive to particular deficits present in mildly aphasic patients.

The purpose of this study was to assess the sensitivity of various measures of narrative discourse for detecting changes in communicative performance throughout the course of recovery in a mildly impaired fluent aphasic patient.

METHOD

Subjects

Aphasic. AJ was a 55-year-old, right-handed male who was 1 month post onset of a single unilateral left thromboembolic cerebrovascular accident

(CVA) at the time this study was initiated. He was a high-school graduate working as a realtor. The *Porch Index of Communicative Ability* (PICA) (Porch, 1967) overall score at 1 month post onset was 12.65, placing him at the 71st percentile. On the four auditory comprehension subtests from the *Boston Diagnostic Aphasia Examination* (BDAE) (Goodglass & Kaplan), he scored at the 86th percentile. The Rating Scale Profile of Speech characteristics from the BDAE was consistent with anomic aphasia.

Normal. Three adult males with a mean age of 56 years, having no history of neurologic disease and matched with AJ on the basis of the Hollingshead Four Factor Index of Social Status (Hollingshead, 1972), served as controls.

Story Elicitation Procedure

Subjects were presented a picture story entitled "The Bear and the Fly" (Winter, 1976) via a filmstrip projector on an 8-by-10-in. screen. The story has 19 frames (with no sound track) showing how a bear inadvertently wrecks his house and abuses his family while attempting to kill a fly. After viewing the filmstrip the subjects were asked to retell the story.

Data Collection

Stories were elicited from the control subjects on one occasion. Stories were elicited from AJ on a monthly basis and, eventually, every other month up to 1 year post CVA. Each story was audiotaped and transcribed verbatim. Transcriptions were distributed into T units prior to analysis. Measurement of story narrative performance was made at three levels: sentence production, intersentential cohesion, and story episode structure.

Sentence Production. A T unit is defined as an independent clause plus any dependent clauses associated with it (Hunt, 1970). T units are roughly equivalent to sentences but are more reliably identified. The primary measure of sentence production was the number of subordinate clauses per T unit (total number of subordinate clauses in each story divided by the total number of T units). This ratio permitted comparisons across stories that varied in length. The frequency of clause use may be considered to measure the complexity of sentence-level grammar.

Intersentential Cohesion. The occurrence of any of Halliday and Hasan's (1976) five cohesive categories (Reference, Lexical, Conjunction, Elipsis, and Substitution) was noted. Each occurrence of a cohesive tie was then judged as to its adequacy using Liles's (1985) procedure. Three categories of adequacy were used:

1. Complete—a tie was judged complete if the information referred to by the cohesive marker was found easily and defined with no ambiguity.

2. Incomplete—a tie was judged to be incomplete if the information referred to by the cohesive marker was not provided in the text.

3. Error—a tie was judged to be an error if the cohesive marker referred the listener to ambiguous information elsewhere in the text.

The measure of intersentential cohesion selected for analysis was the percentage of complete ties relative to the total number of cohesive ties used within each narrative. The percentage of complete ties represents the use of complete ties minus incomplete or error ties and is considered to be a general indicator of cohesive adequacy.

Story Grammar. The number of complete episodes in each story was counted and used as the measure of story grammar performance. According to Stein and Glenn (1979), an episode must consist of (a) an initiating event that causes a character to formulate a goal-directed behavioral sequence; (b) an action; and (c) a direct consequence marking attainment or nonattainment of the goal. These three components must be logically related. An episode was judged complete only if it contained all three components.

Severity of Aphasia

The *Porch Index of Communicative Ability* (PICA) served as a general measure of aphasic impairment. The PICA was administered on a monthly basis and eventually every other month for 12 months.

Reliability

All reliability measures were based on point-to-point scoring. Interexaminer reliability for the sentence-level measures of total number of T units and number of subordinate clauses identified independently by two scorers was 96% and 94%, respectively. Interexaminer reliability was 96% for identification of episodes and 91% for the cohesion measures.

RESULTS

Severity of Aphasia

Figure 1 depicts AJ's aphasia recovery curve as measured by the PICA. From the initial administration at 1 month post onset, AJ's overall score demonstrated a fairly steady recovery, rising from the 71st percentile to the 93rd at 12 months post onset.

Narrative Discourse Performance

Various aspects of AJ's story narrative discourse performance were measured over the same 12-month period, including measures of sentence

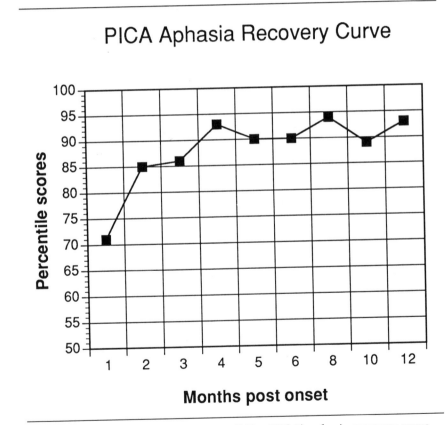

PICA Aphasia Recovery Curve

Figure 1. *Porch Index of Communicative Ability* (PICA) aphasia recovery curve for AJ from 1 to 12 months post onset.

production, intersentential cohesion, and story grammar. AJ's scores on these measures were converted to Z scores for the purpose of comparing them to the average performance of the normal controls.

Sentence Production. The measure selected for sentence production was the ratio of the total number of subordinate clauses in each story divided by the total number of T units. Figure 2 depicts AJ's scores on the story-retelling task. On this task, the complexity of AJ's sentence-level grammar was variable but fairly close to that of the normal controls. In many instances AJ's production of subordinate clauses, throughout the 12-month period it was sampled, surpassed that of two of the control subjects.

Intersentential Cohesion. Intersentential cohesion may be thought of as an organizational system for the content introduced in a narrative. The

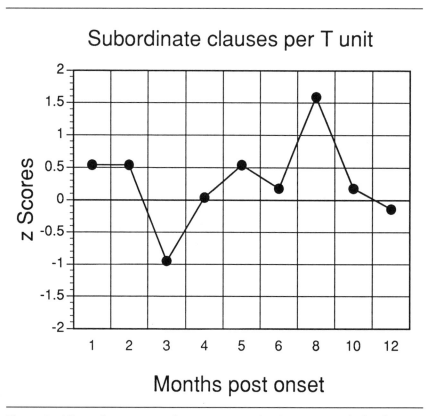

Figure 2. AJ's performance on the sentence production measure (subordinate clauses per T unit in each story) over the 12-month period monitored.

measure of intersentential cohesion selected in this study was the percentage of complete ties per story. Figure 3 illustrates that AJ's performance for the retelling task, although variable, improved steadily over the 12-month period monitored. At 1 year post onset, cohesive adequacy was comparable to that of the normal controls. Therefore, as AJ's language function recovered, his ability to produce a well-organized narrative also improved.

Story Grammar. The production of complete episodes is evidence of story grammar knowledge. Episodes may be considered to be a measure of the integration of a story's content. In the present study, number of complete episodes was selected as the measure of story grammar. Figure 4 depicts AJ's performance on this measure. Initially AJ was unable to generate a single complete episode in the story-retelling task, and he never generated more than two complete episodes over the 12-month period. The normal controls generated four and five complete episodes

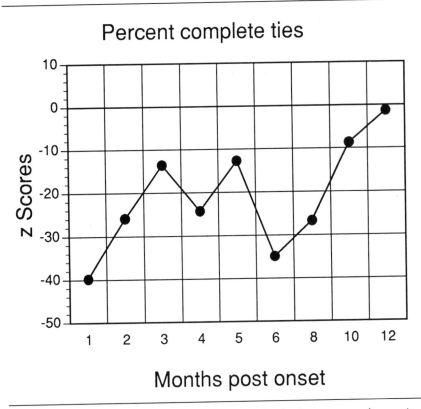

Percent complete ties

Months post onset

Figure 3. AJ's performance on the intersentential cohesion measure (percent complete ties in each story) over the 12-month period monitored.

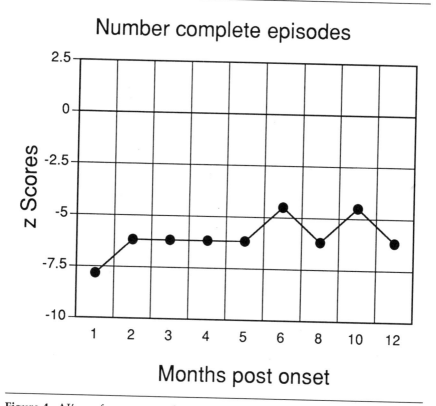

Figure 4. AJ's performance on the story grammar measure (number complete episodes in each story) over the 12-month period monitored.

on the same task. Therefore, in the presence of language recovery, story grammar ability remained relatively impaired and only slightly improved.

DISCUSSION

The findings of this study have both clinical and theoretical implications related to the management of individuals with mild aphasia and to the nature of discourse abilities in patients who have sustained brain injuries.

It is relatively common practice for clinicians, faced with the need to prioritize their limited resources, to discharge those aphasic clients who have either recovered functional language skills or whose language impairments are relatively subtle. Those aphasic clients who are moderately to severely impaired and whose language impairments are more chronic in nature often receive language remediation services that are more intensive and continue for longer periods of time. This is unfortunate, for mildly impaired aphasic individuals may ultimately benefit more from language therapy, in terms of returning to work and resuming near-normal communicative functioning, than more severely involved aphasic patients. If one accepts the notion that mildly aphasic patients should receive at least the same amount of therapy as more severely involved aphasic patients, then clinical measures need to be identified that will delineate the extent and nature of their communicative impairments. Analyses of narrative discourse appear well suited for assessing change in communicative performance over the course of recovery in such patients.

In the present investigation we studied a special form of narrative discourse, that is, story narratives. The use of story narratives permitted an examination not only of sentence-level grammatical ability and inter-sentential cohesion but also of the cognitive abilities underlying the organization and production of a text. Interactions among sentence-level grammar, intersentential cohesion, and story grammar knowledge required to produce a story may place a communicative load on mildly aphasic patients' performance that reveals problems not observable in other forms of discourse. The longitudinal application of these multilevel analyses enabled us to document the differences in AJ's recovery curves for the three measures. Sentence-level grammar, although variable, was relatively normal and showed no significant change over the 12-month trial period. Cohesion yielded a curve similar to that of AJ's aphasia recovery curve, showing some variability but with overall improvement. A flat curve was noted for story grammar, with little apparent change from its moderately impaired status throughout the entire period.

The multilevel analyses also prevented the over- or underestimation of AJ's discourse performance. For example, analysis of just sentence-level grammar or cohesion may have given the impression that AJ's discourse abilities were intact, even though story grammar abilities were moderately depressed. Further, although his cohesion gradually improved, early in the 12-month period it was significantly impaired in the presence of near-normal sentence grammar. Clearly, one could not have predicted the adequacy of AJ's sentence organization from his sentence-level grammar.

With regard to treatment implications, although neither cohesion nor story grammar abilities were directly addressed in the language therapy AJ received, during the 12-month period in which his discourse abilities were monitored, cohesive adequacy appeared to have benefitted from the traditional language-based approach to therapy, whereas story grammar abilities did not. This finding, together with those of previous investigations that have documented improved cohesion in the story narratives produced by normal adults over multiple trials of the same task (Coelho, Liles, & Duffy, 1990), suggests that cohesion may be a promising target for remediation. It should be noted, however, that AJ produced the same one or two episodes in each presentation of the story-retelling task. Over time these episodes became better organized, as indicated by his improved cohesion score. Had he attempted to introduce additional episodes into his retelling of the story we may well have seen a concomitant drop in his cohesive adequacy. It remains to be seen whether therapy, either language-based or cognitively based, directed specifically toward the remediation of story grammar abilities would be effective.

In spite of AJ's recovery of considerable language function by 12 months post onset and his high degree of motivation, he was unable to return to work. Critical elements of language use (perhaps including story grammar ability) not tapped by traditional aphasia batteries remained depressed in AJ, and this affected his functional status. Study of this issue is certainly warranted.

The findings that AJ's intersentential cohesion improved while story grammar abilities remained moderately depressed have theoretical implications as well. Dissociations of microlinguistic (e.g., sentence-level grammar and cohesion) and macrolinguistic (e.g., story grammar) abilities in different groups of brain-injured patients have been hypothesized (see Glosser & Deser, 1990, for a review). For example, fluent aphasics would be expected to have language-specific deficits in the microlinguistic realm but not in the macrolinguistic; patients with Alzheimer's dementia, who demonstrate deficits with higher-order cognitive processes, would be expected to show significant disturbances on macrolinguistic abilities with relative preservation of microlinguistic skills; and patients with closed head injury, with both focal and diffuse brain injuries, would potentially demonstrate deficits in both the microlinguistic and macrolinguistic realms. Our findings are not in agreement with the particular dissociation that has been hypothesized for fluent aphasics, that is, impaired microlinguistic and intact macrolinguistic abilities; in fact, AJ's pattern was just the opposite. Previous studies of this issue have not been based on longitudinally collected discourse samples, and therefore, there is no information available regarding the stability, or the impact, of recovery on such dissociations. Therefore, the notion that specific dissociations are attributable to specific etiologies may be misleading. For example, Coelho, Liles and Duffy (1991) documented distinct dissociations in two patients with closed head injuries, one with relatively intact macrolinguistic abilities (story grammar) and impaired microlinguistic abilities (cohesion), and a second with very poor macrolinguistic abilities and intact microlinguistic abilities. Again, dissociations in discourse abilities may not always be predicted from etiology alone.

Finally, dissociations aside, we suggest two potential explanations for the finding that AJ's cohesive adequacy improved and his story grammar abilities remained depressed, while the severity of his aphasia, as measured by the PICA, decreased: (1) his story grammar impairment may be more attributable to brain injury in general than simply to aphasia, or (2) AJ's pattern may be one example of a variety of discourse deficit patterns that may result in aphasia. Research of these issues is also warranted.

In any event, the clinical application of story narrative analysis holds great potential for assessing brain-injured patients with subtle communicative deficits, as well as for increasing our understanding of the interaction between linguistic and cognitive abilities.

ACKNOWLEDGMENT

This investigation was supported by a grant from the Research Foundation of the National Easter Seal Society.

REFERENCES

Bottenberg, D., Lemme, M. L., & Hedberg, N. (1985). Analysis of oral narratives of normal and aphasic adults. In R. H. Brookshire (Ed.), Clinical aphasiology, Vol. 15 (pp. 241–247). Minneapolis, MN: BRK Publishers.

Coelho, C. A., Liles, B. Z., & Duffy, R. J. (1990). Contextual influences on narrative discourse in normal young adults. Journal of Psycholinguistic Research, 19, 405–420.

Coelho, C. A., Liles, B. Z., & Duffy, R. J. (1991). Discourse analyses with closed head injured adults: Evidence for differing patterns of deficits. Archives of Physical Medicine and Rehabilitation, 72, 465–468.

Gardner, H., Brownell, H. H., Wapner, W., & Michellow, D. (1983). Missing the point: The role of the right hemisphere in the processing of complex linguistic materials. In E. Perecman (Ed.), Cognitive processing in the right hemisphere (pp. 169–191). New York: Academic Press.

Glosser, G., & Deser, T. (1990). Patterns of discourse production among neurological patients with fluent language disorders. Brain and Language, 40, 67–88.

Goodglass, H., & Kaplan, E. (1983). The assessment of aphasia and related disorders (2nd ed.). Philadelphia: Lea & Febiger.

Halliday, M. A. K., & Hasan, R. (1976). Cohesion in English. London: Longman.

Hollingshead, A. B. (1972). Four factor index of social status. Unpublished manuscript, Yale University, Dept. of Sociology, New Haven.

Hunt, K. (1970). Syntactic maturity in school children and adults. Monographs of the Society for Research in Child Development, 35 (Serial No. 134).

Joanette, Y., & Goulet, P. (1990). Narrative discourse in right-brain-damaged right-handers. In Y. Joanette & H. H. Brownell (Eds.), Discourse ability and brain damage: Theoretical and empirical perspectives. New York: Springer-Verlag.

Liles, B. Z. (1985). Narrative ability in normal and language disordered children. Journal of Speech and Hearing Research, 28, 123–133.

Liles, B. Z., Coelho, C. A., Duffy, R. J., & Zalagens, M. R. (1989). Effects of elicitation procedures on the narratives of normal and closed head injured adults. Journal of Speech and Hearing Disorders, 54, 356–366.

Mentis, M., & Prutting, C. A. (1987). Cohesion in the discourse of normal and head-injured adults. *Journal of Speech and Hearing Research, 30,* 88–98.

Porch, B. E. (1967). *Porch Index of Communicative Ability.* Palo Alto: Consulting Psychologists Press.

Stein, N. L., & Glenn, C. G. (1979). An analysis of story comprehension in elementary school children. In R. O. Freedle (Ed.), *New directions in discourse processing* (Vol. 2, pp. 53–120). Norwood, NJ: Ablex.

Ulatowska, H. K., North, A. J., & Macaluso-Haynes, S. (1981). Production of narrative and procedural discourse in aphasia. *Brain and Language, 17,* 345–371.

Winter, P. (1976). *The bear and the fly.* New York: Crown.

Clinical Aphasiology, Vol. 22, 1994, pp. 157–164

PICA Performance Following Left or Right Hemisphere Brain Damage: Influence of Side and Severity

Robert T. Wertz and Nina F. Dronkers

Duffy and Myers (1991) listed several problems in group comparisons across neurologic communication disorders and offered some potential methodologic solutions. One typical problem is that groups with different disorders differ in severity on the measures employed (Halpern, Darley, & Brown, 1973; Wertz, Dronkers, & Shubitowski, 1986). One proposed solution is to equate the samples from different disordered groups for severity. That is the approach we used in this investigation.

One purpose was to compare *Porch Index of Communicative Ability* (PICA) (Porch, 1967) performance by patients who suffered a left hemisphere thromboembolic infarct with performance by patients who suffered a right hemisphere thromboembolic infarct, determine the PICA measures on which the groups differed, and compute a discriminate function analysis to test the PICA's ability to discriminate between groups. A second purpose was to evaluate the influence of severity on group differences by equating the left and right hemisphere groups on overall PICA performance, identify PICA performance differences if they occurred, and compute a discriminant function analysis on the equated groups to test the PICA's ability to discriminate between groups that do not differ in overall severity.

METHOD

Patients met the following selection criteria. They: had suffered a first, single, left or right hemisphere thromboembolic infarct; had suffered no previous neurologic involvement; had no other major medical or psychological disorder; displayed visual acuity adequate to match pictures and copy printing, auditory acuity adequate for conversation, and sensory and motor ability in one upper extremity adequate to gesture and write; and were premorbidly literate in English. Localization of the side of brain damage was confirmed by neurologic evaluation and neuroradiological reports (CT or MRI). All patients who met selection criteria were evaluated with the *Porch Index of Communicative Ability*.

Our initial comparison was done on 70 patients who had suffered a left hemisphere thromboembolic infarct and 30 patients who had suffered a right hemisphere thromboembolic infarct. Descriptive data on these patients are shown in Table 1. The left and right hemisphere groups did not differ significantly ($p < .05$) in age, education, or time post onset. Paired comparisons were conducted on PICA overall, modality, and subtest performance. A discriminant function analysis was computed to determine the PICA's ability to discriminate between patients with left and right hemisphere brain damage. Samples used in these comparisons are referred to as "unmatched" (for severity) groups.

Our second comparison was done on left and right hemisphere patients who were equated for severity. We selected all patients from our original samples who obtained a PICA overall score of 12.00 or above. This yielded 24 patients with left hemisphere lesions and 25 patients with right hemisphere lesions. Descriptive data on these patients are shown in Table 2. There were no significant differences ($p < .05$) between groups for age, education, or months post onset. As before, paired comparisons were conducted on PICA overall, modality, and subtest performance. In addition, a discriminant function analysis was computed to determine the PICA's ability to discriminate between patients with left and right hemisphere brain damage who were "matched" for severity.

Table 1. Descriptive Data for Unmatched Groups of Left Hemisphere and Right Hemisphere Patients

	Group			
	LEFT ($N = 70$)		RIGHT ($N = 30$)	
Variable	*Mean*	SD	*Mean*	SD
Age (in years)	56.10	10.58	54.97	7.11
Education (in years)	11.41	3.01	10.87	2.71
Months post onset	11.21	15.84	10.00	15.44

Table 2. Descriptive Data for Matched Groups of Left Hemisphere and Right Hemisphere Patients

Variable	Group			
	LEFT (N = 24)		RIGHT (N = 25)	
	Mean	SD	Mean	SD
Age (in years)	55.17	12.39	54.36	6.22
Education (in years)	12.54	3.26	11.28	2.56
Months post onset	9.69	11.57	11.38	16.54

RESULTS

A comparison of PICA overall and modality performance for unmatched groups of left and right hemisphere patients, shown in Table 3, indicated the right hemisphere group performed significantly better ($p < .001$) than the left hemisphere group in overall performance and on all modality measures—gestural, verbal, and graphic. Similarly, as shown in Table 4, the right hemisphere group performed significantly better ($p < .01$) on 14 of the 18 PICA subtests. Only visual matching (Subtests VIII and XI) and copying (Subtests E and F) did not differ significantly between groups.

A stepwise discriminant function analysis on the unmatched groups, shown in Table 5, classified 80% of the left hemisphere patients correctly and 93% of the right hemisphere patients correctly. Overall correct classification was 84%. PICA subtests selected by the analysis were Subtest III, pantomime; VIII and XI, visual matching; IX, verbal sentence completion; A, C, and D, writing; and E and F, copying.

Table 6 indicates that when left and right hemisphere groups were matched for overall performance on the PICA, no significant difference ($p < .05$) emerged between groups. Moreover, no significant differences ($p < .05$) occurred in the three PICA modality scores. Comparisons between matched groups on the 18 subtests, shown in Table 7, indicated the right hemisphere group performed significantly better on two—Subtest IV, verbal naming ($p < .05$), and Subtest IX, verbal sentence completion ($p < .01$).

A stepwise discriminant function analysis on the matched groups, shown in Table 8, classified 67% of the left hemisphere patients correctly and 88% of the right hemisphere patients correctly. Overall correct classification was 78%. PICA subtests selected by the analysis were Subtest III, pantomime; VII, reading; IX, verbal sentence completion; XII, verbal repetition; and F, copying.

Table 3. PICA Overall and Modality Performance for Unmatched Groups of Left Hemisphere and Right Hemisphere Patients

| | Group | | | | |
| | LEFT (N = 70) | | RIGHT (N = 30) | | |
PICA Component	Mean	SD	Mean	SD	Mean Difference
Overall	11.12	1.92	13.03	1.21	1.91*
Gestural	12.75	1.55	14.02	.79	1.27*
Verbal	10.48	3.13	13.64	1.15	3.16*
Graphic	9.40	2.54	11.39	2.47	1.99*

*Significant at $p < .001$.

Table 4. Performance on PICA Subtests for Unmatched Left Hemisphere and Right Hemisphere Patients

| | Group | | | | |
| | LEFT (N = 70) | | RIGHT (N = 30) | | |
Subtest	Mean	SD	Mean	SD	Mean Difference
I	8.66	3.06	12.26	1.39	3.60**
II	10.03	2.28	11.73	1.87	1.70**
III	11.11	2.14	12.78	1.61	1.67**
IV	10.12	3.70	13.96	1.07	3.84**
V	11.79	2.60	13.46	1.95	1.67*
VI	13.41	2.21	14.83	.31	1.42**
VII	12.46	2.70	14.55	.74	2.09**
VIII	14.57	1.08	14.90	.28	.33
IX	10.58	3.58	14.25	.97	3.67**
X	13.73	1.66	14.86	.24	1.13**
XI	14.81	1.07	14.98	.08	.17
XII	12.56	3.13	14.55	.91	1.99**
A	6.64	2.21	9.09	2.55	2.45**
B	8.20	3.34	10.99	2.91	2.79**
C	8.89	3.42	10.95	3.13	2.06*
D	9.14	3.25	11.98	2.80	2.84**
E	11.03	3.14	12.07	2.76	1.04
F	12.54	1.74	12.41	2.68	−.13

*Significant at $p < .01$. **Significant at $p < .001$.

Table 5. Classification of Unmatched Left Hemisphere and
Right Hemisphere Patients by Discriminant Function Analysis
of All PICA Subtests

Actual Group	Predicted Group	
	Left	Right
Left (n = 70)		
number of cases	56 (80%)	14 (20%)
Right (n = 30)		
number of cases	2 (7%)	28 (93%)

Note: Percent of all patients classified correctly = 84; subtests selected by the analysis:
F, A, VIII, XI, C, D, IX, E, III.

Table 6. PICA Overall and Modality Performance for Matched
Groups of Left Hemisphere and Right Hemisphere Patients

PICA Component	Group				
	LEFT (N = 24)		RIGHT (N = 25)		
	Mean	SD	Mean	SD	Mean Difference
Overall	13.12	.76	13.43	.77	.31
Gestural	13.99	.43	14.20	.54	.21
Verbal	13.23	1.31	13.84	1.06	.61
Graphic	11.91	1.44	12.21	1.58	.30

DISCUSSION

Our results indicate that Duffy and Myers's (1991) observations about the
influence of severity on comparisons between and among different neurologic communication disorders are correct. Different results are obtained
when severity between groups differs. The importance of this, of course,
depends on the question asked.

Samples unmatched for overall severity indicated that left hemisphere
brain damage results in more severe communication deficits than right
hemisphere brain damage. This is certainly not a new observation. Moreover, right hemisphere patients do not differ significantly from left hemisphere patients in visual matching or copying performance. Again, nothing is new about this observation. Finally, the PICA seems to be a decent
means for differentiating between patients with right hemisphere (93%)
and left hemisphere (80%) brain damage when severity of overall impair-

Table 7. Performance on PICA Subtests for Matched Left Hemisphere and Right Hemisphere Patients

| Subtest | Group | | | | |
| | LEFT (N = 24) | | RIGHT (N = 25) | | |
	Mean	SD	Mean	SD	Mean Difference
I	11.52	2.00	12.36	1.39	.84
II	11.59	1.58	11.95	1.58	.36
III	12.58	1.13	13.12	.96	.54
IV	13.44	1.58	14.26	.77	.82*
V	13.79	1.10	13.90	1.12	.11
VI	14.83	.41	14.93	.18	.10
VII	14.37	.89	14.74	.49	.37
VIII	14.82	.33	14.90	.30	.08
IX	13.68	1.25	14.54	.45	.86**
X	14.76	.50	14.91	.16	.15
XI	14.99	.04	14.99	.04	.00
XII	14.26	1.24	14.77	.43	.51
A	8.95	1.89	9.79	2.12	.84
B	11.43	2.04	11.90	2.13	.47
C	12.10	2.04	11.92	2.27	−.18
D	12.28	1.77	12.75	1.95	.47
E	13.21	1.32	13.06	1.41	−.15
F	13.50	1.10	12.78	2.37	−.72

*Significant at $p < .05$. **Significant at $p < .01$.

Table 8. Classification of Matched Left Hemisphere and Right Hemisphere Patients by Discriminant Function Analysis of All PICA Subtests

| Actual Group | Predicted Group | |
	Left	Right
Left (n = 24)		
number of cases	16 (67%)	8 (33%)
Right (n = 25)		
number of cases	3 (12%)	22 (88%)

Note: Percent of all patients classified correctly = 78; subtests selected by the analysis: IX, F, VII, III, XII.

ment differs between groups. Thus, if the question is whether left and right hemisphere patients differ on a general measure of communicative ability, there appears to be no need for controlling severity.

Samples matched for overall severity indicated only two differences between right and left hemisphere patients, verbal naming and verbal sentence completion. This may imply the presence of persisting "anomic" or word-finding deficits in mildly aphasic (left hemisphere) patients. The PICA's ability to discriminate between left and right hemisphere patients who do not differ in overall severity is reduced for classifying left hemisphere patients (67%) but remains high for classifying right hemisphere patients (88%). Thus, if the question is whether left and right hemisphere patients who display essentially the same overall impairment differ on specific measures of communicative ability, there is a need to control for severity.

The message in methodology may be that a method's value depends on the question asked. This too is not a new observation, but it probably is useful to remember. Thus, we are not advocating the PICA as the best measure for comparing performance between or among different neurologic communication disorders; however, it seems to be a pretty good one. For us, it was a means to explore the influence of severity in group comparisons. Other questions will require different means. The same question may require a better means.

One should exercise caution when interpreting our discriminant function analyses. There is not an exact literature on determining sample size for discriminant function analysis, and there is no prescribed analytical means for deriving appropriate sample size or determining statistical power. A general "rule of thumb" is to include 15 to 20 cases for each variable when using this multivariate procedure. We entered the 18 PICA subtests in the analysis, thus our samples of 100 and 49 are woefully inadequate. The confidence intervals are probably wide, and the probability of a Type II error is high. Nevertheless, correct classification in both analyses was pretty good. More importantly, the purpose of our effort was to examine the influence of severity on comparing left and right hemisphere groups, not to test the PICA's ability to discriminate between groups. Our paired comparisons indicate that severity influences how and how much the groups differ. The discriminate function analyses, interpreted with the limitation of inadequate sample size, suggest the PICA may be a promising means for differentiating between groups.

Duffy and Myers (1991) were prophetic when they observed that "across-group comparison studies are going to be with us as long as we are interested in the classification of communication disorders, their differential diagnosis, and understanding the basic nature of a variety of neurogenic communication deficits" (p. 13). At least 40 papers presented in the Clinical Aphasiology Conferences between 1978 and 1987 made comparisons between or among different brain-injured groups.

We might wonder why we persist in making these comparisons. Duffy and Myers (1991) suggest comparisons may identify similarities and differences among groups, establish the discriminative power of various tests, explore theories about the nature of different communicative deficits, and refine classification systems. These appear to be noble ends; if they are, they require appropriate means.

Our effort examined only one of several problems that may flow from inappropriate means. We examined the influence of severity on group differences, but we may have done this with an inappropriate measure. Moreover, our groups were classified on the basis of side of brain damage. Is that an important classification attribute? Perhaps we should have classified on the basis of side and size of brain damage or on side, size, and site of brain damage. More importantly, we may want to change the question and classify on the presence or absence of specific behaviors, equate severity on other behaviors, and determine what the results tell us about lesion localization. Essentially, how valid is the side of lesion as a criterion for classifying different neurogenic communication disorders? Not all patients with a hole in the left hemisphere are aphasic. Not all patients with a hole in the right hemisphere display what we grossly call right hemisphere communication deficits.

Certainly, our examination of the influence of side and severity on the variety of behaviors measured by a single test has not solved the problems inherent in comparisons across neurologic communication disorders. It does indicate that the severity of impairment in the samples compared will influence conclusions about group differences. Also, it has confirmed an axiom for aphasiologists: "Over the mountain are mountains."

REFERENCES

Duffy, J. R., & Myers, P. S. (1991). Group comparisons across neurologic communication disorders: Some methodological issues. In T. E. Prescott (Ed.), *Clinical aphasiology*, Vol. 19 (pp. 1–14). Austin, TX: PRO-ED.

Halpern, H., Darley, F. L., & Brown, J. R. (1973). Differential language and neurological characteristics in cerebral involvement. *Journal of Speech and Hearing Disorders, 38,* 162–173.

Porch, B. E. (1967). *Porch Index of Communicative Ability.* Palo Alto, CA: Consulting Psychologists Press.

Wertz, R. T., Dronkers, N. F., & Shubitowski, Y. (1986). Discriminant function analysis of performance by normals and left hemisphere, right hemisphere, and bilaterally brain damaged patients on a word fluency measure. In R. H. Brookshire (Ed.), *Clinical aphasiology*, Vol. 16 (pp. 257–266). Minneapolis: BRK Publishers.

Clinical Aphasiology, Vol. 22, 1994, pp. 165–179

The Use of Signal Detection Theory to Evaluate Aphasia Diagnostic Accuracy and Clinician Bias

Donald A. Robin and Malcolm R. McNeil

ERRATUM

In Volume 21 (1993) the article "The Use of Signal Detection Theory to Evaluate Aphasia Diagnostic Accuracy and Clinician Bias," by Donald A. Robin and Malcolm R. McNeil, was printed incompletely. The correct version follows.

Diagnosing aphasia involves differentiating it from other speech-language pathologies that resemble it. This differentiation is difficult because the symptom complex required for most definitions of aphasia include a variety of behaviors shared by other language and communication impairments such as those associated with confusion, dementia, right hemisphere disorders, traumatic brain injury, schizophrenia, malingering, and some forms of motor speech disorders. The validity and reliability of the differential diagnoses among the neurogenic and psychiatric pathologies have been approached from a variety of perspectives. For example, Halpern, Darley, and Brown (1973) used the pattern of performance across a variety of speech, language, and other cognitive tasks to construct a differential profile of performance for confused, demented, and aphasic patients. Wertz and Rosenbek (1971) also profiled differentiation of apraxia of speech from aphasia.

Recently, discriminant function analyses have been used to construct a statistical *profile* for the differentiation of aphasia from conditions resembling it. The *Porch Index of Communicative Ability (PICA)* (Porch, 1971) has been used to differentiate aphasia from malingering (Porch, Frieden, & Porec, 1977), normal (Brauer, McNeil, Duffy, Keith, & Collins, 1990), and from right hemisphere damage (Brauer et al., 1988). The *Revised Token Test (RTT)* (McNeil & Prescott, 1978) has been used to differentiate left hemisphere damaged-aphasic, right hemisphere damaged-nonaphasic and normal individuals using discriminant analyses (McNeil, Brauer, & Prescott, 1988).

While the statistical profile analyses provide useful clinical insight into general areas of impaired and unimpaired functions, they have limited information for generating differential diagnosis standards. The discriminant function studies offer information on the accuracy and bias of a particular test; however, they provide no opportunity to evaluate individual clinicians. It would be useful to have a method of assessing the accuracy and bias (the tendency to favor one outcome over another) for individual clinicians. The theory of signal detection (TSD) quantifies accuracy and response bias for test or individual clinicians. This paper (1) outlines the major tenets of TSD, (2) discusses TST application to diagnosis in aphasia, and (3) presents the results of an initial application of TSD in assessing accuracy and bias in aphasia diagnosis using *PICA* test data.

OVERVIEW OF TSD AND ITS RELATION TO DIAGNOSTICS

The assumption was made that no diagnostic system, test, or clinician is perfectly accurate no matter how **objective** each may be. Moreover, the valid evaluation of the accuracy and bias of diagnostic systems is critical in understanding their potential *clinical value* and diagnostic accuracy must precede the evaluation of treatment efficacy and cost-benefits (Swets, 1988; Swets & Pickett, 1982).

Statistical decision theory, translated into TSD, can be traced to Blackwell in the early fifties (Blackwell, 1953; Blackwell, Prichard, & Ohmart, 1954). For three decades Swets and colleagues (e.g., Green & Swets, 1966; Swets, 1959, 1988; Swets & Pickett, 1982) have pioneered the theory's application to diagnostic systems. Originally developed in World War II to assist in submarine detection, TSD has been used widely in psychophysical experiments (e.g., Gescheider, 1985; Green & Swets, 1966) in order to assess the *true* accuracy of detecting a stimulus.

In any discrimination task there are two possible states: Noise (N) and Signal-plus-Noise (SN). The observer's job is to determine if SN is present or just N. Noise arises from external sources (e.g., the wind, rain, traffic or human noise such as speech or babble) as well as internal sources (e.g., from the observer's physiology). Given these two states (N and SN), there are four possible judgment outcomes at any given time. As

Table 1. Four Possible Outcomes When Presented With Signal Plus Noise (SN) or Noise (N)

		Subject Response	
		SN	N
Actual State	SN	HIT	MISS
	N	FP	TN

shown in Table 1, an observer may say SN when SN is present, a *HIT* (correct detection or true positive). Or the observer may say N when SN is present, a *MISS* (false negative). Likewise, the observer may say SN when N is present, (a *FALSE POSITIVE* [FP] or false alarm) or the observer may say N when N is present, (a *TRUE NEGATIVE* [TN] or correct rejection).

Knowledge of the raw numbers in each of the cells compared to the total number of trials allows one to calculate the probability of each event. As shown in the hypothetical case in Table 2, there are a total of 200 trials: 100 are SN and 100 are N. The observer said SN 60 times and N 40 times in 100 SN trials. Thus, in this example, the probability of a hit, P(hit), is .60 and the probability of a miss, P(miss), is .40. Of the 100 trials in which N was present, the observer said SN 25 times and N 75 times; thus, P(FP) is .25 and P(TN) is .75. P(miss) = 1 - P(hit) and P(TN) = 1 - P(FP). Therefore, the percent of hits and FPs are needed to determine true sensitivity (accuracy) and bias. A point that cannot be overly stressed is that accuracy cannot be assessed based on percent correct (hits) alone; FPs must be accounted for as well. This point will be elaborated below.

Knowledge of hits, misses, FPs, and TNs (hits and FPs) allows for TDS application to evaluate a diagnostic system. Consider SN to be the abnormal case (e.g., an individual with aphasia) and N to be any other state (e.g., normal). How N is defined can be varied systematically to provide different degrees of precision when evaluating a diagnostic system. Given any diagnostic decision, the clinician is faced with the problem of choosing SN or N, and any of the four outcomes (hits, misses, FP, TN) are possible.

A hypothetical example of diagnostic accuracy will serve to demonstrate the need for a better accuracy measure than percent hits alone. Clinician Y is 100% correct in the identification of aphasia when aphasia

Table 2. Hypothetical Data and Response Frequencies When Presented With Signal Plus Noise (SN) or Noise (N)

Subject Response

		SN	N	TOTAL #
Actual State	SN	60	40	100
	N	25	75	100

P (HIT) = .60   P (MISS) = .40   P (FP) = .25   P (TN) = .75
P (MISS) = 1 – P (HIT)   P (TN) = 1 – P (FP)

is present (i.e., P[hit] = 1.0 and P[miss] = 0.0). Clinician Z is only 70% correct in saying aphasia is present when the person actually has aphasia (P[hit] = .70 and P[miss] = .30). Y, under most traditional criteria, would be considered superior. However, if you were also told that Y identified 90% of the normal persons who came into his clinic as aphasic (i.e., P[FP] = .9 and P[TN] = .1) and Z had a FP rate of only 5% (P[FP] = .05 and P[TN] = .95), you might reconsider your evaluation of the adequacy of these individuals and be forced to conclude that Z was a better diagnostician than Y. Thus, the percent correct alone is an inadequate measure of accuracy. One must account for FPs as well as hits. As will be shown, TSD allows one to derive a better measure of accuracy based on hits plus FPs than percent hits alone.

TDS also considers a second importance area, the bias with which one approaches a task. In TSD, *bias* conventionally refers to the tendency to favor a positive outcome (hits). Both tests and individual clinicians have biases. Numerous factors affect these biases, including: (1) a clinician's background and training, (2) the assumptions a clinician or test (or both) brings to a given diagnostic situation, (3) a clinician's environment (e.g., work setting), (4) a clinician's mood, and/or (5) a clinician's cost-benefit assessment of a given situation.

Consider the following hypothetical diagnostic situation. General X is a military radar operator with the job of detecting incoming missiles. General X has family living in the area of his surveillance and wants to make sure that no missiles come close to populated areas, especially those where his family live. Because of his personal and professional situation he adopts a lenient response bias. That is, he wants to make sure that when a missile is detected, he will not miss it. Thus, even though a defensive missile will be launched every time he detects an incoming missile, he launches his defensive missile any time he detects a signal on his radar screen. Because aircraft other than missiles are also detected on the screen, the signal detected may or may not be a missile. As a result, General X has a high FP rate, but never misses an incoming missile. For the General, the cost of missing an incoming missile is greater than the benefit of not taking down an allied or neutral plane. When General X goes off duty, Private A assumes the radar watch. Although the defense of the country from attack is paramount in both General X's and Private A's minds, Private A's family is scheduled to arrive by air some time during his work shift. He knows that every time he launches a defensive missile he is likely to hit his target because they are very accurate. He also reasons that the attack missiles are fairly inaccurate and the chance of hitting a populated area is low. Private A adopts a bias that dictates that he will launch a defensive missile only when he is absolutely positive that the signal detected on the radar screen is an offensive missile. His hit rate is lower than General X's, but so is his rate of FPs. Private A's bias dictates that the cost of a FP far outweighs the benefit derived from identifying every single incoming missile. The distributions of decisions based on N and SN form the data on which TSD is computed.

Figure 1 shows two distributions that represent N on the left and SN on the right. The distributions are similar in shape and their variance is equal. (Note that TSD can handle nonparametric data as well.) Notice that the two curves overlap to some degree. That is, in all situations there are instances where one may report SN when only N is present or only N when SN is present. One main index of accuracy, d', is represented by the difference between the peaks of the N and SN distributions. The greater the overlap of N and SN distributions, the less the distance between the peaks, and the lower the d'. The distributions at the top of Figure 1 have the highest d' and represent the highest accuracy. The bottom distributions with the most overlap have the lowest d' and represent the poorest accuracy. The middle distributions represent some intermediary accuracy level. Accuracy as measured by d' can range from complete overlap of the distributions (d' = 0.00) to as high as about 4.67.

Figure 2 represents theoretical N (top) and SN (bottom) distributions. The perpendicular line represents the response bias which in TSD terms is called ß. Responses to the right of ß are positive for SN (clinician says yes, SN present) whereas those to the left favor N (clinician says no). At the intersection of the two distributions ß is 1, which refers to equal bias for SN and N. As ß decreases, a more lenient criterion is adopted (hits and FPs increase) and as ß increases a more stringent criterion is adopted (hits and FPs decrease). Also note that the areas of the distribution that represent different cells in contingency Table 1 are shown in this figure.

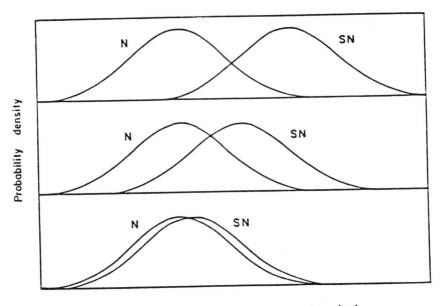

Magnitude of sensory observation (X)

Figure 1. Three different theoretical distributions of noise (N) and signal-plus-noise (SN). Accuracy (d') is defined as the distance between the two peaks of the N and SN distributions. The further the distance between the two peaks, the better the accuracy of and the higher the d'. Thus, the top N and SN distributions represent the highest accuracy and d' is relatively large. The lowest N and SN distributions are almost overlapping and accuracy is poor, d' is close to 0. Reprinted from G. A. Gescheider, *Psychophysics: Method, theory and application* (2nd ed.), p. 87, with permission of Lawrence Erlbaum Associates, Hillsdale, New Jersey.

These probabilities depend on one's bias. Moreover, accuracy does not change as a function of shifts in bias, although the relative percent of hits and FPs do.

One other aspect of TSD needs to be discussed before the data are presented. In order to apply TSD to diagnostic situations, receiver operating characteristic (ROC) curves—a plot of the P(hits) by the P(FP)—need to be developed. The measure d', reflects the distance between the N and SN distributions, which is reflected in the position of the ROC curve on the graph. Figure 3 is a graph of an ROC curve with a d' of 1.0. The diagonal straight line is a d' of zero, where the two distributions have complete overlap. The N and SN distributions that give rise to the position of the ROC curve are shown along with three different biases (ßs)

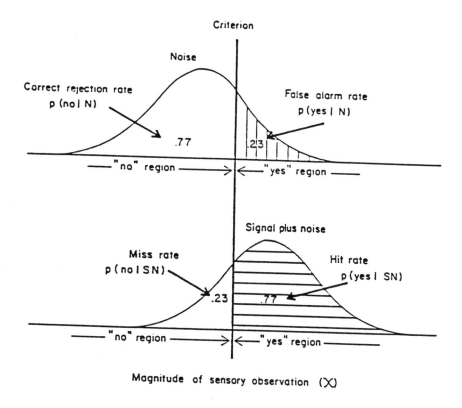

Figure 2. Theoretical distributions of noise (N) on top and signal-plus-noise (SN) bottom. Note that the distance between the peaks represents accuracy or d'. The perpendicular line represents bias (labeled as criterion in the figure) or ß. For responses to the right of the line the clinician says yes, SN present and to the left of the line the clinician says no, SN not present (i.e., N present). Note the areas of overlap between the two distributions. Thus, all four conditions (Hit, FP, miss, and TN) are represented. Hits, (hit rate in figure [P = .77]) are shown by the lined portion of the SN distribution; FPs, false alarm in figure (P = .23), by the lined portion of the N distribution; misses, miss rate in figure (P = .23), by the blank portion of the SN distribution; and TN, correct rejection in figure (P = .77), by the blank portion of the N distribution. As the perpendicular line moves to the left a more lenient bias is adopted, ß goes up. In this case both the hits and FPs increase. As the perpendicular line moves to the right, ß goes down and a more stringent bias is adopted. In this case both hits and FPs decrease. Reprinted from G. A. Gescheider, *Psychophysics: Method, theory and application* (2nd ed.), p. 90, with permission of Lawrence Erlbaum Associates, Hillsdale, New Jersey.

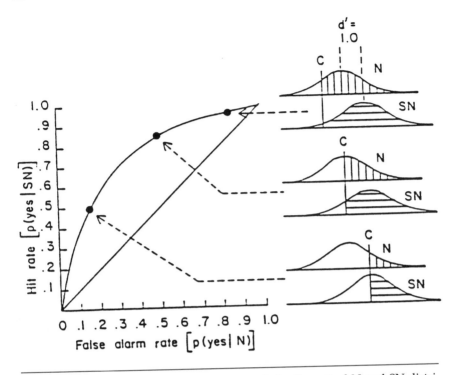

Figure 3. Relation between the ROC curve and the theoretical N and SN distributions that represent a d' of 1.0. The straight diagonal represents a d' of 0 as hits and FPs are equal. Each of the three data points represent a different bias at the same accuracy level (the distance between the peaks of the N and SN distributions is constant), only the perpendicular line moves. The most lenient bias, highest ß is represented by the upper distributions for which both hit and FP rates are high. The most stringent bias, lowest ß is represented by the bottom distributions in which both hit and FP rates are low. Reprinted from G. A. Gescheider, *Psychophysics: Method, theory and application* (2nd ed.), p. 95, with permission of Lawrence Erlbaum Associates, Hillsdale, New Jersey.

that lie along the curve. Different points along the curve represent differences in bias or ß, with the same d'. Thus, d' is an accuracy measure independent of bias. The construction of ROC curves allows an assessment of accuracy *and* bias. The uppermost N and SN distributions have the bias line far to the left, thus indicating a low ß and a lenient bias. Moving down the figure to the lower distributions, ß increases, indicating more stringent biases. Figures 4 and 5 show ROC curves for d's of 2.0 and 0 respectively, each with three bias points.

If diagnostician's data are shown to fit the theoretical curves, then d' and ß may be utilized without developing the entire curve. Convenient

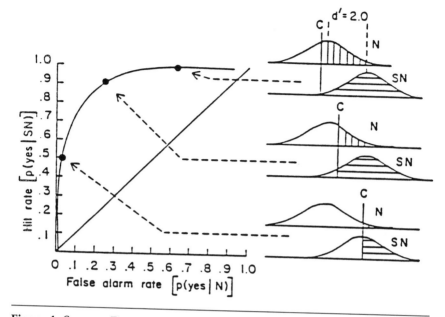

Figure 4. Same as Figure 3, but d' = 2.0. Reprinted from G. A. Gescheider, *Psychophysics: Method, theory and application* (2nd ed.), p. 94, with permission of Lawrence Erlbaum Associates, Hillsdale, New Jersey.

tables for d' and ß exist for any known hit and FP rate. To illustrate TSD application to aphasia diagnostics and to explore its value, ROC curves, d' and ß data for individual clinicians using the *PICA* to diagnose aphasia are presented.

METHOD

Judges

Four individual judges formally trained and experienced in the administration, scoring, and interpretation of the PICA, evaluated item, subtest, and overall scores from 246 different PICA tests. A fifth judge (subject 3) was a PICA-trained, but generally inexperienced graduate student seeking a master's degree in speech-language pathology.

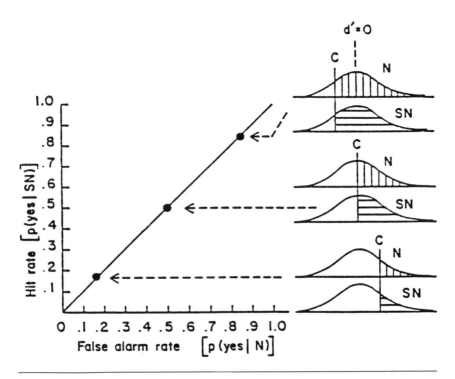

Figure 5. Same as Figure 3, but d' = 0.0. Reprinted from G. A. Gescheider, *Psychophysics: Method, theory and application* (2nd ed.), p. 96, with permission of Lawrence Erlbaum Associates, Hillsdale, New Jersey.

PICA Data

To determine the accuracy of responses, one needs to know, apriori, which *PICA* tests were derived from normal and which were from aphasic individuals. In other words, a *gold standard* for diagnosis is required. Although much theory and philosophy underlies the final categorization, only the general criteria and methods used for making the decisions are discussed. First, the normal subject's PICA performance was provided by Duffy and Keith from their 1980 standardization for normal individuals. Subjects met the criteria for normal as defined in that investigation. The aphasic PICA data were derived from the speech-language pathology patient records at the VA hospital in Madison, Wisconsin. The aphasia diagnosis was made or certified by either Wertz, Rosenbek, or Collins. Although the PICA was used in the patient's diagnosis, in no case was the categorization based solely on PICA data. A variety of other standardized, unstandardized and informal assessment tools, interviews, case histories, and medical records were also utilized to arrive at the final diagnosis. Aphasia was defined in a manner similar to Darley (1982). That is, all aphasic subjects had multimodality language deficits that were disproportionate to other intellective deficits. Onset was sudden and secondary to a focal dominant hemisphere lesion. Of the 246 total *PICA* tests to be evaluated, 103 were from aphasic adults (SN distribution) and 143 were from normal non-brain-damaged individuals (N distribution).

Judges were first required to indicate whether the test presented was from an aphasic or normal individual (subjects said yes for aphasia and no for normal). The clinicians then rated the confidence of their decision on a five-point equal-appearing interval scale from 1 (*not very sure*) to 5 (*very sure*). The rating scale method is a cost effective means of applying TSD to clinical situations in order to generate the ROC curve and to test the validity of the approach (Swets, 1988; Swets & Pickett, 1982). Each point on the rating scale represents a different bias. An individual who is *very sure* of a decision will have a stringent bias (ß will be high) while the bias associated with a rating of *not very sure* will be very lenient (ß will be low). In this manner up to four points along an ROC curve, each with differing bias, were obtained. The maximum number of points is four as the most lenient criterion associated with the rating of 1 will always result in a P(hit) and P(FP) equaling 1.0.

From the rating scale data, the P(hit) and P(FP) for each person at the different biases were determined. ROC curves for each person were plotted and the data were compared to the theoretical curves. From these, accuracy and bias measures were derived. The d' and ß for each person representing their typical levels were determined.[1]

RESULTS AND DISCUSSION

Table 3 shows each subject's d' and ß for the diagnostic decision (yes/no portion of the study). These data generally are thought to reflect the typical accuracy and bias of each judge. High accuracy is indicated by a d' better than 3.5. None of these subjects were close to achieving a high accuracy. The highest d' was 2.78. This judge, subject 5, had the least experience with aphasia and the PICA other than the student. Subject 4 with approximately 12 years of experience with the *PICA*, who uses it as a

---

1. The computer program to calculate the best fit for the data and determine accuracy and bias were kindly provided by Drs. Donald D. Dorfman and Kevin Burnbaum at the University of Iowa in the Departments of Psychology and Radiology, respectively. The original program can be found in Dorfman and Alf (1969).

Table 3. Accuracy (d') and Response Bias (ß) for Each Subject at *Typical* Response Level

SUBJ #	d'	ß
1	1.96	4.10
2	2.66	2.56
3	2.42	3.60
4	1.00	0.46
5	2.79	1.72

Note: Subject 3 was a student.

primary diagnostic tool, had a very low d' of 1.0. At this low level of accuracy, at typical bias, this judge had a P(hit) of .86 and a P(FP) of .62. Thus, this judge identified 86% of the aphasic tests as aphasic but also identified 63% of the normal tests as aphasic. By contrast, subject 5, who had the highest accuracy, had a P(hit) of .89 (89% correct aphasic identification) but a P(FP) of only .06 (6% incorrect identification of normal subjects) at their typical bias. The student clinician (subject 3) had a similar accuracy level to most of the other judges.

Table 3 also shows the bias with which the subjects typically approached the task. While ßs were generally indicative of a relatively stringent bias (>1.0), there was a range of biases among the subjects. Subject 4 had a very lenient bias (ß = .46) while Subject 1 was fairly stringent (ß = 4.10). Thus, some individuals were more willing than others to identify an individual as having aphasia given the *PICA* information they reviewed.

Figure 6 shows the ROC curves for Subjects 4, triangles, and 5, circles. The dotted and solid lines represent the theoretical curves for a d' of 1.00 and 2.79, respectively. The diagonal line is a d' of zero. These data produce a good fit with the theoretical curves; in fact, each of the 5 subjects' data produced a good fit with the theoretical curves. It is interesting to note that Subject 4 reported using a relatively lenient response bias (typical ß = .46) and that this bias caused the high degree of inaccuracy. Recall, however, that d' is independent of bias. At subject 4's most lenient bias (ß = .32), d' was the same as at his more stringent biases (ß = .43, .46, or .70). Subject 5's data illustrate that one may adopt a stringent bias (ß = 6.78) and have only 75% correct, or one may use a lenient bias (ß = .48) and achieve a 96% hit rate but produce the same accuracy. Comparison of Subjects 4 and 5 at the similar bias (ß = .46 and .53, respectively) was independent of their very different accuracy levels (d' = 1.0 and 2.78, respectively). Thus, bias can be assessed independently of accuracy using TSD.

Figure 7 represents the theoretical ROC curves for each of the five subjects. Notice how the position of the ROC curve varies as a function of

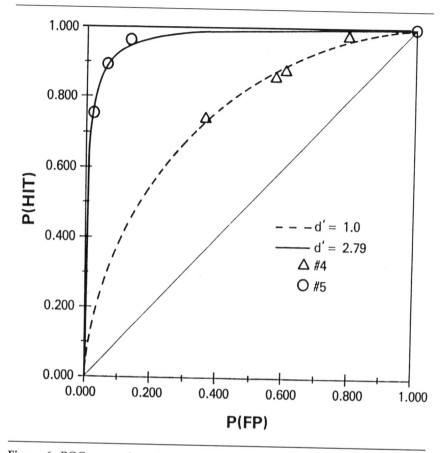

Figure 6. ROC curves for subjects #4 and #5 generated from *actual data* and *theoretical data.*

accuracy. As d' is lowered, the curve approaches the zero line. Different points along each curve represent differing biases. All subjects achieved a hit rate of 80%–90% using their typical bias. Their FPs varied, however, and thus accuracy differed among them.

In summary, TSD provided a method of investigating accuracy and bias in aphasia diagnosis. *PICA* tests alone did not result in acceptable accuracy levels given the extant literature suggesting that a d' greater than 3.5 is achieved in most good diagnostic systems. However, individual clinicians can use TSD to check their own bias and accuracy. Future studies could systematically evaluate accuracy and bias when differing amounts of information are available to the diagnostician. For instance, accuracy and bias could be determined when other standardized aphasia test data are added to those of the PICA. Accuracy and bias could then be

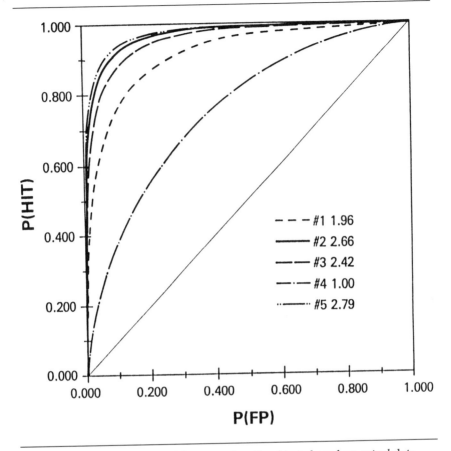

Figure 7. Best fit *theoretical* ROC curves for all subjects based on *actual* data.

determined when a case history or a brain scan is part of the information provided. One could vary *noise* by asking judges to determine if aphasia is present or if the patient is normal, has dementia, or has right hemisphere involvement. Accuracy and bias will vary as a function of the amount of information provided and the amount of noise in the system.

TSD is also useful in cost-benefit assessment. One can objectively determine which measures give the highest accuracy. The minimum amount of information that provides the highest accuracy measures can be determined for any given diagnostic decision.

This paper examined the basic principles of TSD and its application to aphasia diagnosis. Future studies will examine if the assumptions of d' (equal variance of N and SN) hold true. If not, other measures of accuracy may be more appropriate. Moreover, instead of using ß as the bias measure, lnß (natural log of ß) may prove to be a better metric as lenient biases are indicated by ßs between 0 and 1.0 and stringent biases by ß greater than 1.0. The investigation of these and several related methodological issues in the application of TSD to aphasia assessment should assist the clinical aphasiologist in their selection of the most sensitive and specific tools and procedures for their clinical practice.

REFERENCES

Blackwell, H. R. (1953). Psychophysical thresholds: Experimental studies of methods of measurement. *Bulletin of the Engineering Research Institute, No. 53,* University of Michigan.

Blackwell, H. R., Prichard, B. S., & Ohmart, T. G. (1954). Automatic apparatus for stimulus presentation and recording in visual threshold experiments. *Journal of the Ophthalmology Society of America, 44,* 322–326.

Brauer, D., McNeil, M. R., Collins, M. J., Deal, J. L., Duffy, J. R. and Keith, R. (1988). Discriminating normal, aphasic and right hemisphere performance with the PICA. (Abstract) *ASHA,* 30(10), 173.

Brauer, D., McNeil, M. R., Duffy, J. R., Keith R. L., & Collins M. J. (1990). The differentiation of normal from aphasic performance using PICA discriminant function scores. In T. E. Prescott (Ed.), *Clinical Aphasiology, 18,* 117–129.

Darley, F. L. (1982). *Aphasia.* Philadelphia: W. B. Saunders.

Dorfman, D. D. and Alf, E., Jr. (1969). Maximum likelihood estimates of parameters of signal-detection theory and determination of confidence intervals-Rating method data. *Journal of Mathematical Psychology, 6,* 487–496.

Duffy, J. R. & Keith, R. (1980). Performance of non-brain injured adults on the PICA: Descriptive data and a comparison to patients with aphasia. *Aphasia-Apraxia-Agnosia,* 2(2), 1–30.

Gescheider, G. A. (1985). *Psychophysics: Method, theory, and application* (2nd ed.). Hillsdale: Lawrence Erlbaum Associates.

Green, D. M., & Swets, J. A. (1966). *Signal detection theory and psychophysics.* New York: Wiley. (Reprinted 1974, Huntington, NY: Krieger).

Halpern, H., Darley, F. L., & Brown J. R. (1973). Differential language and neurological characteristics in cerebral involvement. *Journal of Speech and Hearing Disorders, 38,* 162–173.

McNeil, M. R., Brauer, D. & Prescott, T. E. (1988). Discriminating normal, aphasic and right hemisphere performance with the RTT. (Abstract) *ASHA,* 30(10), 161.

McNeil, M. R., & Prescott, T. E. (1978). *Revised Token Test.* Austin: PRO-ED.

Porch, B. E. (1971). *Porch Index of Communicative Ability.* Palo Alto: Consulting Psychologists Press.

Porch, B. E., Frieden, T., & Porec, J. (1977). Objective differentiation of aphasic versus nonorganic patients. Paper presented to the International Neuropsychology Association, Santa Fe, NM.

Swets, J. A. (1959). Indices of signal detectability obtained with various psychophysical procedures. *Journal of the Acoustical Society of America, 31,* 511–513.

Swets, J. A. (1988). Measuring the accuracy of diagnostic systems. *Science, 240,* 1285–1293.

Swets, J. A., & Pickett, R. M. (1982). *Evaluation of diagnostic systems: Methods from signal detection theory.* New York: Academic Press.

Wertz, R. T. & Rosenbek, J. C. (1971). Appraising apraxia of speech. *Journal of the Colorado Speech and Hearing Association.* 5, 18–36.

Clinical Aphasiology, Vol. 22, 1994, pp. 181–190

The Construct Validity of the *Limb Apraxia Test* (LAT): Implications for the Distinction Between Types of Limb Apraxia

Robert J. Duffy, James H. Watt, and Joseph R. Duffy

The *Limb Apraxia Test* (LAT) (Duffy, 1974) was developed to meet the need for a comprehensive test of limb apraxia in aphasic individuals. Citing data from several studies that have used the LAT, Duffy and Duffy (1989, 1990) have claimed that it is a reliable and valid test of limb apractic *behavior.* The issue addressed in the present investigation is whether the LAT is a valid test for discriminating ideomotor from ideational apractic *processes.*

The term *limb apraxia* refers to an "impairment of movement control which cannot be explained on the basis of disruptions to afferent and/or efferent sensory-motor systems, poor or absent comprehension of the task in hand, intellectual deficit, inadequate attention or poor co-operation" (Miller, 1986, p. 1). Generally, the term is used to refer not only to the observable impaired motor behaviors but also to two neuropsychological processes construed to be responsible for these behaviors. These two underlying causal constructs are called *ideational apraxia* (IA) and *ideomotor apraxia* (IMA). The existence of these two types of limb apractic processes has been generally accepted since they were conceived by Hugo Liepmann (1900, 1905) in the early 1900s.

DEFINITIONS OF IDEATIONAL APRAXIA (IA) AND IDEOMOTOR APRAXIA (IMA)

Liepmann's model—and most other current models—posits two stages of motor performance: the *idea* of a purposeful act and its *programmed execution.* Liepmann hypothesized that the idea, which he called a "space-time" memory, is aroused in the posterior cortex and transmitted to a frontal area that programs the idea for execution by selected neuromuscular systems. Impairment at either of these two stages produces different symptoms or types of limb apraxia. IA results from damage to the idea in the posterior cortex (or disruption of transmission from it); IMA, from damage to programming in the frontal cortex. Some clinicians and researchers (Kleist, Sittig, & Zangwill, cited in DeRenzi, 1985, p. 47), however, hold that there is only a single causal process responsible for limb apractic behaviors and that IA is simply a more severe form of IMA.

TESTING FOR LIMB APRAXIA

In a comprehensive review of the issues involved in testing limb apraxia, DeRenzi (1985) cites three features that must be considered in any valid test of limb apractic behaviors and their causal processes or types (i.e., IA and IMA). These three features are

1. the types or classes of movements elicited;

2. the modalities used to elicit a response; and

3. the types of error responses.

Types of Movement

According to DeRenzi, a test of limb apraxia should comprise classes of movements that are sensitive to (a) different levels of severity of limb apraxia and (b) differences in IA and IMA. He classifies movements by (a) their *psychological purposes* (to communicate, to manipulate objects, and meaningless movements) and (b) their *physical features* or *shapes* (i.e., whether the movement is sequenced, segmented, simple, complex, or involves the manipulation of objects).

Modality of Elicitation

When selecting the modality of elicitation (e.g., imitation, pictures, verbal command), DeRenzi strongly recommends imitation because it

1. allows the testing of aphasic subjects with comprehension deficits;

2. results in more reliable scoring; and

3. makes possible the inclusion of movements in the "meaning-less" class, which do not lend themselves to elicitation in any other modality.

For these and other reasons, imitation was chosen as the sole mode of elicitation in the LAT. When imitation is used, however, the "communicative" classes (pantomime and intransitive gestures) of movements are necessarily eliminated; although a subject can imitate a movement that simulates the shape of a communicative act, there is no assurance that any imitated motor act is meaningful or communicative to the subject.

On the other hand, using a modality other than imitation (such as verbal command) also has significant disadvantages. Using a nonimitative modality

1. eliminates the meaningless class of movements;

2. risks confounding by aphasic verbal comprehension problems; and

3. confounds motor dysfunction with aphasic symbolic or propositional deficits in communicating meaning.

Even though the use of imitation eliminates communicative classes of movements such as pantomime, there still remain important differences in the shapes of the movements; that is, test task movements can be sequential or segmented, they can be relatively simple or complex, and they can involve manipulated objects or not.

To ensure an adequate sample of classes of movement, the LAT was specifically designed to retain these six shapes (i.e., movement features): Sequenced, Segmented, Simple, Complex, Object, No Object. These six shapes were counterbalanced as three binary feature combinations in the eight subtests of the LAT as shown in Table 1.

The presence of these binary features not only may measure degrees of severity of limb apraxia but also may discriminate IA from IMA. For example, IA (often associated with complex actions) can be contrasted with IMA (often associated with more simple movements). From this standpoint, the Complex subtests of the LAT (3, 4, 7, and 8) may be more sensitive to IA, whereas the Simple subtests (1, 2, 5, and 6) may be more sensitive to IMA. Similarly, the Object subtests (2, 4, 6, and 8) may be more sensitive to IMA. Alternatively, if IA is a consequence of memory, attention, or sequencing ability, as some definitions suggest, the Sequenced subtests (1, 2, 3, and 4) may be more sensitive to IA than are the Segmented subtests (5, 6, 7, and 8).

Table 1. Binary Features and the Eight Subtests of the Limb Apraxia Test (LAT)

LAT subtest	Features		
	Sequenced (+)/ Segmented (–)	Complex (+)/ Simple (–)	Object (+)/ No Object (–)
1	+	–	–
2	+	–	+
3	+	+	–
4	+	+	+
5	–	–	–
6	–	–	+
7	–	+	–
8	–	+	+

LAT Scoring

DeRenzi suggests that distinctions between IA and IMA can be made not only by including various classes of movements but also on the basis of the types of observed response errors. For example, IMA is reportedly characterized by clumsiness and distortion of movements, whereas IA presents itself as omissions, sequencing errors, mislocations, perplexity, and inappropriate object use. To capture these error types and others, the LAT was designed with a comprehensive scoring system capable of quantifying the types of errors that reportedly distinguish IA and IMA. It uses a 21-point, multidimensional, PICA-like scoring scale. (See Duffy & Duffy, 1990, for a detailed description of LAT scoring.)

Therefore, the LAT, even though using only the imitative elicitation modality, may claim to be a valid measure of the constructs of IA and IMA based both on the variety of shapes of the movements it includes and on its method of scoring.

PRESENT INVESTIGATION

The present investigation reviews evidence for the construct validity of the LAT as a test that distinguishes between IMA and IA. Put another way, we investigated whether the data generated by the LAT can support the existence of more than a single construct underlying limb apractic behaviors.

METHOD

Subjects

The LAT has been administered to 77 left-hemisphere-damaged (LHD) aphasic subjects. Fifty-three of the 77 subjects were classified as limb apractic because their overall mean LAT score fell below all 30 non-neurologically impaired control subjects and 2.58 SDs below the controls' overall mean LAT score. These groups of subjects have been described in detail by Duffy and Duffy (1989). The present investigation is concerned with only the 53 LHD aphasic subjects classified as limb apractic and whether they can be discriminated into subgroups evidencing IA or IMA.

RESULTS

Intercorrelations Among LAT Subtests

To obtain evidence of the presence of the constructs of IA and IMA, the intercorrelations among the eight LAT subtests were obtained. This initial analysis is consistent with the recommendation of the American Psychological Association's (APA, 1985) guidelines for the construction of psychological tests: "When several scores are obtained from a single test, each purporting to measure a distinct construct, the intercorrelations among the scores . . . should be reported. . . . Relationships among test scores provide important information regarding the distinctiveness of the constructs being measured" (p. 15). The intercorrelations for the 53 LHD apractic subjects are presented in Table 2, which shows moderate to strong

Table 2. Pearson Product Moment Correlation Matrix for Eight LAT Subtests

LAT subtest	1	2	3	4	5	6	7
2	.67						
3	.69	.53					
4	.64	.52	.81				
5	.70	.64	.76	.80			
6	.51	.81	.47	.50	.68		
7	.62	.63	.75	.76	.78	.68	
8	.43	.47	.77	.78	.65	.52	.76

Note: All coefficients are significant ($p < .05$).

intercorrelations among all pairs of subtests. They range from .43 to .81, with a median of .64, and all are significant ($p < .05$).

These findings do not support the assertion that more than one construct is being measured by the 8 subtests of the LAT.

Cronbach's Alpha

The impression of unidimensionality for the eight subtests is supported by Cronbach's alpha (SPSS, 1988). This coefficient is an index of the internal consistency or reliability of the LAT. In a sense, it treats each LAT subtest as an observer of limb apractic behavior and measures the degree to which the eight subtests are observing the same behavior. The high alpha of .94 indicates that the eight subtests, despite the differences in the shapes of the movements being sampled, are uniformly sensitive to only a single underlying construct.

Factor Analysis

The impression of a single construct underlying performance on the eight LAT subtests was further investigated using a principal components factor analysis (SPSS, 1988). The analysis resulted in the extraction of only one factor with an eigenvalue greater than 1 (which accounts for 70% of the variance in LAT performance). The additional results presented in Table 3 strongly support the assertion that there is only a single factor underlying performance on the LAT.

1. The eight subtests load on a single factor, and the factor loadings for each subtest are high, ranging from .76 to .90.

2. The factor score coefficient matrix shows that each subtest contributes almost identical proportions to the factor being measured (varying slightly between 14% and 16%).

3. The communalities are high for each of the eight subtests. (Communalities are the proportion of variance in the LAT score that each subtest has with all of the other seven subtests.)

In summary, the results of the factor analysis demonstrate that only a single factor was extracted accounting for a major portion of the variance in overall test performance, that all LAT subtests load strongly on the same factor, that each subtest contributes equally to the factor being measured, and that each subtest is strongly related to what is being measured by all the other subtests.

Table 3. Factor Analysis of Eight LAT Subtests

Factor Loadings

	Factor 1
Subtest 5	.90
Subtest 7	.90
Subtest 4	.87
Subtest 3	.87
Subtest 8	.81
Subtest 1	.78
Subtest 2	.78
Subtest 6	.76

Factor Score Coefficient Matrix

	Factor 1
Subtest 1	.14
Subtest 2	.14
Subtest 3	.16
Subtest 4	.16
Subtest 5	.16
Subtest 6	.14
Subtest 7	.16
Subtest 8	.16

Communalities

Subtest 1	.61
Subtest 2	.61
Subtest 3	.76
Subtest 4	.77
Subtest 5	.81
Subtest 6	.58
Subtest 7	.81
Subtest 8	.66

Binary Features Correlational Analyses

Further analysis of the number of factors underlying LAT performance was undertaken by factor analyzing each dichotomous pair of the three binary features represented in the LAT (Sequenced-Segmented; Simple-Complex; Object-No Object). Prior to the actual factor analysis, a composite factor score for each set of four subtests was obtained to represent the construct being measured by those four subtests. For example, a factor score was obtained for the Sequenced subtests (1, 2, 3, and 4) and the

Table 4. Binary Factor Correlational Analyses

Binary Features	LAT Subtests	Pearson r	r^2	$1-r^2$
Sequenced	(1,2,3,4)	.97	.94	.08
Segmented	(5,6,7,8)	.96	.92	.06
Simple	(1,2,5,6)	.93	.87	.13
Complex	(3,4,7,8)	.95	.90	.10
Object	(2,4,6,8)	.96	.92	.04
No Object	(1,3,5,7)	.98	.96	.08

Segmented subtests (5, 6, 7, and 8) (SPSS, 1988). The results of this analysis are presented in Table 4. The steps in the analysis are illustrated for the Sequenced-Segmented binary features:

Step 1: The Sequenced factor score was correlated with the overall LAT score. The *r* was .97.

Step 2: The *r* was squared to obtain a measure of the amount of the variance (i.e., the information) in the overall LAT score that is accounted for by the four Sequenced subtests (1, 2, 3, 4). The r^2 for the Sequenced subtest was (a very large) .94.

Step 3: The next step was to examine the amount of variance (i.e., information) *not* explained by the four Sequenced subtests, that is, by the Segmented subtests (5, 6, 7, and 8). This was obtained by the formula $1 - r^2$. For the Sequenced factor this result was .06. This means that very little (6%) of the variance in LAT not already accounted for by the Sequenced factor was accounted for by the Segmented or some other factor. These steps were then repeated for the Segmented factor score (Subtests 5, 6, 7, and 8). Table 4 shows that the results are virtually identical: The *r* between the Segmented factor score and the overall LAT score was .96; the r^2 was .92; and $1 - r^2$ was .08. Thus, only 8% of variance in LAT was explained by some construct(s) other than Segmented, which means that it is accounting for the same construct as the Sequenced factor score.

Together, these two analyses indicate that whatever construct is being measured by the Sequenced subtests is also being measured equally by the Segmented subtests. The results are strong evidence that only a single construct underlies performance on the Sequenced and Segmented features of the LAT.

These same analyses were done for the other two pair of binary features, and the results for all three binary features are presented in Table 4. The results for the Simple-Complex and the Object-No Object binary features are virtually identical to those of the Sequenced-Segmented binary feature. For each of the three pairs of features, the $1 - r^2$ proportions are small and of similar magnitude, and the conclusions are the same: There is very strong evidence that only one construct is being measured, despite the dichotomous differences in the classes of movement that are represented in the subtests themselves.

Summary

The results of the correlational and factor analyses used in this investigation consistently support the conclusion that the LAT measures only a single underlying construct. The construct validity for the LAT as a test that detects and discriminates IA and IMA was not supported.

DISCUSSION AND CONCLUSIONS

Ventry and Schiavetti (1980), offer the following observation: "The construct validity of a test or measure is borne out if measurements agree with the theoretical prediction, but if the prediction is not verified, it may be the result of an invalid measure, *or* an incorrect theory, *or* both" (p. 90). Applying this statement to the present investigation leads to two possible conclusions about the LAT and limb apraxia. First, the LAT may lack construct validity for detecting distinctions between valid constructs of IA and IMA. The alternative possibility is that the LAT does not detect traditional types of limb apraxia because such types do not exist; that is, the theory about the distinction between IA and IMA is incorrect.

Further Research

Although acceptance of the theory that limb apraxia can be differentiated into two (or more) distinct processes or types has been long-standing, the empirical basis for this theory is surprisingly narrow. Much of the support for it is based on individual case studies. Direct investigations regarding the "modality" effect and "movement type" effect for distinguishing between IA and IMA in a LHD aphasic population are essential to determine whether IA and IMA are qualitatively distinct constructs and clinically discernible types of limb apractic processes in patients with aphasia. One such investigation has been reported by Belanger, Duffy, and Coelho (1992). Consistent with the present investigation, they failed to support the presence of more than a single factor underlying limb apractic behaviors.

The results of the present investigation encourage additional investigations of the validity of the traditional view that IA and IMA are distinct and independent processes.

ACKNOWLEDGMENTS

This investigation was supported by grants from the University of Connecticut Research Foundation and The Gaylord Hospital, Wallingford, CT.

REFERENCES

American Psychological Association (1985). *Standards for educational and psychological testing*. Washington, DC: American Psychological Association.

Belanger, S., Duffy, R. J., & Coelho, C. (1992). An investigation of limb apraxia regarding the validity of current assessment procedures. Paper presented at the Twenty-Second Annual Clinical Aphasiology Conference, Durango, CO.

DeRenzi, E. (1985). Methods of limb apraxia examination and their bearing on the interpretation of the disorder. In E. A. Roy (Ed.), *Neuropsychological studies of apraxia and related disorders* (pp. 45–63). New York: North Holland.

Duffy, J. R. (1974). *Comparison of brain-injured and non-brain-injured subjects on an objective test of manual apraxia*. Doctoral dissertation, University of Connecticut, Storrs.

Duffy, J. R., & Duffy, R. J. (1989). The *Limb Apraxia Test:* An imitative measure of upper limb apraxia. In T. E. Prescott (Ed.), *Clinical aphasiology*, Vol. 18 (pp. 145–159). Austin, TX: PRO-ED.

Duffy, J. R., & Duffy, R. J. (1990). The assessment of limb apraxia: The *Limb Apraxia Test*. In G. R. Hammond (Ed.), *Advances in psychology: Cerebral control of speech and limb movements* (pp. 503–531). Amsterdam: Elsevier.

Liepmann, H. (1900). Das Krankheitsbild der Apraxie "motorischen Asymbolie". *Mschr, Psychiat Neurol.* 8:15–44, 102–132, 182–197.

Liepmann, H. (1905). Die linke Hemisphäre und das Handeln. In Drei Aufsätze aus dem Apraxiegebiet. Berlin: Karger, pp. 17–50.

Miller, N. (1986). *Dyspraxia and its management*. Rockville, MD: Aspen.

SPSS–X user's guide. (1988). Chicago: SPSS.

Ventry, I., & Schiavetti, N. (1980). *Evaluating research in speech pathology and audiology*. Reading, MA: Addison-Wesley.

Clinical Aphasiology, Vol. 22, 1994, pp. 191–201

An Investigation of Limb Apraxia Regarding the Validity of Current Assessment Procedures

Steven A. Belanger, Robert J. Duffy, and Carl A. Coelho

Limb apraxia has been recognized as a distinct manifestation of brain damage since the early 1900s. It is usually defined as a disturbance in the performance of skilled, purposeful motor movements that cannot be attributed to impairments of strength, sensation, coordination, verbal comprehension, or general intelligence (Duffy & Duffy, 1989; Rothi, Ochipa, Leadon, & Meher, 1989). Skilled intentional movements involving either limb are compromised despite the presence of normal reflexes, power, tone, and mobility, as well as seemingly adequate comprehension of the eliciting verbal request. Beyond this general definition, however, there is little agreement. A consensus has yet to emerge regarding observed symptoms, the neuropsychological processes producing the symptoms, or the brain structures involved.

This lack of consensus is reflected in current approaches to clinical assessment. For the most part, the clinical assessment of limb apraxia has been highly subjective and variable. It is currently based on a set of logical distinctions regarding *movement type* (e.g., transitive pantomimes vs. intransitive gestures or meaningful movements vs. nonmeaningful movements) and *eliciting modality* (verbal, visual, and imitative) that have seldom been subjected to rigorous empirical investigation (DeRenzi, 1985). Indeed, even the traditional division of limb apraxia into types—ideational versus ideomotor—has been based on *a priori* distinctions defined by the assessment procedures employed. Ideomotor apraxia (IMA) is usually assessed by observing the production of transitive pantomimes and intransitive gestures elicited in response to verbal commands or imitation (Heilman, Rothi, & Valenstein, 1982; Helm-Estabrooks, 1990). Ideational apraxia (IA), however, is presumed by most investigators necessarily to involve the manipulation of single or multiple objects (DeRenzi & Lucchelli, 1988; Ochipa, Rothi, & Heilman, 1989; Poeck & Lehmkuhl, 1980). In any case, there have been few attempts in the past to verify empirically the validity of this distinction (Duffy & Duffy, 1989).

This state of affairs is unfortunate, for limb apraxia has emerged as a critical issue in the assessment and clinical management of aphasic patients. Helm-Estabrooks and Albert (1991) have written that an early apraxia assessment is crucially important in evaluating aphasic individuals; otherwise, they claim, results of language and cognitive testing may be misleading, because most aphasic examinations require the individual to produce purposeful movement. Furthermore, limb apraxia is the most frequently cited reason for aphasic patients' frequent failure to use nonverbal gestures for communicative purposes (Duffy & Duffy, 1989). Nevertheless, despite its clinical and theoretical significance, the assessment of limb apraxia has been based on distinctions yet to be empirically validated.

PURPOSE OF THE INVESTIGATION

The present investigation was designed to assess the validity of distinctions reported in the literature as important to the assessment IMA and its differentiation from IA. Multiple task comparisons across a group of aphasic subjects were used to make this assessment. The investigation addressed the following specific issues and questions:

1. *The validity of the modality effect:* Does the assessment of IMA through production of transitive pantomimes vary according to the modality used to elicit the response (verbal instructions, visual presentation, or imitation)?

2. *The validity of movement type distinctions:* Do transitive pantomimes versus intransitive gestures or meaningful movements versus nonmeaningful movements represent distinct classes of praxis that may be differentially affected by brain damage?

3. *The validity of types of limb apraxia:* Do the behavioral deficits traditionally associated with IA and IMA reflect different neuropsychological processes, or do they simply reflect a continuum of severity?

METHOD

Subjects

The subjects in this investigation were 20 left-hemisphere-damaged aphasic adults (15 males, 5 females). The mean age of the subjects was 63 years, with a standard deviation of 13.5 and a range of 24 years to 85 years. Mean educational level was 13.5 years, with a standard deviation of 3.53 and a range of 8 years to 19 years. Time post onset averaged 28 months, with a standard deviation of 37.4 and a range from 1 month to 13.5 years. Severity of aphasia, as measured by the overall percentile on the *Porch Index of Communicative Ability* (PICA) (Porch, 1981), ranged from the 12th to the 87th percentile, with the mean occurring at the 53rd. Half of the subjects were above the 50th percentile and half were below. Handedness of the aphasic subjects and hand used in the study were not reported.

The Fluency Rating scale from the *Western Aphasia Battery* (WAB) (Kertesz, 1982) was used to classify subjects as fluent or nonfluent. On this basis, 14 subjects were classified as nonfluent, and 6 were classified as fluent.

Comparison With Neurologically Normal Controls

Ten neurologically normal (NN) subjects were also included in the investigation for comparison purposes. Six of the NN subjects were males, and four were females. All were right-handed by self-report with no previous histories of neurologic or psychiatric illness. The mean age of the NN subjects was 67 years, with a standard deviation of 13.2 and a range of 45 to 82 years. Mean educational level was 12 years, with a standard deviation of of 3.4 and a range of 8 to 17 years.

T-tests indicated that the age and the educational levels of the aphasic and NN subjects did not differ significantly (age: $t = -.90, df = 28, p = .38$; education: $t = 1.03, df = 28, p = .31$).

Procedures

Subjects were administered the following experimental tasks:

1. *The Multiple Object Test (MOT):* Given the necessary objects, subjects were asked to (a) light a candle, (b) open a bottle and pour out its contents, (c) prepare a cup of coffee, (d) pretend to smoke a cigarette, (e) begin to paint a picture, (f) pound a nail into a block of wood, and (g) beat an egg. Tasks of this type are generally accepted as valid elicitation measures of IA (DeRenzi, 1985; Poeck & Lehmkuhl, 1980). A modification of a scoring procedure reported by DeRenzi and Lucchelli (1988) was employed to assess performance on the MOT. Each subject's score was the total number of errors made across the seven individual test items. Possible error types included mislocation errors, misuse errors, sequencing errors, and perplexity errors.

2. *Three transitive pantomime tasks (TP-VIS, TP-VER, TP-IM):* The three transitive pantomime tasks were identical except for the modality used to

elicit the response: TP-VIS was visual; TP-VER was verbal; and TP-IM was imitative. Test items for the transitive pantomime tasks consisted of pantomiming the function of 15 common objects. For the transitive pantomime tasks, as well as for all subsequent tasks, subject performances were judged using a multidimensional scoring procedure adapted from that employed on the PICA.

3. *Two intransitive gestural tasks (IG-IM and IG-C):* The first intransitive gestural task was imitative; the second involved eliciting the target gestures using verbal commands. Test items for the intransitive gestural tasks consisted of eight well-known symbolic gestures such as waving good-bye and making the victory sign.

4. *A single measure of the ability to imitate nonmeaningful movements (IM-NMM):* This measure consisted of the first subtest of the *Limb Apraxia Test* (LAT) (Duffy & Duffy, 1989).

Tasks 2 through 4 are generally accepted measures of IMA (Heilman et al., 1982; Helm-Estabrooks, 1990; Wang, 1990). All scoring was done on the basis of videotapes made at the time of task administration.

Reliability

Intraexaminer reliability coefficients were obtained for all measures and ranged from .93 to .99. Interexaminer reliability coefficients were not reported. Test-retest reliability coefficients for 10 aphasic subjects ranged from .81 to .97.

RESULTS

Comparison of Aphasic and NN Subjects

Table 1 presents the results of a series of t-tests between performances of aphasic and NN subjects on all experimental tasks. The results demonstrate that the aphasic subjects performed significantly less well than the NN subjects on six of the seven tasks. Only on the intransitive gestures–imitation (IG-IM) task were the mean performances of the aphasic and NN subjects *not* significantly different ($p = .05$).

The Modality Effect

The hypothesis that the aphasic subjects' production of transitive pantomimes might vary depending on the eliciting modality was not sup-

Table 1. Comparison Between Aphasic and Neurologically Normal (NN) Subjects' Mean Performances on Experimental Tasks

Value	Tasks						
	MOT	TP-VIS	TP-VER	TP-IM	IG-IM	IG-C	IM-NMM
Mean							
Aphasics	3.2	10.6	10.4	10.4	13.6	11.7	12.4
NN	0.5	13.5	13.7	14.0	14.4	14.4	13.8
SD							
Aphasics	3.4	2.7	2.6	2.6	1.6	2.8	1.7
NN	0.7	0.8	0.8	0.8	0.7	0.6	0.5
t	3.42*	−4.40*	−5.09*	−5.81*	−1.88	−4.15*	−3.37*

Note: The mean MOT score is the total number of errors recorded on this measure averaged across subjects. All other means are mean PICA scores. MOT = multiple object test; TP-VIS = transitive pantomimes–visual modality; TP-VER = transitive pantomimes–verbal modality; TP-IM = transitive pantomimes–imitation modality; IG-IM = intransitive gestures–imitation; IG-C = intransitive gestures on command; IM-NMM = imitation of nonmeaningful movements.
*$p < .01$.

Table 2. Aphasic Subjects' Means, Standard Deviations, and Ranges for Each of the Transitive Pantomime Tasks

Values	Tasks		
	TP-VIS	TP-VER	TP-IM
Mean	10.6[a]	10.4[a]	10.4[a]
SD	2.7	2.6	2.6
Range	4.7–14.4	5.5–14.6	6.3–14.5

Note: TP-VIS = transitive pantomimes–visual modality; TP-VER = transitive pantomimes–verbal modality; TP-IM = transitive pantomimes–imitation modality.
[a]F—not significant ($p > .05$)

ported. As indicated in Table 2, mean scores across the three transitive pantomime tasks (TP-VIS, TP-VER, and TP-IM) were nearly identical (10.6, 10.6, and 10.4, respectively). Standard deviations and ranges were also comparable. Moreover, examination of the Pearson r correlation coefficients among the variables indicated extremely strong intercorrelations. The correlation between TP-VIS and TP-VER was .92; between TP-VIS and TP-IM, .92; and between TP-VER and TP-IM, .91. Finally, Cronbach's alpha, a measure of internal consistency, was .98 when the three measures were analyzed as a single 45-item scale.

These findings support the assertion that, for a randomly selected group of aphasic subjects, the modality effect does not exist. The aphasic subjects performed similarly when asked to produce transitive panto-mimes regardless of whether the corresponding object was shown, verbal instructions were given, or subjects were asked to imitate the target move-ments of the examiner. It therefore appears that when transitive panto-mimes are used as a measure of IMA, similar results will be obtained irrespective of the eliciting modality.

Type of Movement Distinctions

Because there were no differences in mean performance on each of the three transitive pantomime tasks, a new variable was created to represent transitive pantomime performance. This new variable, TP-3, is a compo-site variable created by averaging scores across the three transitive panto-mime tasks.

Table 3 shows the means, standard deviations, and ranges for the variables TP-3, IG-IM (intransitive gestures–imitation), IG-C (intransitive gestures on command), and IM-NMM (imitation of nonmeaningful move-ments). Each of these variables was employed as a measure of IMA. With one exception, pairwise multiple t-tests indicated that the mean scores among the four variables were significantly different from each other at the .05 level (adjusted for Type I error). The exception was the difference between IG-C and IM-NMM.

Table 4 presents the correlation coefficients (Pearson r) among the four IMA variables. The data indicate strong correlations among all four vari-ables: Four of the six correlation coefficients are above .72, and both remaining coefficients are above .60.

Table 3. Aphasic Subjects' Means, Standard Deviations, and Ranges for Measures of IMA (Ideomotor Apraxia)

	Measures			
Values	TP-3	IG-IM	IG-C	IM-NMM
Mean[a]	10.5$_a$	13.6$_b$	11.7$_c$	12.4$_c$
SD	2.6	1.6	2.8	1.7
Range	5.7–14.5	8.5–15.0	7.0–14.7	8.9–14.9

Note: TP-3 = transitive pantomimes; IG-IM = intransitive gestures–imitation; IG-C = intransitive gestures on command; IM-NMM = imitation of nonmeaningful movements.
[a]Means with different subscripts are significantly different at the .05 level.

Table 4. Pearson _r_ Correlation Coefficients Among Measures of IMA (Ideomotor Apraxia)

Measures	TP-3	IG-IM	IG-C
IG-IM	.73*		
IG-C	.87*	.77*	
IM-NMM	.73*	.62*	.66*

Note: TP-3 = transitive pantomimes; IG-IM = intransitive gestures–imitation; IG-C = intransitive gestures on command; IM-NMM = imitation of nonmeaningful movements.
*p < .01.

Table 5. Results of Factor Analysis of IMA (Ideomotor Apraxia) Variables

Variables	Factor 1
TP-3	.934
IG-C	.924
IG-IM	.813
IM-NMM	.750

Note: TP-3 = transitive pantomimes; IG-C = intransitive gestures on command; IG-IM = intransitive gestures–imitation; IM-NMM = imitation of nonmeaningful movements.

Table 5 displays the results of a factor analysis of the four IMA variables; principle factors was used as the method of extraction (Dixon, Brown, Engelman, & Jennrich, 1990). Only a single factor was extracted. By itself, this single factor, which had an eigenvalue of 2.95, explained 98% of the common variance attributable to all four IMA variables.

These findings suggest that movement-type distinctions reported in the literature regarding IMA assessment are _not_ representative of distinct classes of praxis. Although different types of movements appear to involve different degrees of difficulty (i.e., overall mean scores for the IMA tasks were, with one exception, significantly different from one other), factor analysis yielded only a single underlying factor. Indeed, it is worth noting that performances across the different movement types (transitive pantomimes, intransitive gestures, and nonmeaningful limb movements) were so strongly correlated that multicollinearity was detected when an attempt was made to examine the relationships among the IMA variables through multiple regression (Belanger, 1992).

Types of Limb Apractic Processes: Ideomotor (IMA) and Ideational (IA)

Tasks involving the manipulation of multiple objects and simple acts not involving the manipulation of real objects (i.e., transitive pantomimes, intransitive gestures, and nonmeaningful limb movements) were used to assess the traditional distinction between ideational and ideomotor limb apraxia. Table 6 displays the results of a factor analysis (Principle factors; Dixon et al., 1990) using MOT (the investigation's measure of IA) and three of the four IMA variables. (Intransitive gestures–imitation was not included in the analysis to preserve the five-to-one ratio between subjects and variables that Tabachnick and Fidell, 1989, suggest is necessary for reliable factor analysis. This variable was excluded because, of the four IMA tasks, it was the only one on which mean performances between aphasic and NN subjects were not significantly different.) As Table 6 indicates, only a single underlying factor was extracted; by itself, it explained 98% of the shared variance among the variables.

A single composite score was also obtained for all the IMA variables. This score was generated by factor analysis (see Table 5) and served to represent IMA performance. The correlation between this score and MOT performance was .83 ($p < .01$).

These findings support the assertion that measures of IA and IMA are best viewed as reflecting a single underlying disorder along a continuum of severity. If IA and IMA were distinct disorders representing unique underlying neuropsychological impairments, more than one factor should have been generated through a factor analysis of the IA and IMA variables.

SUMMARY AND CONCLUSIONS

Current procedures in the diagnosis and assessment of limb apraxia typically reflect the assumption that important distinctions in elicited performance can be obtained by using tests that (a) differ in the modality of elicitation, (b) differ in the type of movement, and (c) reflect two distinct and independent impaired neuropsychological processes traditionally identified as ideomotor and ideational apraxia. A group of 20 left-hemisphere-damaged aphasic adults underwent a battery of tests of limb movements, and the results were analyzed to determine whether the assumption of differences in motor performance related to these three factors is valid and whether any differences in performance across tasks can be accounted for by two or more independent underlying casual factors.

Table 6. Results of Factor Analysis of IA (Ideational Apraxia) and IMA (Ideomotor Apraxia) Variables

Variables	Factor 1
IG-C	.932
TP-3	.931
MOT	.871
IM-NMM	.746

Note: IG-C = intransitive gestures on command; TP-3 = transitive pantomimes; MOT = multiple object test; IM-NMM = imitation of nonmeaningful movements.

Modality Effect

Does the production of transitive pantomimes differ with the modality used (verbal, visual, or imitation) to elicit the response? The three mean scores for transitive pantomimes (TP-VER, TP-VIS, TP-IM) were not significantly different from one another. The assertion of a modality effect on pantomime performance thus is not supported.

Type of Movement Distinctions

Does motor performance differ across different classes of movement (transitive pantomimes, intransitive gestures, and nonmeaningful limb movements)? Statistically significant differences were obtained between tasks that differed in the classes of movement used. There was a modality difference for intransitive gestures elicited by imitation (IG-IM) and by verbal command (IG-C); performance on both intransitive gestures tests (IG-IM, IG-C) differed significantly from a measure of transitive pantomime (TP-3) performance; and nonmeaningful imitated movements (IM-NMM) differed significantly from transitive pantomimes (TP-3) and imitated intransitive gestures (IG-IM). The only performances that did not differ significantly were intransitive gestures elicited by verbal command (IG-C) and nonmeaningful movements (IM-NMM).

Our results, therefore, support the assertion that motor performance differs with the class of movement that is being tested. Such differences in the accuracy of performance should not, however, be interpreted as reflecting distinct or different types of limb apractic processes. The strong correlations obtained between all four movement types and the extraction of only a single factor from a factor analysis of the four types of movement support the assertion that the differences across tests reflect different levels of task difficulty rather than distinct types of underlying practic processes.

Types of Limb Apractic Processes: Ideomotor (IMA) and Ideational (IA)

Do the two types of apractic behaviors commonly identified as IA and IMA reflect different and independent impaired neuropsychological processes? A multiple object manipulation test (MOT) was used as a test of IA, and a composite single object pantomime score (TP-3), an intransitive gesture test (IT-C), and an imitative test of nonmeaningful movements (IM-NMM) were used as measures of IMA. The relationship between the IA and IMA measures was examined using correlational and factor analyses. Only a single factor was extracted from the IA and three IMA measures. A very high correlation coefficient (.83) was also obtained between the measure of IA (MOT) and a composite factor score representing the four IMA tasks (TP-3, IG-C, IG-IM, IM-NMM). These results fail to support the assertion that differences in performance on IMA and IA tests reflect deficits in different and distinct underlying neuropsychological processes. Our results are similar to those of Duffy, Duffy, and Watt (1994) in failing to confirm the independence of IA and IMA processes. The results of our study support the need for additional investigations to examine the validity of distinctions that have generally been believed to exist among types of limb apraxia.

ACKNOWLEDGMENTS

This investigation was supported by grants from the University of Connecticut Research Foundation and The Gaylord Hospital, Wallingford, CT.

REFERENCES

Belanger, S. A. (1992). *An investigation of limb apraxia typology: The validity of the distinction between ideational and ideomotor apraxia.* Unpublished doctoral dissertation, University of Connecticut, Storrs.

DeRenzi, E. (1985). Methods of limb apraxia examination and their bearing on the interpretation of the disorder. In E. A. Roy (Ed.), *Neuropsychological studies of apraxia and related disorders* (pp. 45–63). New York: North Holland.

DeRenzi, E., & Lucchelli, F. (1988). Ideational apraxia. *Brain, 111,* 1173–1185.

Dixon, W. J., Brown, M. B., Engelman, L., & Jennrich, R. I. (Eds.). (1990). *BMDP Statistical Software Manual* (Vol. 1). Berkeley: University of California Press.

Duffy, J. R., & Duffy, R. J. (1989). The Limb Apraxia Test: An imitative measure of upper limb apraxia. In T. E. Prescott (Ed.), *Clinical aphasiology,* Vol. 18 (pp. 145–159). Austin, TX: PRO-ED.

Duffy, R. J., Duffy, J. R., & Watt, J. H. (1994). *The construct validity of the Limb Apraxia Test (LAT): Implications for the distinction between types of limb apraxia.* In M. L. Lemme (Ed.), *Clinical aphasiology,* Vol. 22 (pp. 181–190). Austin, TX: PRO-ED.

Heilman, K. M., Rothi, L. J., & Valenstein, E. (1982). Two forms of ideomotor apraxia. *Neurology, 32,* 342–346.

Helm-Estabrooks, N., (1990). *Test of Oral and Limb Apraxia: Standardization Edition.* San Antonio, TX: Special Press.

Helm-Estabrooks, N., & Albert, M. L. (1991). *Manual of aphasia therapy.* Austin, TX: PRO-ED.

Kertesz, A. (1982). *The Western Aphasia Battery.* New York: Grune & Stratton.

Ochipa, C., Rothi, L. J. G., & Heilman, K. M. (1989). Ideational apraxia: A deficit in tool selection and use. *Annals of Neurology, 25,* 190–193.

Poeck, K., & Lehmkuhl, G. (1980). Ideatory apraxia in a left-handed patient with a right-sided brain lesion. *Cortex, 16,* 273–284.

Porch, B. (1981). *Porch Index of Communicative Ability.* Palo Alto, CA: Consulting Psychologists Press.

Rothi, L. J. G., Ochipa, C., Leadon, M. R., & Meher, L. M. (1989). Limb apraxia: A neuropsychological approach. A miniseminar presented at the annual convention of the American-Speech-Language-Hearing-Association, St. Louis, Missouri.

Tabachnick, B. G. & Fidell, L. S. (1989). *Using multivariate statistics* (2nd ed.). New York: Harper & Row.

Wang, L. (1990). *The nature of impaired pantomime performance in aphasic patients.* Unpublished doctoral dissertation, Boston University, Boston.

Clinical Aphasiology, Vol. 22, 1994, pp. 203–218

Acoustically Derived Perceptual Evidence for Coarticulatory Errors in Apraxic and Conduction Aphasic Speech Production

Malcolm R. McNeil, Michiko Hashi,
and Helen Southwood

INTRODUCTION

Deficits in the temporal and spatial coordination of speech have been suggested by many (Itoh, Sasanuma, & Ushijima, 1979; Kent & Rosenbek, 1983; Rosenbek, Kent, & LaPointe, 1984; Wertz, LaPointe, & Rosenbek, 1984) to explain the mechanisms underpinning apraxia of speech. Data have been amassed from acoustic, physiologic, and perceptual studies to support these suggestions and to attribute the observed speech deficits to a phonetic/motoric level of the speech production system (see McNeil & Kent, 1990, for a review of this evidence). Recent evidence from acoustic (Kent & McNeil, 1987; McNeil, Liss, Tseng, & Kent, 1990), kinematic (McNeil & Adams, 1991; McNeil, Weismer, Adams, & Mulligan, 1990; McNeil, Hashi, & Tseng, 1991) and perceptual (Odell, McNeil, Rosenbek, & Hunter, 1990, 1991) studies have also supported the idea that at least some individuals with conduction aphasia may also present phonetic/motoric deficits in addition to, or instead of, their assumed phonologic-level speech errors.

Among the more salient sources of evidence for temporal and spatial coordination speech production deficits in the apraxia of speech population are data provided from a perceptual approach used first with this population by Ziegler and Von Cramon (1985). In this paradigm, normal listeners judge the presence of a particular vowel in CV or CCV sequences when the vowel has been systematically reduced (computer edited) in a right-to-left fashion. This approach eliminates portions of the sound ranging from only a few milliseconds to the entire vowel. In the Ziegler and Von Cramon study, utterances from normal and apraxic subjects' productions were judged by normal listeners. These judges were required to identify or predict the vowel that followed each stimulus. Each utterance was "gated" at five different durations, and the listener selected responses from three vowels. The premise underlying this procedure is that, even if a listener hears only part of a vowel—or in some cases, none of it—the consonant carries sufficient information about lip-retracted (/i/) or -protruded (/U/) vowels to predict the vowel that follows. This premise is supported by acoustic analyses of normal speech (Ohman, 1966; Sereno, Baum, Marean, & Lieberman, 1986; Soli, 1981) wherein a spectral peak in the region of the second formant of the following vowel has been identified in the consonant portion of the CV sequence that is believed to carry the cue for the vowel. This assumes that in normal speakers, the speech plan (the selection and ordering of the phonological units) and the motor speech program (the conversion of the phonological information into instructions for movement) prepare the articulators in advance of their execution. Further assumed is that an impaired speech motor program would be indicated by the production of consonants that do not carry sufficient information about the **correctly selected vowel** for their accurate prediction.[1] In such a task, the amount of acoustic information available to the listener is a function of the gating, and the accuracy of vowel identification represents the efficiency of coarticulation as well as the integrity of the motor speech programmer (assuming that the speech plan has been assembled properly). Results for Ziegler and Von Cramon's normal speakers confirmed that only the lip retracted or protruded consonantal acoustic information, and little or none of the vowel, was needed to accurately predict the vowel. Results for two apraxic speakers, however, revealed that more of the vowel was needed for correct identification from their productions. This result was interpreted as a reflection of a delayed onset of anticipatory vowel gestures and an impaired motor speech programmer in the apraxic speakers.

A partial replication of the Ziegler and Von Cramon study by Katz (1987) failed to locate coarticulatory deficits among normal "anterior" and "posterior" aphasic subjects using acoustic analyses. A second replication by Katz (1988), however, did report coarticulatory deficits in anterior aphasic subjects. Several acoustic analyses of aphasic subjects—"anterior,"

---

1. Sussman, Marquardt, MacNeilage, and Hutchinson (1988) point out that analyses restricted to "on-target" productions omit important data and sources of evidence that are available with the analysis of error data. However, in the present study, it is imperative that the experimenters' target vowel was also the subject's target vowel; the source of the deficit in the speech production process thus must be attributed to the motor-programming level rather than to the speech-planning level (a level often implicated in many aphasic phonologic errors and in normal "slips of the tongue.")

"posterior," "fluent," and "nonfluent"—and normal subjects by Katz (1987), Katz, Machetanz, Orth, and Schonle (1990a), and Tuller and Story (1987) revealed inconsistent patterns of anticipatory lingual and labial coarticulation for the aphasic populations compared to the normal control subjects. A kinematic study of anticipatory coarticulation in two anterior aphasic subjects (Katz, Machetanz, Orth, and Schonle, 1990b) revealed coarticulatory patterns that were more variable than the same patterns of two control subjects. This variability was found in displacement and not in the temporal aspects of the movement.

Because of the inconsistent results across both perceptual and acoustic studies of anticipatory coarticulation, the present study was designed as a replication in apraxic speakers and an extension of these analyses to the speech of conduction aphasic subjects. This extension is of particular interest because speech problems in conduction aphasia have traditionally been assigned exclusively to the phonological level of speech production. Although some challenges to this assignment have been proposed (Kent & McNeil, 1987; McNeil, Liss, Tseng, & Kent, 1990; McNeil, Hashi, & Tseng, 1991; Tseng, McNeil, Adams, & Weismer, 1990), there is insufficient evidence to argue conclusively for a phonetic assembly, motor-programming, or execution mechanism deficit in this population.

METHOD

Subjects

The speech samples for this study were taken from one normal speaker, two subjects with apraxia of speech uncomplicated by dysarthria or aphasia, and two subjects diagnosed as having conduction aphasia without concomitant apraxia of speech or dysarthria.[2] The selection criteria for all subjects have been summarized elsewhere (e.g., McNeil & Adams, 1991) and are not repeated here. These subjects were chosen from the pool of subjects used in a series of studies, and their biographic characteristics, speech, language, and cognitive performance on a variety of measures are summarized in Table 1.

Six normal adults served as judges for this study. They were considered sophisticated listeners in that they: (1) had successfully completed a college-level course in phonetics and a graduate-level course in motor speech disorder; (2) had at least 1 year of research or clinical experience in neuro-

2. The subjects used in this investigation have been used in a series of studies. The following scheme identifies the subjects used in both the present study (first designation) and the original one (second designation): $N_1 = N_1$, $A_1 = A_3$, $A_2 = A_2$, $C_1 = C_4$, $C_2 = C_3$.

Table 1. Summary of Biographical and Descriptive Data for Normal Control, Apraxic, and Conduction Aphasic Speakers

Subject Characteristics	N_1	A_1	A_2	C_1	C_2
Gender	M	M	M	M	M
Age (in years)	67	54	62	62	60
Structural-functional exam.[a]	WNL	WNL	WNL	WNL	WNL
Total RCPM[b]	32	30	28	27	32
Overall PICA[c]	14.73	14.53	14.33	14.87	14.13
Overall RTT[d]	14.35	12.23	12.08	13.94	13.04
BDAE Aud. Comp.[e]	119	118	113	114	117
BDAE speech rating					
Artistic agility	7	3	4	5	5
Phrase length	7	4	4	5	5
Melodic line	7	4	4	5	7
BDAE total sent. repetitions w/o errors	8	1	7	3	1
Apraxia battery for adults					
Total limb	48	48	50	50	50
Total oral	50	49	47	49	49

[c]*Porch Index of Communicative Ability* (Porch, 1967). [d]*Revised Token Test* (McNeil & Prescott, 1978). [e]*Boston Diagnostic Aphasia Examination* (Goodglass & Kaplan, 1983). S-F Exam. Structural-Functional Examination.

WNL There was a questionable right-sided lingual weakness on clinical examination that was not confirmed with additional testing for this subject.

Total RCPM Total number correct on the Raven Coloured Progressive Matrices.

Total WFM Total Word Fluency Measure score.

O.A. PICA Overall score on the *Porch Index of Communicative Ability* (see text for method of calculation).

O.A. RTT Overall score on the *Revised Token Test*.

BDAE Aud. Comp. total number correct on all four auditory comprehension subtests of the *Boston Diagnostic Aphasia Examination*.

BDAE Spch. Rtg. Ratings assigned for articulatory agility, phrase length, and melodic line from the rating of speech characteristics section of the *Boston Diagnostic Aphasia Examination*.

BDAE Total Sent. Rep. w/o Errors Total number of sentences repeated without articulatory errors from the sentence repetition subtest of the *Boston Diagnostic Aphasia Examination*.

Apraxia Bat. for Adults Total score on the limb and oral apraxia subtests from the Apraxia Battery for Adults. (A score of 50 represents error-free performance.)

WNL There was a question of oral sensory diminution on clinical examination in this subject.

genic communication disorders or in developmental phonological disorders; (3) had no speech or language problems; (4) were native speakers of American English; and (5) had normal hearing by self-report.

Stimuli

The single normal and four pathologic speakers' productions of 10 single words (*six, sixteen, stop, stopping, build, building, big, bigger, bob,* and *bobby*), with either an /S/, /ST/, or /B/ consonant preceding either the lip-retracted vowel /I/ (as in *six*) or the lip neutral vowel /a/ (as in *Bob*), were used as stimuli. Only utterances judged as *on target* at the word level, using a broad phonetic transcription reference, were employed as stimuli. This selection of data allowed the elimination of obvious phonemic-level errors and increased the interpretability of the data relative to the assignment of phonetic/motoric mechanisms for any observed effects. Five repetitions of each utterance from each speaker were digitized at a 20-kHz sampling rate using a 10-kHz low-pass filter. The stimuli from each speaker were computer edited (gated) at five different durations and were randomized and rerecorded onto audiotape. Figure 1 shows the acoustic waveform for one utterance (*six*) used in this study. The five different gates that were presented to each normal judge are shown. Gate 5 represents the consonant plus the entire vowel and should be identified correctly, beyond chance-level errors, in all instances of correct production.

Judge's Task

The judges listened to all 250 stimuli and selected, from among five choices (/a/, /I/, /i/, /ae/, and /ǝ/—the schwa), the vowel that followed each consonant. A probability of identifying the correct vowel by chance was 20%, or 1 in 5, if the judges believed that all five vowel choices were present (though only the /I/ and /a/ vowels were present in the stimuli). All listening sessions were conducted in a sound-treated chamber, the tapes were presented in a sound field, and the listeners selected the volume with which they felt most comfortable. Listeners were required, and frequently encouraged, to guess when they were not certain.

Analysis

All responses were tabulated by speaker and utterance. Binomial probabilities were calculated for each combination of subject, utterance, and

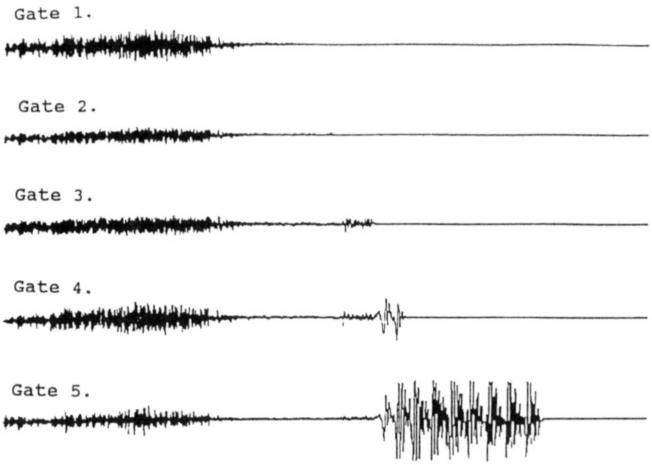

Gate 1.

Gate 2.

Gate 3.

Gate 4.

Gate 5.

Figure 1. Acoustic waveform for the utterance "six" showing complete signal for gate 5, with successive portions of the signal removed (gaited) to gate 1, where only the /s/ was retained for perceptual judgment.

gate. The alpha level was set at .05 for each comparison and was calculated as a one-tailed test.

RESULTS AND DISCUSSION

The general results of this investigation are illustrated in Figures 2 through 11. These figures represent the data for each subject for each of the 10 stimuli used in this study and show the probability at which the correct vowel was identified. The horizontal line at the bottom of each figure represents the .05 confidence level. Symbols falling below this level represent instances in which the vowel was identified *correctly* at a rate significantly beyond chance level for that subject on that particular utterance. Symbols falling above this line represent vowels that were judged *incorrectly* or exceeded the .05 confidence level for that particular subject. The ordinate in these figures, then, represents the alpha level achieved for that subject on that particular stimulus at each gate. Gate 5 contained the consonant plus the entire vowel and should in all instances be identified correctly beyond chance level for all subjects whose productions were perceived accurately by these judges. There were instances in which the stimulus at Gate 5 was not identified significantly beyond chance level

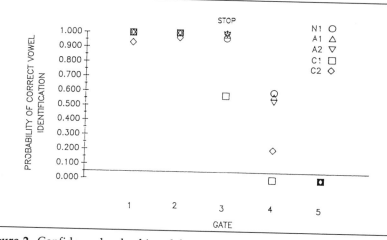

Figure 2. Confidence level achieved for each individual subject's judgments at each of the five gaited stimuli for the normal and pathologic subject's productions of the word "STOP." Judgments falling below the horizontal line in the figure at the .05 alpha level (probability of correct vowel identification) represent significantly correct vowel identification. Symbols falling above this line represent nonsignificant vowel identification.

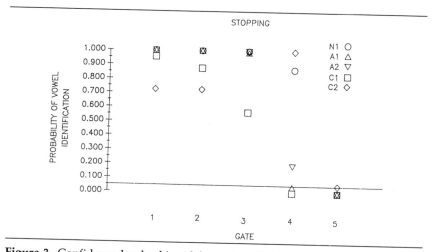

Figure 3. Confidence level achieved for each individual subject's judgments at each of the five gaited stimuli for the normal and pathologic subject's productions of the word "STOPPING." Judgments falling below the horizontal line in the figure at the .05 alpha level (probability of correct vowel identification) represent significantly correct vowel identification. Symbols falling above this line represent nonsignificant vowel identification.

(as was the case with subjects C_2 and A_1 for the utterance *six*; see Figure 4). In these cases, it is difficult to interpret the data as evidence that the vowels identified at earlier gates represent coarticulatory effects rather than the selection of the incorrect vowel and, hence, a speech-planning (i.e., phonologic-level) error for these particular subjects on that particular utterance. However, in some instances, as is the case with subject A_1 in the same trial, the vowel was identified correctly beyond chance levels at all gates preceding Gate 5. It might be argued that alterations in the vowel itself caused the listener to perceive abnormalities when the entire vowel was produced; consequently, an incorrect vowel was identified with an *increase* in acoustic information.

Figure 6 (the utterance *build*) shows that the vowel productions for the N_1 and C_1 were judged accurately at all gates. However, A_1 and C_2 were judged inaccurately for Gates 1 through 3 and 1 through 4, respectively. It should be noted, however, that because A_2 was judged inaccurately at Gate 5, the result is difficult to interpret as a coarticulatory error for this particular subject and utterance.

Figure 7 shows the results for the utterance *building*. As with the utterance *build*, the vowels for N_1 and C_1 were judged accurately at all gates (save Gate 2 for N_1), whereas A_2 and C_2's vowels were not identified accurately until considerably more of the vowel was present. With the correct identification of the vowel when it was acoustically present, the differences can more readily be assigned to the effects of coarticulatory differences in the speech of the two apraxic and one conduction aphasic subjects. Results for the remainder of the utterances are shown in Figures 8 through 11. In general, they paralleled those for the previous two utterances.

Overall, it was found that the neutral vowel /a/ in *stop* and *stopping* did not provide sufficient acoustic cues in the consonant for any of the subjects (including the normal subject) to predict the vowel above chance level until all or nearly all of the vowel was heard. This is interpreted as support for the notion that there are coarticulatory cues imbedded in the consonantal portion of the signal for some phonetic contexts, such as lip-retracted vowels, and that this experiment was in line with the experimental paradigm.

With the exception of those in the utterances *stop* and *stopping*, C_1's vowels were identified correctly at a rate significantly beyond chance for all words at all gates. Likewise, the normal subject's vowels were generally identified correctly at all gates for all utterances, and in all instances in Gates 4 and 5. A_1, A_2, and C_2 all demonstrated productions in which the vowel could not be identified correctly beyond chance level for any of the utterances (though not at every gate for all utterances).

These results are of interest in two ways. First, the coarticulation deficits in apraxia of speech demonstrated by Ziegler and Von Cramon (1985) were replicated in the present study, though with less consistency than

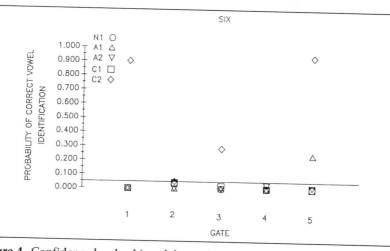

Figure 4. Confidence level achieved for each individual subject's judgments at each of the five gaited stimuli for the normal and pathologic subject's productions of the word "SIX." Judgments falling below the horizontal line in the figure at the .05 alpha level (probability of correct vowel identification) represent significantly correct vowel identification. Symbols falling above this line represent nonsignificant vowel identification.

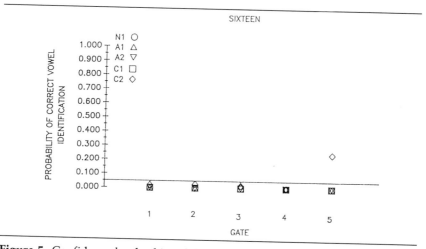

Figure 5. Confidence level achieved for each individual subject's judgments at each of the five gaited stimuli for the normal and pathologic subject's productions of the word "SIXTEEN." Judgments falling below the horizontal line in the figure at the .05 alpha level (probability of correct vowel identification) represent significantly correct vowel identification. Symbols falling above this line represent nonsignificant vowel identification.

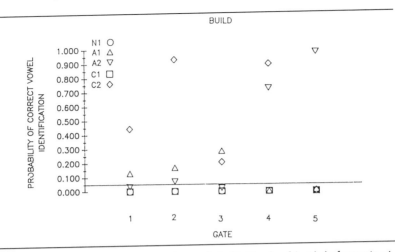

Figure 6. Confidence level achieved for each individual subject's judgments at each of the five gaited stimuli for the normal and pathologic subject's productions of the word "BUILD." Judgments falling below the horizontal line in the figure at the .05 alpha level (probability of correct vowel identification) represent significantly correct vowel identification. Symbols falling above this line represent nonsignificant vowel identification.

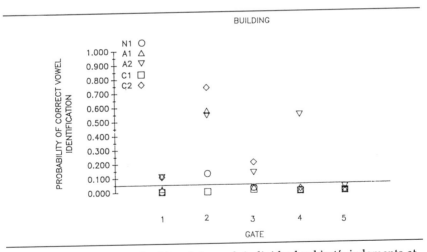

Figure 7. Confidence level achieved for each individual subject's judgments at each of the five gaited stimuli for the normal and pathologic subject's productions of the word "BUILDING." Judgments falling below the horizontal line in the figure at the .05 alpha level (probability of correct vowel identification) represent significantly correct vowel identification. Symbols falling above this line represent nonsignificant vowel identification.

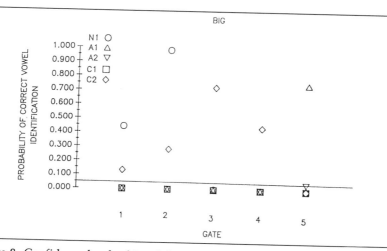

Figure 8. Confidence level achieved for each individual subject's judgments at each of the five gaited stimuli for the normal and pathologic subject's productions of the word "BIG." Judgments falling below the horizontal line in the figure at the .05 alpha level (probability of correct vowel identification) represent significantly correct vowel identification. Symbols falling above this line represent nonsignificant vowel identification.

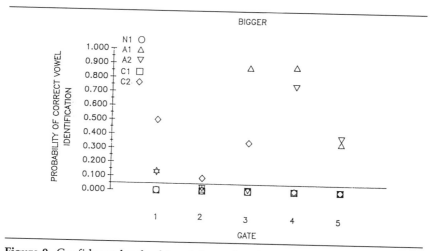

Figure 9. Confidence level achieved for each individual subject's judgments at each of the five gaited stimuli for the normal and pathologic subject's productions of the word "BIGGER." Judgments falling below the horizontal line in the figure at the .05 alpha level (probability of correct vowel identification) represent significantly correct vowel identification. Symbols falling above this line represent nonsignificant vowel identification.

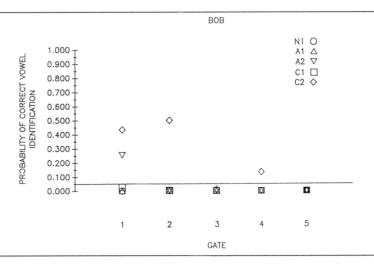

Figure 10. Confidence level achieved for each individual subject's judgments at each of the five gaited stimuli for the normal and pathologic subject's productions of the word "BOB." Judgments falling below the horizontal line in the figure at the .05 alpha level (probability of correct vowel identification) represent significantly correct vowel identification. Symbols falling above this line represent nonsignificant vowel identification.

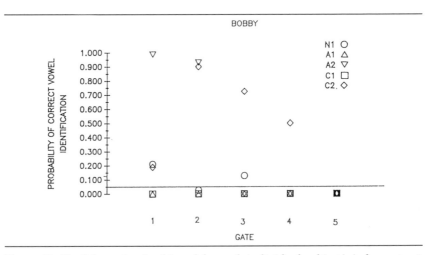

Figure 11. Confidence level achieved for each individual subject's judgments at each of the five gaited stimuli for the normal and pathologic subject's productions of the word "BOBBY." Judgments falling below the horizontal line in the figure at the .05 alpha level (probability of correct vowel identification) represent significantly correct vowel identification. Symbols falling above this line represent nonsignificant vowel identification.

reported by those authors. Second, the results demonstrated abnormalities of coarticulation in one of the two conduction aphasic speakers. Vowels from C_1 were identified correctly to the same extent as those from the normal speaker. This is interpreted to imply that this admittedly limited test of anticipatory coarticulation did not show C_1 to have problems in that area. Conversely, vowels from A_2 were identified no better than those from the apraxic speakers, suggesting the existence of coarticulatory problems in this particular subject. Taken together, the results suggest that conduction aphasic speakers may well vary in their speech production ability, and some of them may demonstrate anticipatory coarticulatory deficits similar to apraxia of speech.

It might be speculated that the anticipatory coarticulatory deficits found in this conduction aphasic speaker are in some way related to lesion location. C_1, who demonstrated normal coarticulation, had a widespread lesion that included part of Broca's area; pre- and postcentral gyri; the superior parietal, supramarginal, and angular gyri; Wernicke's area; part of middle temporal gyrus; and part of the insula. In contrast, C_2, who demonstrated coarticulatory deficits similar to the apraxic subjects, had a lesion in the supramarginal, part of superior parietal, and angular gyri; Wernicke's area; part of middle temporal gyrus; and part of the insula. No lesion was found in either the precentral gyrus or in Broca's area in this conduction aphasic subject. Such clinicoanatomical relations contradict the subclassification of conduction aphasia proposed by several aphasiologists such as Kertesz (1979), suggesting instead a motor component in conduction aphasic subjects with *anterior* lesions. They also call to question the classification systems used in previous anticipatory coarticulation studies, such as the anterior/posterior dichotomy and perhaps the fluent/nonfluent dichotomy, for neither of these two conduction aphasic subjects would have been classified as nonfluent aphasic subjects using the criteria of the *Boston Diagnostic Aphasia Examination* (Goodglass & Kaplan, 1983). This result is also difficult to reconcile with disconnection and phonologic accounts for the speech of conduction aphasic subjects and suggests a more complex explanation for the speech production errors of these subjects than such models provide. The findings also highlight the inadequacy of the classification system employing conduction aphasia for representing the underlying nature (linguistic vs. motoric) for some of the deficits on which the classification is based (i.e., *phonologic* speech errors that are more frequent on repetition than in spontaneous speech or in reading).

Adding to this classification dilemma, Valdois, Joanette, Nespoulous, and Poncet (1988) have questioned whether some subjects typically classified as conduction aphasic are not actually afferent motor aphasic subjects or, alternatively, whether afferent motor aphasia is not a subform of conduction aphasia. Given the lack of established validity for this category in any classification system, the lack of established criteria for selecting afferent motor aphasic subjects, and the lack of knowledge as to whether linguistic or motoric mechanisms underlie the speech production errors in this population, these alternatives add little to a clinically useful application or theoretical explanation for the behaviors observed in the conduction aphasic subjects in this investigation.

The lack of anticipatory coarticulation effects in the conduction aphasic subject whose performance matched the normal subject's could be explained as a matter of severity of deficit rather than as a difference in the nature of the mechanisms generating the errors or the lack thereof. The problem with this potential explanation is that there is no clear, unbiased (with respect to level of analysis), and preferred method for determining the severity of the speech production deficit. In spite of these problems, the subjects from this study are in agreement with this hypothesis. The conduction aphasic subject who demonstrated no evidence of an anticipatory coarticulatory deficit, C_1, repeated fewer sentences without errors and had a higher score on the melodic line rating of the *Boston Diagnostic Aphasia Examination* (Goodglass & Kaplan, 1983) and less aphasia as measured by the *Porch Index of Communicative Ability* (Porch, 1967) and the *Revised Token Test* (McNeil & Prescott, 1978) than C2, who *did* demonstrate an anticipatory coarticulation deficit. This extremely small sample size does not allow a conclusion from this observation; however, there may be reason to formulate and test this hypothesis. A confirmation of this notion has implications that reach far beyond the mere involvement of a motor speech mechanism in some or all of the speech errors of apraxic and conduction aphasic individuals.

The data from this investigation are consistent with the attribution to at least some conduction aphasic subjects a motor-speech-level deficit responsible for at least some of their errors. These findings also are consistent with others demonstrated by perceptual, acoustic, and physiologic studies by our research group, although we obviously need additional subjects in this and other analyses before we can generalize these findings. It is clear, however, that the diagnosis of conduction aphasia does not require the speech production errors to be a matter of forming slots, selecting phonologic elements, or filling the slots with phonologic information that has been properly selected and sequenced (in the model of Shattuck-Hufnagel, 1979, 1983, 1987).

REFERENCES

Goodglass, H., & Kaplan, E. (1983). *Boston Diagnostic Aphasia Examination* (2nd ed.). Philadelphia: Lea and Febiger.

Itoh, M., Sasanuma, S., & Ushijima, T. (1979). Velar movements during speech in a patient with apraxia of speech. *Brain and Language, 7,* 227–239.

Katz, W. F. (1987). Anticipatory labial and lingual coarticulation in aphasia. In J. H. Ryalls (Ed.), *Phonetic approaches to speech production in aphasia and related disorders* (pp. 221–242). Boston: College-Hill.

Katz, W. F. (1988). Anticipatory coarticulation in aphasia: Acoustic and perceptual data. *Brain and Language, 35,* 340–368.

Katz, W. F., Machetanz, J., Orth, U., & Schonle, P. (1990a). A kinematic analysis of anticipatory coarticulation in the speech of anterior aphasic subjects using electromagnetic articulography. *Brain and Language, 38,* 555–575.

Katz, W. F., Machetanz, J., Orth, U., & Schonle, P. (1990b). Anticipatory labial coarticulation in the speech of German-speaking anterior aphasic subjects: Acoustic analyses. *Journal of Neurolinguistics, 5*(2/3), 295–230.

Kent, R. D., & McNeil, M. R. (1987). Relative timing of sentence repetition in apraxia of speech and conduction aphasia. In J. Ryalls (Ed.), *Phonetic approaches to speech production in aphasia and related disorders* (pp. 181–220). Boston: College-Hill.

Kent, R. D., & Rosenbek, J. C. (1983). Acoustic patterns of apraxia of speech. *Journal of Speech and Hearing Research, 26,* 231–249.

Kertesz, A. (1979). *Aphasia and associated disorders: Taxonomy, localization and recovery.* New York: Grune & Stratton.

McNeil, M. R., & Adams, S. (1991). A comparison of speech kinematics among apraxic, conduction aphasic, ataxic dysarthric, and normal geriatric speakers. In T. E. Prescott (Ed.), *Clinical aphasiology,* Vol. 19 (pp. 279–294). Austin, TX: PRO-ED.

McNeil, M. R., Hashi, M., & Tseng, C-H. (1991, October). *Effects of concurrent finger tapping on bilabial kinematics in conduction aphasia.* Paper presented to the Academy of Aphasia, Rome.

McNeil, M. R., & Kent, R. D. (1990). Motoric characteristics of adult aphasic and apraxic speakers. In G. R. Hammond (Ed.), *Advances in psychology: Cerebral control of speech and limb movements* (pp. 349–386). New York: Elsevier/North Holland.

McNeil, M. R., Liss, J., Tseng, T-H., & Kent, R. D. (1990). Speech timing in apraxia and conduction aphasia: A phonetic-motoric disorder. *Brain and Language, 38,* 135–158.

McNeil, M. R., & Prescott, T. E. (1978). *Revised Token Test.* Austin, TX: PRO-ED.

McNeil, M. R., Weismer, G., Adams, S., & Mulligan, M. (1990). Oral structure nonspeech motor control in normal, dysarthric, aphasic and apraxic speakers: Isometric force and static position control. *Journal of Speech and Hearing Research, 33*(2), 255–268.

Odell, K. H., McNeil, M. R., Rosenbek, J. C., & Hunter, L. (1990). Perceptual characteristics of consonant productions by apraxic speakers. *Journal of Speech and Hearing Disorders, 55*(2), 345–359.

Odell, K. H., McNeil, M. R., Rosenbek, J. C., & Hunter, L. (1991). Perceptual characteristics of vowel and prosody production in apraxic, aphasic and dysarthric speakers. *Journal of Speech and Hearing Research, 34*(1), 67–80.

Ohman, S. E. G. (1966). Coarticulation in VCV utterances: Spectrographic measurements. *Journal of the Acoustical Society of America, 39,* 151–168.

Porch, B. E. (1967). *Porch Index of Communicative Ability.* Palo Alto: Consulting Psychologists Press.

Rosenbek, J. C., Kent, R. D., & LaPointe, L. L. (1984). Apraxia of speech: An overview and some perspectives. In J. C. Rosenbek, M. R. McNeil, & A. E. Aronson (Eds.), *Apraxia of speech: Physiology, acoustics, linguistics, management* (pp. 1–72). Boston: College-Hill Press.

Sereno, J. A., Baum S. R., Marean, G. C., & Lieberman, P. (1986). Acoustic analysis and perceptual data on anticipatory labial coarticulation in adults and children. *Journal of Acoustical Society of America, 81*(2), 512–519.

Shattuck-Hufnagel, S. (1979). Speech errors as evidence for a serial ordering mechanism in sentence production. In W. E. Cooper & E. C. T. Walker (Eds.), *Sentence processing: Psycholinguistic studies presented to Merril Garrett* (pp. 295–342). Hillsdale, NJ.: Lawrence Erlbaum.

Shattuck-Hufnagel, S. (1983). Sublexical units and suprasegmental structure in speech production planning. In P. F. MacNeilage (Ed.), *The production of speech* (pp. 109–136). New York: Springer-Verlag.

Shattuck-Hufnagel, S. (1987). The role of word-onset consonants in speech production planning: New evidence from speech error patterns. In E. Keller & M. Gopnik (Eds.), *Motor and sensory processes of language* (pp. 17–51), Hillsdale, NJ.: Lawrence Erlbaum.

Soli, S. D. (1981). Second formants in fricatives: Acoustic consequences of fricative-vowel coarticulation. *Journal of Acoustical Society of America, 70*(4), 976–984.

Sussman, H. M., Marquardt, T. P., MacNeilage, P. F., & Hutchinson, J. A. (1988). Anticipatory coarticulation in aphasia: Some methodological considerations. *Brain and Language, 35,* 369–379.

Tseng, C-H., McNeil, M. R., Adams, S., & Weismer, G. (1990). Effects of speaking rate on bilabial (a)synchrony in neurogenic populations. Paper presented to the annual convention of the American-Speech-Language-Hearing Association, Seattle.

Tuller, B., & Story, R. S. (1987). Anticipatory coarticulation in aphasia. In J. H. Ryalls (Ed.), *Phonetic approaches to speech production in aphasia and related disorders* (pp. 243–260). Boston: College-Hill.

Valdois, S., Joanette, Y., Nespoulous, J-L., & Poncet, M. (1988). Afferent motor aphasia and conduction aphasia. In H. A. Whitaker (Ed.), *Phonological processes and brain mechanisms* (pp. 60–92). New York: Springer-Verlag.

Wertz, R. T., LaPointe, L. L., & Rosenbek, J. C. (1984). *Apraxia of speech in adults: The disorder and its management.* Orlando: Grune & Stratton.

Ziegler, W., & Von Cramon, D. (1985). Anticipatory coarticulation in a patient with apraxia of speech. *Brain and Language, 26,* 117–130.

Clinical Aphasiology, Vol. 22, 1994, pp. 219–229

Oral Motor Tracking in Normal and Apraxic Speakers

Carlin F. Hageman, Donald A. Robin,
Jerald B. Moon, and John W. Folkins

INTRODUCTION

Apraxia of speech has been a topic of much controversy. Arguments have focused on whether the underlying pathogenesis of the disordered behaviors described as apraxic is linguistic or motoric. Although debate continues, the extant, though limited, data suggest that apraxia of speech is a disorder of speech motor control (e.g., McNeil, Weismer, Adams, & Mulligan, 1990). A second controversy surrounding apraxia of speech that has been the focus of recent literature (e.g., Luschei, 1991; Weismer & Liss, 1991) concerns whether apraxia of speech also affects nonspeech movement control. Robin (1992) has argued that apraxia of speech is a disorder of motor control that manifests itself in both speech and nonspeech movements of the articulators.

Although it was once thought that apraxic speakers had abnormal control of peak velocity during speech (e.g., Kent & Rosenbek, 1983), it is abundantly clear that no relation exists between apraxic speakers and the control of peak velocity (McNeil et al., 1990; Robin, Bean, & Folkins, 1989). Robin et al. (1989) hypothesized that apraxia of speech might best be understood as a problem of coordination within and between articulators. Along these lines, McNeil and colleagues (1990) reported that apraxic speakers had greater instability (poorer control) of the articulators during nonspeech fine force and position control tasks than did normal or aphasic speakers.

McClean, Beukelman, and Yorkston (1978) used a visuomotor tracking task to measure the coordination of movement for individual articulators. Tracking tasks have a number of important advantages over fine force or position control tasks, the most important of which is that they are dynamic rather than static. Thus, the control and coordination of articulator movement can be assessed. Also, subjects may be required to track predictable and nonpredictable signals. Finally, one can require subjects to track predictable signals at different speeds or frequencies.

Normal subjects tracking predictable targets use a different strategy than do those tracking nonpredictable targets. Tracking a predictable target successfully requires a model of the target motion. That is, subjects track the target based on an internal representation of target motion and attend to the external target only intermittently to ensure that the model is accurate. Support for this mode of tracking comes from the fact that in both speech and nonspeech systems (Flowers, 1978; Moon, Zebrowski, Robin, & Folkins, 1992), subjects typically phase-lead a predictable target, whereas if they were *following* the external signal, they would phase-lag the target. The use of an internal model or predictive mode allows for smooth movement transitions. By contrast, tracking a nonpredictable signal requires subjects to attend to the target constantly and *not* to rely on an internal model. Thus, subjects must adjust their movement patterns online. As a result, subjects show significant phase lag during nonpredictable tracking tasks, and their movements are more jerky as they continually adjust to error. The result is that overall tracking of nonpredictable targets is poorer than that found for predictable tracking as measured by cross-correlation. (It is also the case that tracking performance decreases as the frequency of the predictable signal increases, but this may be because more rapid predictable targets require more frequent checks, and thus performance decreases [Noble, Fitts, & Warren, 1955]).

In the course of a large study aimed at understanding speech motor control and its impairments, we extended the visuomotor tracking paradigm of McClean et al. (1978) to include predictable targets of different frequencies and a nonpredictable target condition. The present study reports data from apraxic and non-brain-damaged (NBD) speakers on phase relationship and cross-correlation of tracking. It was expected that apraxic speakers would have lower correlations than would normal speakers in all conditions. It also was hypothesized that apraxic speakers would phase-lag predictable targets, whereas NBD speakers would evidence phase synchrony or lead. Finally, it was anticipated that all subjects would show phase lag during nonpredictable tracking.

If apraxic subjects performed poorly on both predictable and nonpredictable tracking, then one could argue that motor control, regardless of tracking mode (internal or external), was impaired. If apraxic speakers performed better on predictable tracking than they did on nonpredictable tracking, it could be hypothesized that they were able to develop an internal model or plan but had difficulty executing the movements in a coordinated manner. If, however, apraxic speakers performed better on nonpredictive tracking than predictable tracking, then one could hypothesize that these subjects did not generate an internal plan to predict movement outcomes but were able to follow an external target that required no such predictive strategy. Thus, the motor control problem would be at the planning or predictive stage of movement execution, and the movements for predictable targets would be jerky rather than smooth.

METHOD

Subjects

Five apraxic and 23 NBD speakers participated. All NBD speakers reported normal speech, language, and hearing and had no known evidence of neurologic or uncorrected vision disorders. The apraxic subjects ranged in age from 20.9 to 79.5 years with a mean of 52.5 years. The NBD subjects ranged in age from 17.2 years to 44.3 years with a mean of 28.2 years. Four of the apraxic subjects have been described in detail by Robin et al. (1991). The remaining subjects fit the same selection criteria as that study (Kent & Rosenbek, 1983). Of these apraxic subjects, four were relatively "pure" in that they had no concomitant language problems, save one who had anomia.

Procedures

The specific procedures used in this investigation have been described in detail by Moon, Zebrowski, Robin, and Folkins (1992). A summary follows.

Visual Feedback and Instructions. A horizontal bar (1.5 in. wide) was displayed on an oscilloscope screen as a target for tracking. The bar moved vertically up to 5 cm. Transduced articulator signals from either the lower lip, jaw, or fundamental frequency (F_o) of sustained phonation were displayed as a dot centered horizontally on the bar. Subjects were instructed to keep the dot on the target bar throughout the extent of the bar's vertical movement.

Lower lip and jaw movements were transduced using a standard strain-gauge cantilever system (Barlow, Cole, & Abbs, 1983; Muller & Abbs, 1979). Subjects were seated in a dental chair and their heads were immobilized using a wall-mounted cephalostat. The strain-gauge cantilevers were fixed to the lower lip and the underside of the jaw at the midline with pieces of double-sided tape. A bite block was used to stabilize the jaw during lower lip tracking.

Control of the laryngeal system was assessed by having subjects modulate the fundamental frequency (F_o) of sustained phonation. Each subject

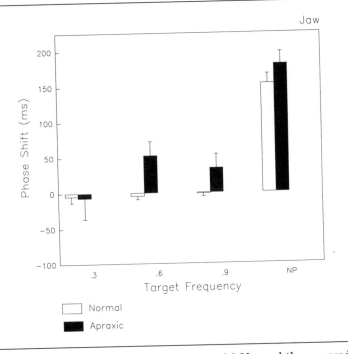

Figure 1. Phase shift in milliseconds for 0.3, 0.6, 0.9 Hz, and the nonpredictable signal for the jaw.

voiced a prolonged /a/, and the voice signal was transduced with a microphone, amplified, and input to a custom-built online F_o extraction module. This module produced an output voltage varying as a function of the F_o that was fed back to the subject.

Tasks. The range of target excursion for the lower lip and jaw was 10 mm. The strain-gauge offsets were adjusted for each subject so that the 10-mm target excursion occurred in the middle of the individual's maximum movement range. The range of target excursion for F_o tracking was 40 Hz. The output of the fundamental frequency extractor was offset so that the lower limit of the 40 Hz excursion was at a comfortable pitch set by the subject.

Four tracking conditions were employed for each articulator. These included sinusoids of 0.3, 0.6, and 0.9 Hz, which made up the predictable target, and a nonpredictable signal composed of ten equal amplitude frequencies ranging from 0.1 to 1.0 Hz in 0.1 Hz steps. Presentation order was counterbalanced.

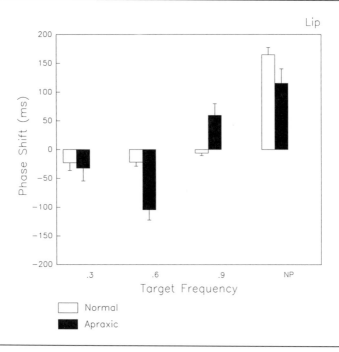

Figure 2. Phase shift in milliseconds for 0.3, 0.6, 0.9 Hz, and the nonpredictable signal for the lip.

Data analysis. Target and tracking signals were recorded using a Sony (PC-108) digital recorder and were subsequently digitized at 50 Hz for analysis. Within each condition, six 10-sec tracking blocks were extracted from the digitized signals for analysis. For the purposes of this preliminary report, only the best cross-correlation and phase shift were examined.

RESULTS

The first question addressed phase relationships between the target and tracking behavior. Figures 1, 2, and 3 show phase relationships for the apraxic and NBD groups for each tracking condition. Results are shown for each tracking frequency (0.3, 0.6, 0.9) and the nonpredictable condition. Negative phase values indicate phase lead and positive values indicate phase lag.

For the jaw (Figure 1), NBD speakers showed essentially no phase difference for the predictable targets (sinusoids). The apraxic trackers showed phase lag at 0.6 and 0.9 Hz. That means that for the faster sinu-

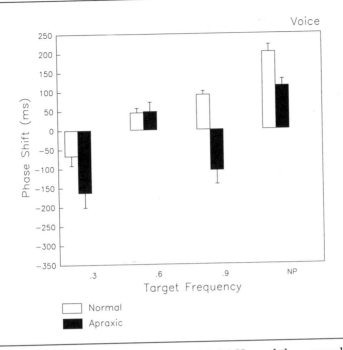

Figure 3. Phase shift in milliseconds for 0.3, 0.6, 0.9 Hz, and the nonpredictable signal for the voice.

soids, apraxic trackers were not anticipating the target motion. For the unpredictable signal, significant phase lag characterized both groups.

For the lip (Figure 2), the NBD trackers again demonstrated essentially no phase difference in all conditions. The apraxic trackers showed significant phase lead at 0.6 Hz and no difference at 0.3 Hz and 0.9 Hz. Both groups showed large phase lag for the unpredictable signal.

For voice tracking (Figure 3), significant phase advance at .3 Hz was present for both groups with no phase difference at 0.6 Hz and 0.9 Hz. Both groups showed phase lag for the nonpredictable signal, but apraxic trackers showed the most. Apraxic trackers found the voice-tracking task extremely difficult. No apraxic tracker completed all voice-tracking trials, whereas all normal speakers completed them.

In general, apraxic trackers did not always present the longest lag times. However, apraxic trackers were more often behind the target (phase lag) than were the NBD speakers. It is important to note that when only those phase relationships characterized by reasonable cross-correlations were examined, the apraxic trackers did not differ from the NBD trackers.

Tracking performance accuracy is displayed as cross-correlations between the target and the tracker's performance. When cross-correlations are

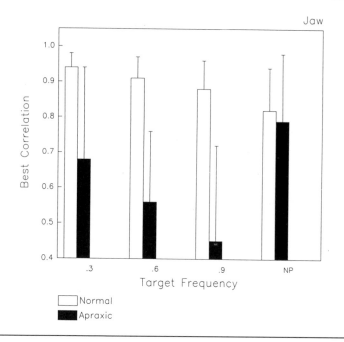

Figure 4. Best cross-correlation for 0.3, 0.6, 0.9 Hz, and the nonpredictable signal for the jaw.

low, however, phase relationships are difficult to interpret. Figure 4 shows best cross-correlation for both groups for jaw tracking. For both groups, jaw-tracking accuracy decreased across the predictable target signals, with the poorest performance at the fastest target speed, 0.9 Hz. Apraxic trackers' performances were poorer, and much more variable than NBD trackers'. However, apraxic trackers' performed best on the nonpredictable task whereas NBD trackers performed poorest on that task.

Lip tracking is shown in Figure 5. Again, tracking performance decreased across predictable target signals, with the poorest performance for both groups on the fastest signal. Apraxic trackers performed more poorly than NBD trackers. Again, apraxic trackers showed their best performance with the unpredictable signal, whereas NBD trackers showed their poorest performance on that trial.

For voice tracking, shown in Figure 6, a similar pattern of performance was obtained. Predictable tracking by both groups was poorest at the highest target speeds, with the apraxic trackers performing more poorly than NBD trackers for all speeds. However, for the nonpredictable signal the apraxic trackers showed their best performance and NBD trackers their poorest.

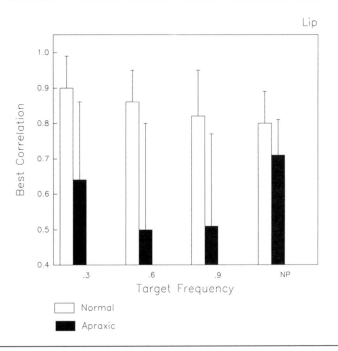

Figure 5. Best cross-correlation for 0.3, 0.6, 0.9 Hz, and the nonpredictable signal for the lip.

DISCUSSION

For the predictable tracking tasks, the apraxic trackers always performed more poorly than the NBD subjects. For the nonpredictable task, however, apraxic trackers demonstrated their best performance, which was nearly as good as the normal trackers'. In other words, the unpredictable tracking task brought out the best in the apraxic trackers. In addition to these quantitative differences, there also were qualitative differences between subject groups. Figure 7 contrasts the smooth versus jerky tracking performances of two subjects. The apraxic tracker's performance is shown in the lower graph, and a brain-damaged nonapraxic tracker's performance is shown in the upper one. The target is the smooth sine wave; the subject's performance is the waveform with noise components. The apraxic tracker's path was jerky, showing constant adjustment to error, whereas the nonapraxic tracker's path was smoother, showing an infrequent need to adjust the tracking path.

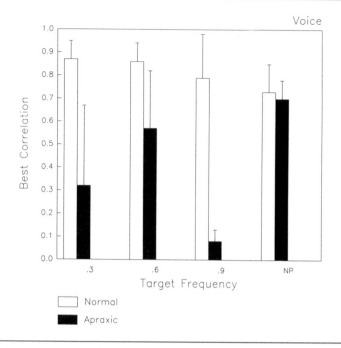

Figure 6. Best cross-correlation for 0.3, 0.6, 0.9 Hz, and the nonpredictable signal for the voice.

It is apparent from these data that there are no easy answers to help us understand the mechanisms underlying apraxia of speech. However, several points need to be made. First, these data support the notion that movement control for nonspeech tasks is impaired in apraxia of speech. Further, these impairments are discernible when only one articulatory system is being controlled (e.g., the lip). Second, as hypothesized by Robin et al. (1989), intraarticulator coordination was impaired, particularly for predictable signals. Third, we had hypothesized several possible outcomes of tracking performance, one of them being that a performance by apraxic trackers on the nonpredictable target superior to their performance on the predictable ones, would suggest that the apraxic speakers did not develop an accurate internal model of target motion. We also hypothesized that tracking performance for the predictable target would be jerky rather than smooth. Apraxic trackers performed exactly in these ways.

Because the apraxic trackers were poor predictors of the target movement, we propose that the apraxic speakers may have problems developing an internal model or plan of intended movement patterns. Several hypotheses concerning the nature of this planning problem are possible. First, apraxic trackers may be unable to develop a plan. However, this

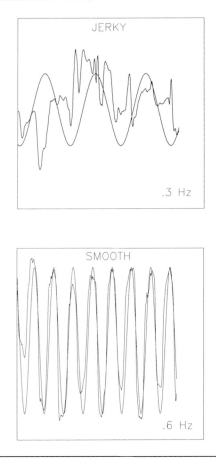

Figure 7. Tracking performance of two subjects (one apraxic speaker, AS, top, and one brain-damaged nonapraxic speaker, NAS, bottom) illustrating smooth and jerky tracking performance.

explanation may be obviated by the finding that their phase relationship to the target was not consistently behind the target. Again, we note the difficulty in interpreting phase relationships when the cross-correlation values are low. A second hypothesis would be that apraxic speakers develop a model of movement, but the model is inaccurate or poorly defined. Another potential explanation is that the apraxic speakers develop a plan, but the model occurs online and does not allow for prediction of the upcoming movements. Finally, it could be hypothesized that the movement model is in place, but the apraxic tracker has difficulty accessing the plan during online tasks. The results of this study do not allow us to address any of these possibilities, adequately. However, because the apraxic speakers performed as well as the normal speakers when tracking unpredictable targets, we suggest that apraxia of speech results from a breakdown at some level of the planning stage of movement rather than a breakdown in motor execution. Further studies will address each of these hypotheses to advance our understanding of oral motor tracking in apraxic and normal speakers.

REFERENCES

Barlow, S., Cole, K., Abbs, J. (1983). A new head-mounted lip-jaw movement transduction system for the study of motor speech disorders. *Journal of Speech and Hearing Research, 26*, 283–288.

Flowers, K. (1978). Some frequency response characteristics of parkinsonism on pursuit tracking. *Brain, 101*, 19–34.

Kent, R. D., & Rosenbek, J. C. (1983). Acoustic patterns of apraxia of speech. *Journal of Speech and Hearing Research, 26*, 231–249.

Luschei, E. S. (1991). Development of objective standards of nonspeech oral strength and performance: An advocate's view. In C. A. Moore, K. M. Yorkston, & D. Beukelman (Eds.), *Dysarthria and apraxia of speech: Perspectives on management* (pp. 3–14). Baltimore: Paul H. Brookes.

McClean, M., Beukelman, D., & Yorkston, K. (1978). Speech-muscle visuomotor tracking in dysarthric and nonimpaired speakers. *Journal of Speech and Hearing Research, 30*, 276–282.

McNeil, M. R., Weismer, G., Adams, S., & Mulligan, M. (1990). Oral structure nonspeech motor control in normal, dysarthric, aphasic, and apraxic speakers: Isometric force and static position control. *Journal of Speech and Hearing Research, 33*, 255–268.

Moon, J. B., Zebrowski, P., Robin, D. A., & Folkins, J. W. (1992). Visuomotor tracking ability of young adult speakers.

Muller, E., & Abbs, J. (1979). Strain gauge transduction of lip and jaw motion in the midsagittal plane: Refinement of a prototype system. *Journal of the Acoustical Society of America, 65*, 481–486.

Noble, M., Fitts, P., & Warren, C. (1955). The frequency response of skilled subjects in a pursuit tracking task. *Journal of Experimental Psychology, 4*, 249–256.

Robin, D. A. (1992). Developmental apraxia of speech: Just another motor problem. *American Journal of Speech-Language Pathology: A Journal of Clinical Practice, 1*, 19–22.

Robin, D. A., Bean, C., & Folkins, J. W. (1989). Lip movement in apraxia of speech. *Journal of Speech and Hearing Research, 32*, 512–523.

Weismer, G., & Liss, J. (1991). Reductionism is a dead-end in speech research: Perspectives on a new direction. In C. A. Moore, K. M. Yorkston, & D. Beukelman (Eds.), *Dysarthria and apraxia of speech: Perspectives on management* (pp. 15–28). Baltimore: Paul H. Brookes.

Clinical Aphasiology, Vol. 22, 1994, pp. 231–243

Treatment for Acquired Apraxia of Speech: A Review of Efficacy Reports

Julie L. Wambaugh and Patrick J. Doyle

There have been numerous reports on a wide array of strategies used to treat acquired apraxia of speech (Dabul & Bollier, 1976; Deal & Florance, 1978; Dworkin, Abkarian, & Johns, 1988; Raymer & Thompson, 1991; Rubow, Rosenbek, Collins, & Longstreth, 1982). The purpose of this paper was to review treatment investigations that have been reported over the past twenty years.

The following journals and published proceedings were searched from 1972 (or from the first volume) through 1991: *Archives of Physical Medicine and Rehabilitation, Brain and Language, Clinical Aphasiology, Cortex, Journal of Communication Disorders, Journal of Speech and Hearing Disorders,* and *Journal of Speech and Hearing Research.* Reports cited in studies from these sources and those included in texts on apraxia of speech, were also considered for potential inclusion in the review.

Following identification of treatment reports, two basic inclusion criteria were employed: (a) the investigators had to specify that the treatment was for acquired apraxia of speech or that the impact of treatment on apraxia of speech was being measured, and (b) data from at least one subject had to be presented.

A total of 28 treatment reports met inclusion requirements for this review and are summarized in Table 1. In two cases, the same treatment investigation had been reported in an earlier publication with only slightly different information (Square-Storer & Hayden, 1989; Stevens, 1989); for the purposes of this review, the overlapping reports were treated as a single report.

All reports were compared on a number of variables related to subject description, methodologic information, and treatment efficacy. Suggestions for procedural changes in future research are provided.

Table 1. Investigations of Treatment of Apraxia of Speech

Author(s)	Number of Subjects	Severity of Apraxia	Type of Aphasia	Months Post Onset	Design	Behaviors Measured
Dabul and Bollier 1976	2	Not described	PICA %:[a] S1:75th S2:70th	S1:192 S2:108	Uncontrolled case studies	Unclear; or reading or word repetition
Deal and Florance 1978	4	Severe	Unclear	S1:17 S2:14 S3:1 wk. S4:12	Uncontrolled case studies	Production simple sentences
Dowden, Marshall, and Tompkins 1981	2	Both severe	S1:severe S2:mod.– severe	S1:216 S2:14	Case studies with repeated measures	PICA score production gestures du ing CADL[b] and in response to pictures
Dworkin, Abkarian, and Johns 1988	1	Moderate	None (some anomia noted)	16	Multiple probe	Nonspeech oromotor movements articulation alternate motions; multisyllab words and sentences
Florance, Rabidoux, and McCauslin 1980	3	S1:unclear S2:severe S3:severe	S1:none S2:nonfluent S3:fluent	5–6	Uncontrolled case studies	MLU[c] in spontaneou utterances; communica tive success unclear
Holtzapple and Mar-shall 1977	1	Unclear	Present, but type unclear	3	Uncontrolled case study	Production of error phonemes
Keith and Aronson 1975	1	Severe	Severe	1	Uncontrolled case study	PICA[a] scor
Lane and Samples 1981	4	All severe	All moderate	S1:42 S2:96 S3:3 S4:48	Uncontrolled case studies	Pointing to symbol anc naming symbol

Treatment Methods	Response General- ization	Stimulus General- ization	Results	Relia- bility Data	Speech Analysis Procedures	Maintenance
Combination of sound place- ment, sound drill, and graphic stimulation	Not reported	Not reported	Positive results reported	No	Not described	Unclear if measured
Flexible treat- ment hierarchy combined with home programs	Not reported	Not reported	Positive results reported	No	Clinician judgement of overall utterance intelligibility	Not reported
Hierarchy: Object manipu- lation, imita- tion, graphic and auditory stimulation	To untrained gestures	Not reported	No significant increase in PICA[a] scores	No	N/A	Received additional treatment dur- ing "mainte- nance" phase– positive results
Metronome pacing accom- panying drill of all behaviors	Mea- sured, but unclear	To con- textual speech	Positive	Yes	Accept- able/ unaccept- able ratings	Yes; of previ- ously trained behaviors during subse- quent training
Significant others trained in interviewing techniques; training in self- regulation	Not reported	Anecdotal	Dramatic increases in MLU[c]	No	Unclear	Not reported
Multiphonemic rtic. therapy: visual, audi- ory; Phonetic lacement –undefined other" treatment)	Not reported	Not reported	Positive	No	Unclear	Not reported
inging	Not reported	Not reported	Positive	No	N/A	Not reported
issymbol aining	Not reported	Not reported	Positive for 3 of 4	No	Unclear	No

(Continued)

Table 1. (continued)

Author(s)	Number of Subjects	Severity of Apraxia	Type of Aphasia	Months Post Onset	Design	Behaviors Measured
LaPointe 1984	1	Initially severe	Nonfluent	3	Multiple baseline across behaviors	Single word naming
McNeil, Prescott, and Lemme 1976	4, 1 not apraxic	2 moderate, 1 mild	Unclear; PICA %:[a] 58–98th	10–71	Small group	PICA[a] scores, RTT[d] scores, Standard speech samp
Rabidoux, Florance, and McCauslin 1980	3	Severe	Minimal to severe	4+	Uncontrolled case studies	MLU;[c] communicative success (unclear)
Raymer and Thompson 1991	1	Severe	Severe Broca's	10	Multiple baseline across behaviors	/s,f,t,l/ in words
Rosenbek et al. 1973	3	Moderate	Present (type unclear)	12+	Uncontrolled case studies	5 utterances (1–7 words)
Rubow, Rosenbek, Collins, and Longstreth 1982	1	Moderate	Mild-Moderate (not agrammatic)	14	Modified ATD[e]	A = plosive words, B = fricative words
Simmons 1978	1	Marked	PICA %:[a] 37th (at 3mpo.)	14	Uncontrolled case study	Performance on PICA[a]
Simmons 1980	1	Moderate	Nonfluent with agrammatism; PICA %:[a] 51st	8+	ABCBCA[g]	Sentence formulation
Skelly et al. 1974	6	All severe	2 with 4 without	S1:24 S2, S3:36, S4 S6:36, S5:1	Uncontrolled case study	PICA[a] scores
Southwood 1987	2	S1-mild S2-moderate	Some residual not agrammatic	Both 6	Withdrawal, changing criterion	Articulation in oral reading; rate in oral reading

Treatment Methods	Response Generalization	Stimulus Generalization	Results	Reliability Data	Speech Analysis Procedures	Maintenance
Package: modeling, integral stim., phonetic placement, multiple repetitions	Limited	Not reported	Positive	Yes	Plus/minus based on all phonemes	Positive for previously trained set 1; during training of set 2
Electromyographic biofeedback (re: tension)	N/A	N/A	Significant increases in PICA[a] gestural and verbal and RTT[d]	Yes	Qualitative	Not reported
Use of Handi Voice	Not reported	Anecdotal	Positive results for all subjects	No	N/A	Not reported
Verbal plus gestural	Limited to repetition	To oral-reading, naming, and repetition	Improvement limited to repetition	Yes	10-point scale	Measured during treatment of subsequent sounds
4-step continuum modeling, integral stim., graphic stim.	Not reported	Not reported	Positive	No	Modified PICA[a]	Not reported
A =imitation B = imitation + vibrotactile stress/rhythm	Not reported	Not reported	Pre-, posttreatment scores only positive results	Yes	16 point rating of entire word	Not reported
Finger counting combined with graphic cues in sentence production	Not reported	Not reported	Increased PICA[a] scores and positive anecdotal reports	No	N/A	Not reported
Hierarchy: unison production, repetition, responding to questions, use of braille	Not reported	Not reported	Positive acquisition results stronger when braille included in treatment	No	PICA 15 point scoring system	Positive in final A phase
AMERIND paired with speech	Not reported	Not reported	Positive for verbalizations and sign use	No	N/A	Not reported
Prolonging rate and reducing rate during reading	Not reported	To one-minute monologues, minimal	Decreased rate and articulation errors; no generalization	Yes	On-line error frequency counts	Not reported

(Continued)

Table 1. (continued)

Author(s)	Number of Subjects	Severity of Apraxia	Type of Aphasia	Months Post Onset	Design	Behaviors Measured
Square, Chumpelik, and Adams 1985 (abstract)	1	Severe	Moderate Broca's aphasia	Probably "chronic"	Uncontrolled case study	Phrases and minimal pai of words
Square, Chumpelik, Morningstar, and Adams 1986 and Square-Storer and Hayden 1989	3	All severe	All Broca's WAB[f] AQ: 23.2–52.8	All at least 12	Uncontrolled case studies	Minimally contrastive phonemes: polysyllabic words; func tional phras
Stevens, E. R. 1989 and Stevens, E. 1986	10	Severe	Unclear	At least 6	2 group comparison and case studies	Verbal pro- duction dur ing a variety of activities one total sco
Stevens and Glaser 1983	5	All severe	Severe to mild- moderate	2–36	Uncontrolled case studies	Verbal expre sion (unclea
Thompson and Young 1983	1	Moderate	Mild Broca's	4	Multiple baseline across behaviors	/s,r,l/-cluste and /o/ in words
Warren 1977	5	Unclear	All mode- rate Broca's	S1:16, S2:65, S3:10, S4:67, S5:26	Modified ATD[e]	Production (bisyllabic nouns
Wertz 1984	19:Apraxia of speech 10:possible AOS	Varied	Varied	1	Retrospec- tive 2 groups 2 treatments	Ratings of severity of apraxia
Wertz et al. 1984	Report several single-case experiments illustrating various approaches to treatmen reports are somewhat brief, but appear to be experimentally sound; replications lackin					

Note: PICA = *Porch Index of Communicative Ability*   ATD = Alternate Treatment Desig
  CADL = *Communicative Abilities of Daily Living*   WAB = *Western Aphasia Battery*
  RTT = *Revised Token Test*   AOS = Aphasia of Speech

...atment ...thods	Response General- ization	Stimulus General- ization	Results	Relia- bility Data	Speech Analysis Procedures	Maintenance
...MPT ...tem and ...gral ...ulation	Not reported	Not reported	Positive results reported	No	Not described	Measured over 5 mo. period declining per- formance noted
...MPT ...okinesthetic ...ulation ...h some rate ...trol	To untrained exemplars	Not reported	Positive acqui- sition results; minimal gen- eralization results	Yes	Correct/ incorrect for entire word or sound pair and 3-pt. scoring (1989 report)	Not reported
...up 1: multi- ...input phon. ...apy (deri- ...on of new ...ds from stereo- ...es); Group 2: ...efined tradi- ...al therapy	Not reported	Not reported	Positive increases reported for multiple input phon. therapy but not tradi- tional; results unclear	No	Not reported	Not reported
...ivation of ...words ...n stereo- ...d utter- ...es; unclear	Not reported	Not reported	Anecdotal positive results reported	No	Not reported	Not reported
...deling, imi- ...on, use of ...usive schwa	Limited within class; neg- ligible across class	Not reported	Positive acqui- sition; limited generalization	Yes	Plus/minus based on target phoneme	Measured during treat- ment of sub- sequent sounds
...imitation ...rehearsal	Not reported	Not reported	Positive; no real difference between con- ditions	Yes	Phonetic transcrip- tion	Yes
...undefined ...itional ...general ...uage ...ulation	Not reported	Not reported	Positive for group A sub- jects only	Yes	Rating on 7 point scale based on 3–5 minute conversation	Not reported

SUMMARY OF REPORTS

Subject Description

The number of subjects studied in each investigation ranged from 1 to 19, with the modal number being 1 (40% of the reports). The number of apraxic subjects studied across all reports was 84.

The severity of the apraxia of speech was indicated for 56 of the 84 subjects (67%). Of those 56 subjects, 84% had marked/severe apraxia, 12.5% had moderate apraxia, and 3.5% had mild apraxia.

The majority of the subjects were chronic apraxic speakers, with 52 of the 84 subjects (62%) being 6 months postonset (MPO) or greater. Of those 52 subjects, 32 were at least 12 MPO. Of the remaining 32 subjects who were less than 6 MPO, 23 were less than 3 MPO.

All but 6 of the subjects were reported to have some degree of aphasia. The amount of information provided regarding co-occurring aphasia varied across studies, but in general it was quite limited.

Suggestions for describing subjects with adult neurogenic disorders have been offered by Brookshire (1983) and Tompkins, Jackson, and Schulz (1990). In reviewing this group of apraxia treatment studies, it was found that the majority of investigators had reported information on subjects' age, gender, MPO, and etiology, as suggested by Brookshire. However, other characteristics that Brookshire suggested be reported, such as education, handedness, and source of referral, were most often not included in these investigations.

Tompkins et al.'s (1990) more recent suggestions of including measures of subjects' nonchronological age, estimated premorbid intelligence, auditory processing, personality or additudinal factors, and social support have not been included in apraxia treatment reports. Clearly, these subject characteristics may influence response to treatment and should be considered in future research.

Additionally, in light of the evolving picture we have of apraxia of speech (AOS) (Odell, McNeil, Rosenbek, & Hunter, 1990; Square-Storer & Apeldoorn, 1991), it is important to provide more information specific to apraxic subjects' diagnoses, overall severity, speech output, and aphasic impairments. Specifically, the criteria used in making the diagnosis of AOS should be reported, as should the background and experience of the diagnosticians. Because some cases of AOS may be particularly difficult to diagnose, consensus diagnosis should be employed when possible.

The procedures used to determine AOS severity ratings should be described in sufficient detail to allow for replication and comparisons across studies. Because speech production skills vary considerably across apraxic speakers, investigators should provide a summary sound error analysis based on narrow phonetic transcription, along with basic temporal measures of speech production (e.g., speaking rate, sound/word durations).

Finally, because AOS is frequently accompanied by aphasia, a thorough description of apraxic subjects' language skills should be provided. This should include standardized aphasia subtest scores, measures of auditory processing, and data regarding mean length and complexity of subjects' spoken utterances.

Methodologic Information

In terms of methodologic issues, we examined (a) type of experimental design, (b) description of dependent measures, (c) method of speech/communication analysis, (d) description of treatment, and (e) reports of reliability measures.

Fifty-six percent of the treatment reports were uncontrolled case studies. However, several single-subject experimental designs were employed, including a multiple probe design, three multiple baseline designs, two modified alternating treatments designs, and two reversal designs. In addition, three group designs were used.

Dependent measures varied across investigations and often were not operationally defined. They included measures of mean length of utterance, communicative success, production of error sounds, production of word/phrases/sentences, rate of nonspeech movements, gestures, and standard test scores. The most frequently measured behaviors were productions of whole words and utterances (40% of all measured behaviors).

The manner in which speech production was analyzed was difficult to determine in most cases and could not be determined for 36% of the reports. Twenty percent of the investigations employed correct/incorrect scoring of sounds or entire utterances, 12% used scaled scoring, another 12% employed nonspecific subjective ratings of the *adequacy* of productions, and 4% used error frequency counts. The remaining 16% of the reports measured behaviors inappropriate for speech analysis (e.g., gesturing).

Intervention programs also varied across studies. Most investigators used some type of treatment package or hierarchy. One of three basic approaches appeared to underlie most techniques: (a) improving speech production itself through direct means (e.g., imitation, integral stimulation, or multiple repetitions); (b) reorganizing speech indirectly through relatively intact nonspeech systems (e.g., singing, vibrotactile stimulation, or gesturing); or (c) training an alternate/augmentative system of communication. Treatments often appeared to be specifically tailored to meet an individual subject's needs, which accords with the large number of single-subject reports.

Reliability data of any kind were reported for only 60% of the investigations.

The methodologic issues that should be addressed in future AOS treatment research center on the concerns of internal and external validity, procedural replicability, and reliability.

In examining the types of experimental designs employed, it was apparent that a lack of design was the most common. However, because this review covered 20 years of research, this predominance of case studies was not surprising. The more recent reports of AOS treatment have used some type of controlled experimental design, so that internal validity concerns pertain primarily to the older reports.

However, even with the more recent studies, direct and systematic replications have been lacking; such replications are necessary to "establish the reliability of previous findings" and to "determine the generality of findings" (Barlow & Hersen, 1984, p. 325). As indicated previously, many AOS treatments appeared to be designed specifically for an individual subject. This may be why many investigators have not attempted to replicate their findings. However, although direct replications may not always be possible with AOS subjects, systematic replications should be attempted.

An important consideration in this regard has to do with the description of treatment techniques. Most of the reviewed reports did not provide enough detail about their treatment procedures for other researchers to attempt replications. Dworkin, Abkarian, and Johns (1988) suggested that treatment descriptions specify (a) the nature of the task, (b) the type and sequences of the steps in treatment, (c) the criterion for progression in treatment, and (d) the number of trials and the time required to complete intermediate goals.

Similarly, detailed descriptions of dependent measures were frequently lacking in the reports we reviewed and are equally important for purposes of replication. Operational definitions should specify (a) the behaviors being measured, (b) the specific conditions under which measurements were obtained, and (c) any instrumentation employed.

With respect to reliability, reports should include descriptions of who performed the measures, how reliability was calculated, and any reliability training that was involved. It is suggested that at least three basic types of reliability data be reported in future AOS treatment research: (a) reliability of scoring of the dependent measures, (b) reliability of administration of the treatment (particularly when treatment hierarchies are employed), and (c) reliability of phonetic or orthographic transcription.

Treatment Efficacy

Almost all the reviewed studies reported positive results. However, claims that treatment resulted in improved performance were often unsubstantiated because of lack of experimental control, as evidenced by the large percentage of uncontrolled case studies.

Measures of generalization and maintenance of treatment effects were usually not reported. Response generalization (to untrained exemplars of trained behaviors) was reported in only 24% of the studies and was limited in most cases. Stimulus generalization (to other measurement conditions) was reported in only 12% of the investigations and was also limited.

Maintenance measures were reported in 32% of the studies. In six reports, maintenance of a previously trained behavior was measured during subsequent training of another behavior. In only two reports was maintenance measured at time intervals following cessation of all treatment. Findings of maintenance effects were varied.

Social validation findings were not included in any of the reports.

Future AOS treatment research should include measures of generalization, maintenance, and social validity to further our understanding of the full impact of treatment on subjects' communication skills.

SUMMARY

A wide variety of interesting and apparently promising treatments have been reported for AOS. Unfortunately, basic methodologic problems were frequently encountered in this review of the literature, thus limiting our confidence in reported findings. Inroads have been made in more recent years with regard to design and generalization issues (LaPointe, 1984; Raymer & Thompson, 1991, Wertz, LaPointe, & Rosenbek, 1984). Future AOS treatment research should include more comprehensive descriptions of subjects and treatment procedures, and promising findings should be replicated across subjects and research sites.

ACKNOWLEDGMENTS

Preparation of this article was supported by the Department of Veterans Affairs, Rehabilitation, Research and Development Grant C69-2RA, awarded to the Highland Drive VA Medical Center, Pittsburgh, Pennsylvania.

We gratefully acknowledge the assistance of Karen Oleyar in the preparation of the summary table.

REFERENCES

Barlow, D. H., & Hersen, M. (Eds.). (1984). *Single case experimental designs: Strategies for studying behavior change.* New York: Pergamon.

Brookshire, R. H. (1983). Subject description and generality of results in experiments with aphasic adults. *Journal of Speech and Hearing Disorders, 48,* 342–346.

Dabul, B., & Bollier, B. (1976). Therapeutic approaches to apraxia. *Journal of Speech and Hearing Disorders, 41,* 268–276.

Deal, J. L., & Florance, C. L. (1978). Modification of the eight-step continuum for treatment of apraxia of speech in adults. *Journal of Speech and Hearing Disorders, 43,* 89–95.

Dowden, P. A., Marshall, R. C., & Tompkins, C. A. (1981). Amer-Ind sign as a communicative facilitator for aphasic and apraxic patients. In R. H. Brookshire (Ed.), *Clinical Aphasiology Conference proceedings* (pp. 133–140). Minneapolis: BRK.

Dworkin, J. P., Abkarian, G. G., & Johns, D. F. (1988). Apraxia of speech: The effectiveness of a treatment regime. *Journal of Speech and Hearing Disorders, 53,* 280–294.

Florance, C. L., Rabidoux, P. L., & McCauslin, L. S. (1980). An environmental manipulation approach to treating apraxia of speech. In R. H. Brookshire (Ed.), *Clinical Aphasiology Conference proceedings* (pp. 285–293). Minneapolis: BRK.

Holtzapple, P., & Marshall, N. (1977). The application of multiphonemic articulation therapy with apraxic patients. In R. H. Brookshire (Ed.), *Clinical Aphasiology Conference proceedings* (pp. 46–58). Minneapolis: BRK.

Keith, R. L., & Aronson, A. E. (1975). Singing as therapy for apraxia of speech and aphasia: Report of a case. *Brain and Language, 2,* 483–488.

Lane, V. W., & Samples, J. M. (1981). Facilitating communication skills in adult apraxics: Application of blissymbols in a group setting. *Journal of Communication Disorders, 14,* 157–167.

LaPointe, L. L. (1984). Sequential treatment of split lists: A case report. In J. Rosenbek, M. McNeil, & A. Aronson (Eds.), *Apraxia of speech: Physiology, acoustics, linguistics, management* (pp. 277–286). San Diego: College-Hill.

McNeil, M. R., Prescott, T. E., & Lemme, M. L. (1976). An application of electromyographic biofeedback to aphasia/apraxia treatment. In R. H. Brookshire (Ed.), *Clinical Aphasiology Conference proceedings* (pp. 151–171). Minneapolis: BRK.

Odell, K., McNeil, M. R., Rosenbek, J. C., & Hunter, L. (1990). Perceptual characteristics of consonant production by apraxic speakers. *Journal of Speech and Hearing Disorders, 55,* 345–359.

Rabidoux, P., Florance, C., & McCauslin, L. (1980). The use of a Handi Voice in the treatment of a severely apractic nonverbal patient. In R. H. Brookshire (Ed.), *Clinical Aphasiology Conference proceedings* (pp. 294–301). Minneapolis: BRK.

Raymer, A. M., & Thompson, C. K. (1991). Effects of verbal plus gestural treatment in a patient with aphasia and severe apraxia of speech. In T. E. Prescott (Ed.), *Clinical aphasiology,* Vol. 20 (pp. 285–298). Austin, TX: PRO-ED.

Rosenbek, J. C., Lemme, M. L., Ahern, M. B., Harris, E. H., & Wertz, R. T. (1973). A treatment for apraxia of speech in adults. *Journal of Speech and Hearing Disorders, 38,* 462–472.

Rubow, R. T., Rosenbek J. C., Collins, M. J., & Longstreth, D. (1982). Vibrotactile stimulation for intersystemic reorganization in the treatment of apraxia of speech. *Archives of Physical Medicine Rehabilitation, 63*, 150–153.

Simmons, N. N. (1978). Finger counting as an intersystemic reorganizer in apraxia of speech. In R. H. Brookshire (Ed.), *Clinical Aphasiology Conference proceedings* (pp. 174–179). Minneapolis: BRK.

Simmons, N. N. (1980). Choice of stimulus modes in treating apraxia of speech: A case study. In R. H. Brookshire (Ed.), *Clinical Aphasiology Conference proceedings* (pp. 302–307). Minneapolis: BRK.

Skelly, M., Schinsky, L., Smith, R. W., & Fust, R. S. (1974). American Indian Sign (AMERIND) as a facilitation of verbalization for the oral verbal apraxic. *Journal of Speech and Hearing Disorders, 39*, 445–456.

Southwood, H. (1987). The use of prolonged speech in the treatment of apraxia of speech. In R. H. Brookshire (Ed.), *Clinical Aphasiology Conference proceedings* (pp. 277–287). Minneapolis: BRK.

Square, P. A., Chumpelik, D., & Adams, S. (1985). Efficacy of the PROMPT system of therapy for the treatment of acquired apraxia of speech. In R. H. Brookshire (Ed.), *Clinical Aphasiology Conference proceedings* (pp. 319–320). Minneapolis: BRK.

Square, P. A., Chumpelik, D. A., Morningstar, D., & Adams, S. (1986). Efficacy of the PROMPT system for the treatment of acquired apraxia of speech: A follow-up investigation. In R. H. Brookshire (Ed.), *Clinical Aphasiology Conference proceedings* (pp. 221–226). Minneapolis: BRK.

Square-Storer, P., & Hayden, D. C. (1989). PROMPT treatment. In P. Square-Storer (Ed.), *Acquired apraxia of speech in aphasic adults* (pp. 190–219). Hove and London: Lawrence Erlbaum.

Square-Storer, P. A., & Apeldoorn, S. (1991). An acoustic study of apraxia of speech in patients with different lesion loci. In C. Moore, K. M. Yorkston, and D. R. Beukelman (Eds.), *Dysarthria and apraxia of speech: Perspectives on management* (pp. 271–288). Baltimore: Paul H. Brooks.

Stevens, E. (1986). Efficacy of multiple input phoneme therapy in the treatment of severe expressive aphasia. *Journal of Rehabilitation Research and Development—Rehabilitation R & D Progress Reports, 24*, 338.

Stevens, E. R. (1989). Multiple input phoneme therapy. In P. Square-Storer (Ed.), *Acquired apraxia of speech in aphasic adults* (pp. 220–238). Hove and London: Lawrence Erlbaum.

Stevens, E., & Glaser, L. (1983). Multiple input phoneme therapy: An approach to severe apraxia and expressive aphasia. In R. H. Brookshire (Ed.), *Clinical Aphasiology Conference proceedings* (pp. 148–155). Minneapolis: BRK.

Thompson, C. K., & Young, E. C. (1983). A phonological process approach to apraxia of speech: An experimental analysis of cluster reduction. Paper presented at the meeting of the American Speech and Hearing Association, Cincinnati, Ohio.

Tompkins, C. A., Jackson, S. T., & Schulz, R. (1990). On prognostic research in adult neurologic disorders. *Journal of Speech and Hearing Research, 33*, 398–401.

Warren, R. L. (1977). Rehearsal for naming in apraxia of speech. In R. H. Brookshire (Ed.), *Clinical Aphasiology Conference proceedings* (pp. 80–90). Minneapolis: BRK.

Wertz, R. T. (1984). Response to treatment in patients with apraxia of speech. In J. Rosenbek, M. McNeil, & A. Aronson (Eds.), *Apraxia of speech: Physiology, acoustics, linguistics, management* (pp. 257–276). San Diego: College Hill.

Wertz, R. T., LaPointe, L. L., & Rosenbek, J. C. (1984). *Apraxia of speech in adults: The disorder and its management.* Orlando, FL: Grune & Stratton.

Clinical Aphasiology, Vol. 22, 1994, pp. 245–256

Feature Analysis for Treatment of Communication Disorders in Traumatically Brain-Injured Patients: An Efficacy Study

Maryellen Massaro and Connie A. Tompkins

According to Szekeres, Ylvisaker, and Cohen (1987), disturbances in organization interfere with extensive searches of the knowledge base after traumatic brain injury and, therefore, compound retrieval problems. Feature Analysis (Szekeres et al., 1987) is a protocol designed to promote organization of verbal output and increase the amount of information retrieved.

The Feature Analysis treatment (see Appendix A) involves considering any familiar concept and describing it in terms of six predefined descriptors (Group, Action, Use, Location, Properties, and Associations). Patients are taught to use the procedure as a strategy for facilitating the retrieval of additional information about a concept. Feature Analysis is based on a semantic network theory of storage and retrieval (Anderson, 1983). Prior to this study, the program had not been operationally specified, and its efficacy had not been established.

This investigation was designed to develop a systematic protocol for Feature Analysis training and to determine its efficacy in treating communication disorders of two patients with traumatic brain injury.

METHOD

Subjects

Subject 1 was a 24-year-old male, 5 years post injury, with 14 years of premorbid education. Subject 2 was a 28-year-old female, 12 years post injury, with 11 years of premorbid education. Both were diagnosed as sustaining severe traumatic brain injury, the result of a fall and of a motor vehicle accident, respectively. Spoken output was telegraphic in nature and resembled that of Broca's aphasia. Details regarding selected clinical characteristics appear in Appendix B (see Massaro, 1991, for specific inclusion criteria).

Stimuli

Subjects ranked various topics for interest and knowledge, and those rated high across both dimensions were used for training. Three superordinate categories (e.g., Animals) with six subtopics each (e.g., Dogs) were identified for each subject. Topics were arranged in pairs according to their semantic features. One member of each pair was randomly selected as a training topic, and the other served as a generalization topic (see Table 1).

Table 1. Training and Generalization Stimuli

Superordinate	Training	Generalization
Subject 1		
Animal	Rabbit	Hamster
	Turtle	Fish
	Cat	Dog
Exercise	Jogging	Walking
	Swimming	Yoga
	Aerobics	Dancing
Leisure	Reading	Photography
	Picnicking	Dining
	Concerts	Movies
Subject 2		
Animal	Rabbit	Hamster
	Cat	Dog
	Turtle	Fish
Leisure	Picnicking	Dining
	Concerts	Movies
	Shopping	Dancing
Sports	Hockey	Baseball
	Soccer	Football
	Golf	Tennis

Experimental Design

A multiple baseline design across superordinate categories was used. Responses were analyzed for number of semantic features listed and number of semantic descriptors accessed per topic. Probe data were collected in an identical fashion across baseline, training, and maintenance phases (see Massaro, 1991, for probe schedule). The subjects were asked to state all they knew about the topic presented. Two trials were always given: an unstructured trial followed by a structured trial in which a blank Feature Analysis format was provided.

Stimulus Generalization

To assess stimulus generalization, each subject was probed with two unfamiliar listeners (one male, one female, both about 50 years of age) on two separate occasions prior to baseline. On each occasion, one unfamiliar listener introduced a training topic from the superordinate ranked as highest interest and knowledge, and the other unfamiliar listener introduced a generalization topic from the same superordinate. The subjects were asked to state all they knew about each topic. This same procedure was repeated with the same unfamiliar listeners immediately after training. Two weeks after training ended, the subjects were probed with the same topics by their speech-language pathologist, a familiar listener who was unaffiliated with the Feature Analysis training.

Training Procedures

Each of the three training topics for a given superordinate category was trained each session. If cuing was necessary to elicit appropriate responses, cues were systematically provided (see Table 2 for hierarchy). Cues were given after a 15-second delay, requests for help, rejection of the task, or incorrect responses. Training proceeded until all six semantic descriptors were accessed or the complete set of cues was presented without success.

During the final three training sessions, the Feature Analysis chart was shrunk to credit card size to promote compensatory use of Feature Analysis as a self-cuing system.

Social Validation

To determine whether persons unfamiliar with the subjects and the targeted behaviors could detect changes in verbal output, four speech-language

Table 2. Cuing Hierarchy With Example Cues for Target Response

Cue Type	Example
Redefinition of category	The location is where the movie is found.
Sentence completion	You watch the movie in the . . . .
Writing initial letter	t . . .
Producing initial phoneme	/th/ . . .
Binary choice question	Is it a theater or a stadium?
Yes/no question	Is it a theater?
Requesting imitation	Say, "Theater"

Note: Target response = *theater,* in the descriptive category *Location,* under the topic *Movie.*

pathologists listened to tape-recorded samples of the subjects' performances. Samples were randomly selected from structured trials within the baseline and maintenance conditions for each subject. Judges rated the samples along the dimensions of organization, cohesion, and completeness, using the following operational definitions: *organization*—the sample has an inherent structure (a beginning, middle, and ending); *cohesion*—each individual unit of the sample has a relationship to other units; *completeness*—the topic is discussed in full detail. A direct magnitude estimation procedure was employed (Campbell & Dollaghan, 1992).

RESULTS

Training Data

Table 3 summarizes the number of cues used during training. As training progressed, the amount of cuing decreased for both subjects, but Subject 2 required more cues per trial than Subject 1.

Treatment Effects

Probe data for mean number of features listed by each subject are presented in Figures 1 and 2. Results are not provided for number of descriptors accessed because the trends are identical (see Massaro, 1991).

Data for training and generalization topics were collapsed for baseline and training conditions, because the number of probes per session was not the same for each type of topic and the data could not be converted to

Table 3. Summary of Cues Used During Training

Subject 1		Subject 2	
Session	No. of Cues	Session	No. of Cues
Exercise		Animals	
1	27	1	21
2	14	2	14
3	11	3	13
4	0	4	9
5	3	5	8
6	3	6	9
7	1	7	7
8	3	8	5
9	0	9	8
Animals		Leisure	
10	8	10	17
11	2	11	17
12	5	12	7
13	1	13	8
14	0	14	5
15	0	15	5
Leisure		Sports	
16	4	16	12
17	3	17	6
18	1	18	7
19[a]	2	19[a]	3
20[a]	2	20[a]	4
21[a]	0	21[a]	1
Total	90	Total	186

[a]Denotes sessions in which prosthesis-sized Feature Analysis chart was used for training.

a common scale. However, performance was highly similar across training and generalization topics. Training and generalization data are graphed separately for maintenance probes because the number of trials per session was the same for each type of topic.

As indicated in Figure 1, Subject 1 displayed variable performance during baseline. The rising baseline is dramatic for Superordinate 2 (Animals), suggesting a possible loss of experimental control. If this were the case, however, we would predict an even more dramatic pattern during baseline for Superordinate 3, which did not occur.

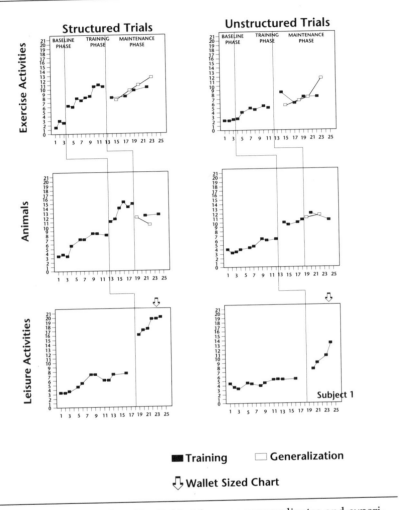

Figure 1. Mean features listed by Subject 1 across superordinates and experimental phases.

Treatment effects were demonstrated during the training phases. Subject 1 performed optimally on structured trials during training and maintained performance at levels comparable to or greater than training. As the open boxes show, response generalization to untrained topics was achieved.

Figure 2 shows that Subject 2's baseline performance was more stable. Treatment effects were demonstrated, and Subject 2 also performed optimally on structured trials during training. Subject 2's performance decreased during maintenance yet remained above baseline levels. Again, response generalization was achieved.

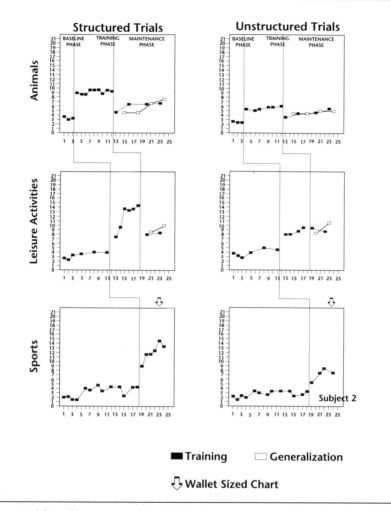

Figure 2. Mean features listed by Subject 2 across superordinates and experimental phases.

Stimulus Generalization

Although both subjects demonstrated generalization to untrained topics, neither made notable improvement from before to after therapy with unfamiliar listeners (see Table 4). Subject 1's performance improved with his speech-language pathologist, who is a familiar listener. No notable change occurred for either subject when the miniaturized Feature Analysis chart was provided as a self-cue.

Table 4. Summary of Conversational Generalization Measurements

Measurement	Total No. of Features	
	Subject 1	Subject 2
Pretherapy probes (unfamiliar listener)[a]	2.5	2.0
Posttherapy probes (unfamiliar listener)[a]	2.8	3.5
Follow-up with speech-language pathologist (unstructured trials)[b]	8.0	5.5
Follow-up with speech-language pathologist (structured trials—prosthesis-sized chart)[b]	9.0	5.0

[a]Data are averages obtained with two different listeners on two separate occasions.
[b]Data are averages for two probes with one familiar therapist.

Social Validation

As noted in Table 5, Subject 1's verbal output was judged to improve in organization, but cohesion was noted to deteriorate slightly from baseline to maintenance. Completeness was rated somewhat more favorably for the maintenance probes. Subject 2's samples were judged as having decreased in organization; however, cohesion was rated much higher during maintenance. Ratings of completeness were equivalent across conditions.

DISCUSSION

The results indicate clear treatment effects, maintenance, and response, generalization for both subjects. Stimulus generalization was disappointing, but this is not especially surprising, because training trials were massed without variation and neither trainer nor setting were varied. Social validation ratings were also modest and inconsistent. Most perplexing were the ratings of completeness, which were not perceived to improve even though each subject listed many more features during maintenance probes. Listeners may have been distracted by the poor organization and cohesion of the samples they heard, as well as by the telegraphic nature of the subjects' verbal output.

Results of this study have several clinical implications. Feature Analysis may be a useful tool for tapping existing semantic networks. Subjects with severe verbal memory deficits retrieved many more semantic features of a topic after being trained. Subjects performed optimally during

Table 5. Social Validation Ratings

Organization

| | SUBJECT 1 | | SUBJECT 2 | |
Rater	Baseline	Maintenance	Baseline	Maintenance
1	2	5	2	1,1[a]
2	3	7	3	2,1[a]
3	3	5	5	1,2[a]
4	2	4	3	0,0[a]

Cohesion

| | SUBJECT 1 | | SUBJECT 2 | |
Rater	Baseline	Maintenance	Baseline	Maintenance
1	2,2[a]	1	0	3
2	2,2[a]	1	1	5
3	4,3[a]	2	1	3
4	3,3[a]	2	0	2

Completeness

| | SUBJECT 1 | | SUBJECT 2 | |
Rater	Baseline	Maintenance	Baseline	Maintenance
1	2	4	2,2[a]	3
2	3	4	3,4[a]	3
3	3	4	4,3[a]	3
4	3	5	3,3[a]	3

[a]Denotes sample repeated for intrarater reliability.

structured trials in which they were provided with a Feature Analysis chart; thus, Feature Analysis may be useful as a model procedure for patients who respond well to visual cuing systems. Future research should aim to promote generalization to novel settings and conversational partners by using loose training procedures (Thompson, 1989) and by varying treatment settings, trainers, and even the position of the descriptors on the Feature Analysis chart. The utility of training with a miniature format and of teaching subjects to self-cue in conversational contexts also needs to be examined in a more comprehensive fashion. With proper training in the use of a self-cuing system, patients with traumatic brain injury who benefit from visual cues may be able to adopt a procedure like Feature Analysis as a compensatory aid.

REFERENCES

Anderson, J. R. (1983). *The architecture of cognition.* Cambridge: Harvard University Press.

Campbell, T. F., & Dollaghan, C. (1992). A method for obtaining listener judgments of spontaneously produced language: Social validation through Direct Magnitude Estimation. *Topics in Language Disorders, 12,* 42–55.

Goodglass, H., & Kaplan, E. (1983). *The Boston Diagnostic Aphasia Examination.* Philadelphia: Lea and Febiger.

Massaro, M. (1991). *Feature Analysis for treatment of communication disorders in traumatically brain-injured patients: An efficacy study.* Unpublished manuscript.

Szekeres, S. F., Ylvisaker, M., & Cohen, S. B. (1987). A framework for cognitive rehabilitation therapy. In M. Ylvisaker & E. M. Gobble (Eds.), *Community reentry for head injured adults* (pp. 87–136). Austin, TX: PRO-ED.

Thompson, C. K. (1989). Generalization research in aphasia: A review of the literature. In T. E. Prescott (Ed.), *Clinical aphasiology,* Vol. 18 (pp. 195–222). Boston: Little, Brown.

Wechsler, D. (1987). *Wechsler Memory Scale–Revised.* New York: Psychological Corporation.

APPENDIX A

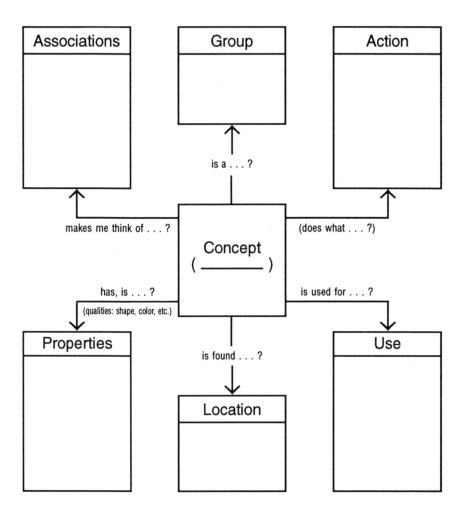

Associations

Group

Action

is a . . . ?

makes me think of . . . ?

(does what . . . ?)

Concept

(————)

has, is . . . ?

(qualities: shape, color, etc.)

is used for . . . ?

Properties

is found . . . ?

Use

Location

APPENDIX B

1. To rule out severe comprehension deficits, the auditory comprehension subtests of the *Boston Diagnostic Aphasia Examination* (Goodglass & Kaplan, 1983) were administered.

Auditory Comprehension Summary Profile

Test Component	Subject 1	Subject 2
Word Discrimination	100	100
Body Part Identification	60	70
Commands	70	90
Complex Ideational Material	70	80

Note: Data are percentiles based on aphasic adults' performance.

2. Various subscales of the *Wechsler Memory Scale–Revised* (WMS–R) (Wechsler, 1987) were administered to obtain a baseline of each subject's memory capabilities. Visual memory was superior to verbal memory for both subjects.

Wechsler Memory Scale–Revised Summary Profile

Subscale	Subject 1	Subject 2
Verbal Memory (74 maximum) Story retelling Verbal paired associates	32	16
Visual Memory (69 maximum) Figural memory Visual paired associates Visual memory span Visual reproduction	69	60
General Memory (143 maximum) Verbal and visual Profiles combined	101	76
Attention/ (82 maximum) Concentration Digit span forward and Digit span backward	36	34

Clinical Aphasiology, Vol. 22, 1994, pp. 257–264

Differential Performance of Traumatic Brain Injury Subjects and Non-Brain-Injured Peers on Cognitive Tasks

Brenda L. B. Adamovich and
Thomas A. Hutchinson

The *Scales of Cognitive Ability for Traumatic Brain Injury* (SCATBI) (Adamovich & Henderson, 1992) is a test designed to assess cognitive-linguistic status after closed head injury (CHI) and to describe the extent of changes during and following rehabilitation. This test measures performance on five scales, each representing a general area of ability that may be impaired after CHI and is necessary to function in day-to-day life. The five scales are (1) Perception and Discrimination, (2) Orientation, (3) Organization, (4) Recall, and (5) Reasoning. Each scale is made up of a series of small tests, or "testlets" (Thissen, Steinberg, & Mooney, 1989). Testlets are collections of similar items designed to measure a common trait or subdomain. The testlets for each scale are summarized in Table 1.

In general, items within each testlet progress from easier to more difficult. The item scores are summed to produce a testlet score, and the testlet scores are summed to produce a total score for each of the five scales. The total raw score for each of the scales can be converted to normed scores (percentile ranks or standard scores). A severity score can be computed from the total composite score. The standardization form of the test was administered to 322 subjects over a period of approximately 1 year. The subjects included 244 CHI and 78 non-brain-injured individuals drawn from 26 sites in the United States and Canada. The scores of the non-brain-injured subjects were used to estimate the average difficulty of the test as a kind of upper bound of expectations for head-injured subjects.

The SCATBI standardization sample is reported by age intervals in Table 2. Approximately half of the head-injured patients were between 15

Table 1. Five SCATBI Scales and Their Associated 41 Testlets

I. Perception and Discrimination
1. Sound recognition
2. Shape recognition
3. Word recognition (no distraction)
4. Word recognition (with distraction)
5. Color discrimination
6. Shape discrimination
7. Size discrimination
8. Discrimination of color, shape, size
9. Discrimination of pictured objects
10. Auditory discrimination (real words)
11. Auditory discrimination (nonsense)

II. Orientation
1. Premorbid questions
2. Postmorbid questions

III. Organization
1. Identifying pictured categories
2. Identifying pictured category members
3. Word associations (word categories)
4. Sequencing objects (size)
5. Sequencing words (alphabetical)
6. Sequencing events (time of year)
7. Sequencing events (pictured task steps)
8. Sequencing events (recall task steps)

IV. Recall
1. Memory for graphic elements
2. Naming pictures (word retrieval)
3. Immediate recall of word strings
4. Delayed recall of word strings
5. Cued recall of words
6. Cued recall of words in discourse
7. Word generation
8. Immediate recall of oral directions
9. Recall of oral paragraphs

V. Reasoning
1. Figural reasoning: matrix analogies
2. Convergent thinking: central theme
3. Deductive reasoning: elimination
4. Inductive reasoning: opposites
5. Inductive reasoning: analogies
6. Divergent thinking: homographs
7. Divergent thinking: idioms
8. Divergent thinking: proverbs
9. Divergent thinking: verbal absurdities
10. Multiprocess reasoning: task insight
11. Multiprocess reasoning: analysis

and 30 years of age, and the median age was 30. The sample contained more than twice as many males as females, a proportion typical of the head-injured population. As indicated in Table 3, approximately two-thirds of the patients in the sample were tested between 30 days and 1 year post injury, and the percentage tested within 30 days post injury was nearly equal to the percentage tested more than one year post injury. The groups were similar with regard to years of education, years of employment, and primary language.

Table 2. SCATBI Standardization Sample by Age

Age Range (Years)	Brain-Injured		Non-Brain-Injured	
	n	%	n	%
15–19	26	13.3	7	10.0
20–29	67	34.2	26	37.1
30–39	46	23.5	23	32.9
40–49	25	12.8	8	11.4
50–59	14	7.1	2	2.9
< 59	18	9.2	4	5.7
Total reporting	196	100.1	70	100.0
Not reporting	48		8	

Note: Copyright 1991 by the Riverside Publishing Company. Used with permission of the publisher.

Table 3. SCATBI Standardization Sample
(Brain-Injured Only) by Time Post Injury

Time Post Injury	n	%
< 30 days	32	18.2
31–60 days	26	14.8
61–90 days	19	10.8
91–120 days	12	6.8
121–180 days	23	13.1
181–365 days	34	19.3
12–18 months	26	14.8
> 18 months	4	2.3
Total reporting	176	100.1
Not reporting	68	

Note: Copyright 1991 by the Riverside Publishing Company. Used with permission of the publisher.

Pearson product moment correlations were computed between each of the raw scores on the five SCATBI scales and the level scores on *Rancho Los Amigos Levels of Cognitive Functioning* (Malkmus, Booth, & Kodimer, 1980). As shown in Table 4, the correlations for 125 selected subjects were moderate, ranging from a low of .50 (Perception and Discrimination) to a high of .60 (Reasoning). This moderate agreement between the two instruments supports the validity of each as a measure of cognitive functioning, but it also suggests that they are complementary measures rather than substitutes for each other. The internal consistency reliability of the SCATBI was assessed using Cronbach's alpha. The alphas for the SCATBI,

Table 4. Correlations Between Scores for Five SCATBI Scales and Rancho Severity Level, Standardization Sample (n = 125)

	Rancho Level with SCATBI Raw Scores*	Rancho Level with SCATBI Standard Scores*
Perception/discrimination	.50	.40
Orientation	.58	.50
Organization	.51	.46
Recall	.59	.57
Reasoning	.60	.57

Note: Copyright 1991 by the Riverside Publishing Company. Used with permission of the publisher.
*p < .001.

Table 5. SCATBI Scale Raw Score Means, Standard Deviations, Interitem Consistency Reliability Coefficients (alphas), and Standard Errors of Measurement, Standardization Sample (n = 164)

	M	SD	r	SEM
Perception/discrimination	49.2	10.9	.95	2.4
Orientation	16.6	5.1	.90	1.6
Organization	22.4	7.2	.92	2.0
Recall	32.1	10.8	.90	3.4
Reasoning	31.9	13.8	.93	3.7

Note: Copyright 1991 by the Riverside Publishing Company. Used with permission of the publisher.

reported in Table 5, reflect high interitem consistency for the raw scores on the five scales.

Perhaps the most important question for users of test instruments such as the one under study is how effectively the scores differentiate between head-injured and non-brain-injured subjects. The CHI subjects in the standardization sample evidenced a wide range of ability and impairment, whereas the non-brain-injured subjects exhibited a somewhat narrower range of abilities. A discriminant analysis of the standard scores of the five scales classified 96% of the non-brain-injured subjects as non-brain-injured and 79% of brain-injured subjects as brain-injured. These relatively high levels of agreement with the previously made classifications positively support the predictive validity of the SCATBI (see Table 6).

The purpose of this investigation was to examine the differences among three groups for each of the 41 individual testlets that make up the SCATBI's five scales.

Table 6. Classification of Brain-Injured Patients and Matched Samples of Non-Brain-Injured Peers Using Standard Scores of Five SCATBI Scales

Match variables	Non-Brain-Injured Accurately Classified		Brain-Injured Accurately Classified	
	n	%	n	%
Site, Age	55	84.6	93	86.9
Site, Age, Sex	46	88.5	56	84.9
Site, Age, Sex, Education	33	91.7	33	86.8
Site, Age, Sex, Education, Years Worked	22	95.7	19	79.2

Note: Copyright 1991 by the Riverside Publishing Company. Used with permission of the publisher.

METHOD

Three groups were studied: 78 non-brain-injured subjects who had been selected from peer groups of head-injured patients in each standardization site; 80 CHI subjects who had obtained a composite score below the mean for the total CHI group (low CHI); and 84 CHI subjects who had obtained a composite score at or above the mean for the CHI group (high CHI). These were subjects from the previously described standardization sample. Mean scores were computed for each group on each of the 41 testlets and five scales. An effect size (Cohen, 1988) was obtained to determine the magnitude of the differences between means of the three experimental groups.

RESULTS

The means and standard deviations for each scale for each group, reported in Table 7, show a consistent pattern of higher scores for non-brain-injured subjects across all five scales; in most cases, mean scores of non-brain-injured subjects were within a few points of the maximum possible score. The low CHI group exhibited greater variability, as reflected in the larger standard deviations, than did the non-brain-injured subjects. The high CHI group had higher mean scores than the low CHI group, and both head-injured groups had lower mean scores than the non-brain-injured group. Because a simple difference between each pair of means for each

Table 7. Mean Testlet Scores and Standard Deviations for Selected Subgroups of Closed-Head-Injured (CHI) Subjects and Non-Brain-Injured Peers

Scale Totals	CHI High[a] Mean	SD	CHI Low[b] Mean	SD	Noninjured[c] Mean	SD	Total Possible Points
Perception and discrimination	54.4	3.0	43.9	13.3	55.7	3.9	58
Orientation	19.3	1.3	13.7	6.0	19.8	0.7	20
Organization	26.2	1.2	18.6	8.1	26.3	2.5	30
Recall	39.4	4.3	24.4	10.3	44.7	6.4	52
Reasoning	41.0	6.5	22.3	12.9	47.2	7.9	55

[a]$N = 84$. [b]$N = 80$. [c]$N = 78$.

of the three groups would not reflect the difference variances of the three groups, an effect size was computed for each difference. An effect size represents the difference between two means divided by the average standard deviation (that is, the square root of the sum of the squared standard deviations for the two groups). Not only does effect size reflect the variances of the groups, but there are also conventional guidelines for judging the meaningfulness of its various magnitudes. Cohen (1988) has suggested a three-level classification—small, medium, and large, corresponding to effect sizes of .2, .5, and .8, respectively. Cohen gives the following examples: "A small effect size is not visible to the naked eye. A medium effect size is conceived as one large enough to be visible to the naked eye. That is, in the course of normal experience, one would become aware of an average difference in IQ between clerical and semi-skilled workers or between members of professional and managerial occupational groups" (1988, p. 27). A difference with a large effect size "is represented by the mean IQ difference estimated by the difference between holders of the Ph.D. degree and typical college freshmen" (Cohen, 1988, p. 27).

Table 8 reports effect sizes for the differences between scale means of three groups: high CHI minus low CHI, non-brain-injured minus high CHI, and non-brain-injured minus low CHI. Effect sizes greater than .5 are indicated by an asterisk, and those greater than .8 are indicated by two asterisks. The data in Table 8 reflect the substantial differences observed between non-brain-injured subjects and subjects with closed-head-injury. The effect size for each testlet within each of the five scales was also computed. In a comparison of CHI subjects below the mean with CHI subjects above the mean, 38 of 41 testlets yielded medium or large effect sizes. In the comparison of CHI subjects below the mean with non-brain-

Table 8. Effect Sizes of Differences Between Mean Testlet Scores for Selected Subgroups of Closed-Head-Injured (CHI) Subjects and Noninjured Peers

Scale Totals	CHI High/ CHI Low	Non-Brain-Injured/ CHI High	Non-Brain-Injured/ CHI Low
Perception and discrimination	1.09**	0.40	1.21**
Orientation	1.30**	0.51*	1.44**
Organization	1.31**	0.09	1.30**
Recall	1.90**	0.99**	2.37**
Reasoning	1.83**	0.85**	2.33**

*Effect size > .5. **Effect size > .8.

injured subjects, 37 of 41 testlets yielded medium or large effect sizes. The comparison between non-brain-injured subjects and CHI subjects above the mean produced medium or large effect sizes for 10 of 41 testlets.

DISCUSSION

Significant differences were observed between non-brain-injured subjects, CHI subjects scoring above the mean, and CHI subjects scoring below the mean. Significant differences were also observed between high CHI subjects and low CHI subjects.

The comparison of the high CHI group and the low CHI group yielded large effect sizes (> .8) for all five scales. The comparison of the non-brain-injured group and the high CHI group yielded a medium effect size (> .5) for the Orientation scale and a large effect size (> .8) for the Recall and Reasoning scales. The comparison of the non-brain-injured group and the low CHI group yielded large effect sizes for all five scales.

The non-brain-injured subjects and high CHI subjects produced mean or large effect sizes for only 10 of 41 testlets. The fact that the majority of these differences were in the Recall and Reasoning testlets and scales suggests that tasks from those domains are the most critical in differentiating higher functioning CHI subjects from their non-brain-injured counterparts. These differences have important implications for both assessment and treatment. Although this study grouped patients above and below the SCATBI mean, there are pervasive deficits even at the mild level of head injury, and these deficits are reflected over a wide variety of tasks. However, mildly injured persons often do not receive treatment, even though they report significant changes in all aspects of their life, including divorce and loss of employment. Years after their injury they are frequently obsessed with their inability to process and remember information, only to be told by their physician and others that what they need is a good psychiatrist. It is to be hoped that this test will provide information regarding the specific deficits of mildly impaired patients, as well as the moderate and severe deficits seen in more seriously impaired patients. In any event, the results warrent further investigation of the SCATBI performance of patients with minor head injury, as defined by conventional criteria (e.g., initial Glasgow Coma scale scores above 12).

REFERENCES

Adamovich, B. B., & Henderson, J. (1992). *Scales of Cognitive Ability for Traumatic Brain Injury* (SCATBI). Chicago: Riverside.

Cohen, J. (1988). *Statistical power analysis for the behavioral sciences* (2nd ed.). Hillsdale, NJ: Lawrence Erlbaum.

Malkmus, D., Booth, B., & Kodimer, G. (1980). *Rehabilitation of the head-injured adult: Comprehensive management.* Downey, CA: Professional Staff Association of Ranchos Los Amigos Hospital.

Thissen, D., Steinberg, L., & Mooney, J. A. (1989). Trace line for testlets: A use of multiple-categorical-response models. *Journal of Educational Measurement, 26,* 161–176.

Clinical Aphasiology, Vol. 22, 1994, pp. 265–273

A Theory of the Deficit: A Prerequisite for a Theory of Therapy?

Sally Byng

"If we are to serve aphasic patients better . . . and to turn clinical art into clinical science, then we must begin to develop explicit and falsifiable theories of treatment, to test their assumptions and contrast various theoretically-driven forms of treatment."–Holland (1991)

The relationship between theory and therapy has become a subject of increased discussion in recent years, as volumes of *Clinical Aphasiology* can attest. Nonetheless, are we in agreement about why we need to develop theoretically driven forms of treatment? My assumption is that theories are necessary to relate the nature of the disability or impairment to what we are trying to do about it. This means that we need first to provide a clear statement or hypothesis about the nature of a deficit before we can then develop theories about what forms of therapy or intervention are appropriate and effective and why. Becoming an adult with aphasia produces many and various effects, of course. It therefore follows that, to address a range of effects, we will need to compare not only different theoretical accounts of the same phenomena but also different types of theories.

It does not matter that we may have different theories. What does matter is that we are explicit about them and explicit about why a particular therapy should be appropriate. The only falsifiable theories are explicit ones, as Holland (1991) makes clear: "If clinicians and clinical researchers simply demand from themselves a written justification of why they believe such and such will work in treatment and why something else might not, a major step will be taken in the development of testable hypotheses about the process of treatment in aphasia." In this paper, I suggest one approach to making an explicit hypothesis about why a specific treatment for a specific aspect of the language impairment should or should not work. This is far from comprehensive; the theoretical basis that I describe here does *not* address many of the aspects or variables involved in providing therapy for someone with aphasia—it deals only with the language impairment itself.

My premise is that any treatment that can address the language deficit in aphasia must begin with a theory about the *nature* of the deficit. Another basic premise, and one on which the previous premise is prefaced, is that the deficit cannot be inferred from observing or examining the surface symptomatology, as is suggested by much current research (Berndt, 1991; Howard & Patterson, 1989). This means that treatment cannot be planned only on the basis of the observed presence or absence of a particular linguistic feature in the language of a person with aphasia. Therefore, any treatment for the language deficit requires a prior hypothesis about the underlying nature of an individual's language impairment that explains why a particular pattern of symptoms might be observed. This hypothesis can be derived from a number of converging sources, for example, from informed observation of the person with aphasia communicating in a variety of contexts or from performance on tests of a range of specific language tasks suggested by the observation (Byng, in press).

The crucial question here is what informs the observations and what motivates the testing that shapes the hypothesis. A current approach is to draw on the basic architecture of the language-processing system offered by cognitive neuropsychological models along with a logical way of thinking about the deficit. In addition to the basic architecture, psycholinguistic concepts about representations and processes that may be involved in comprehending and producing language are used (e.g., Coltheart, Sartori, & Job, 1987).

Toward the end of the 1970s, cognitive experimental psychologists were becoming interested in testing empirically based architectural models of the normal language-processing system by investigating whether damage to one or more of the components of these models could account for different disorders of language processing (Coltheart, Patterson, & Marshall 1980). This methodology has developed into a discipline known as cognitive neuropsychology. The basic approach is to try to identify where the deficit underlying the impaired language arises within these empirically based, multicomponent, modular representations of language processing. Current models usually represent the component modules of the language-processing system through box-and-arrow diagrams, in which the boxes represent stores of information and the arrows represent processes linking them. These models offer a logical, coherent framework with which to approach a basic account of a language impairment. A patient's performance pattern can be elucidated in terms of a pattern of both the impaired and preserved components of the language-processing system.

Using concepts about, and the architecture of, the normal language-processing system has a number of benefits that can affect the design of a therapeutic procedure and the interpretation of the outcome (Howard & Patterson, 1989). One of the benefits of this approach is that it can provide some theoretically motivated predictions of the outcome of therapy. Because the models try to make explicit the relationships between different components of the language system, it is possible to hypothesize about what should happen to one component when a different component is treated. Thinking through the implications of the architecture of the language-processing system can assist in making predictions about the effects of a therapy. This in turn can help to measure the effectiveness of intervention; if we can demonstrate that our therapy has affected those aspects of the language system that we anticipated should be affected, but not those that we did not anticipate should be affected, we are in a stronger position to claim that our intervention was influential in bringing about the change. Alternatively, if the therapy does not produce the expected outcome, then we are in a better position to ask why.

This suggests that pre- and posttherapy measurement of not only treated but untreated items must be carried out, as has become well established. Additionally, there should be measures of untreated language functions, some of which are related to the function being treated and some of which are not. The relationships between the functions must be specified so that predicted improvements in related but untreated functions can be measured, providing yet more evidence for the efficacy of the therapy. In this paper, I will illustrate this aspect of theoretically driven therapy at length.

In a sequence of studies with a small number of people with agrammatic Broca's aphasia, the sentence processing deficits demonstrated by these people on a number of specific assessments were interpreted to be in line with the "mapping deficit hypothesis" of Schwartz, Linebarger, and Saffran (1985). This hypothesis suggests that patients with symptoms of agrammatism cannot assign, or map, appropriate semantic (or thematic) roles onto Noun Phrases in particular structural positions; that is, they are unable to coordinate sentence form and sentence meaning to interpret even simple sentences. The hypothesis suggests that this might affect not only sentence comprehension but also sentence production. Current linguistic theories suggest that this kind of mapping is not a single process but involves two types of information and procedures: lexical information and general procedures that apply to specific sets of thematic roles. The lexical representation of a lexical item (e.g., a verb) specifies which thematic roles are involved and how they are assigned to particular positions within the sentence structure. In addition, as there are systematic regularities in the assignment of thematic roles (e.g., Agents are usually mapped onto Subject NP positions), mapping may also involve procedures that are not item specific (Byng & Black, 1989).

This hypothesis about our patients was made on the basis of specific features of sentence comprehension and production; namely, that the patients were unable to comprehend reliably simple reversible sentences, either active declarative, passive, or locative sentences. Additionally, their sentence production was structurally limited, with the patients relying on simple utterances, either holophrastic or at least minimally structured. Some of the patients also made errors assigning thematic roles in a comprehension task for single words, suggesting that their problems in comprehending sentences were not because of failure to parse the syntax.

With the first patient, BRB (Byng, 1988), a therapy task was devised that focused only on enhancing the comprehension of one set of thematic roles and on input. We adopted this approach on the premise that if an aspect of the language system is being changed (in this case, we hypothesized this to be the procedure that maps thematic roles and grammatical relations), then the effects of that change should not be confined to items practiced but should be observed in any task involving the changed procedure. Therefore, if a therapy affects a process or a set of processes involved in mapping sentence form and sentence meaning, any language task involving these processes should show benefit, provided there are no other deficits remaining that would further interfere with that process. In this way we can plan for and anticipate theoretically specified generalization. The rationale underlying this therapy, then, was that if the hypothesis about the mapping deficit was correct, then remediation of the mapping deficit in one modality should bring about improvement in the untreated modality and in untreated thematic roles.

The results of the therapy demonstrated that BRB had made a statistically significant improvement in comprehending all sentences where he had to map thematic roles onto syntactic relations to interpret the sentence correctly. This included not just the sentence types used in therapy but also reversible simple active sentences and passive sentences. BRB had therefore learned more than just a strategy for interpretation of sentences, such as that the most agentlike entity will be in the subject NP position, which would facilitate comprehension of active sentences. Because application of that strategy would not have allowed BRB to interpret locative or passive sentences any better, he must have learned some principle about mapping thematic relations.

After the therapy, a statistically significant shift was measured in the production of narrative speech, away from producing single words or phrases and toward combining nouns and verbs to form structured utterances. It therefore seemed that the hypothesis about the deficit underlying his problems in one aspect of both sentence comprehension and production might have been correct—treatment effects had generalized beyond the treated sentence types both to untreated sentence types and to a different modality after treatment of only a limited number of specific exemplars. Other aspects of BRB's impaired language that were not related to the therapy did not improve, however, so that although there is generalization, it is only a specific one related to the therapy.

The same therapy was attempted unsuccessfully with a second patient, JG (Byng, 1988), which then prompted the use of a **further** therapy procedure. This therapy was then replicated with another severely agrammatic patient, AER (Nickels, Byng, & Black, 1991), to investigate its effects in more detail and to reexamine the hypothesis about the underlying disorder in more detail. The basic purpose of the therapy task was to increase the patient's awareness of the roles that the different entities involved in an event play and how those roles are represented in the structure of the sentence. The therapy was designed not to get the patients to practice comprehending and producing sentences of various types but rather to convey to them some aspects of predicate-argument structure (Nickels, Byng, & Black, 1991; Byng, 1992).

Both JG and AER demonstrated statistically significant gains both in comprehension of simple active agentive sentences and in production of structured utterances. This improvement in production was not confined to picture description tasks but also included gains in production of narrative speech and, according to observations and reports from relatives, in spontaneous day-to-day speech. After the therapy both AER and JG were able to produce utterances with more structure and greater content, showing a particular improvement in producing verbs. They were not just producing sentences practiced in therapy better than previously, but they were also generating their own language more effectively. Their ability to comprehend specific sentences did not show such marked improvement, however, as BRB's had; improvement was confined to the sentence type used in therapy, but not just to the lexical items used in therapy. It seems that they had learned a principle about how to interpret that type of sentence. Additional tasks were performed pre- and post-therapy using processes that were predicted not to be involved in therapy and therefore served to act as controls for those aspects of the language that were predicted to be positively affected. In both patients, these control measures showed that the improvements were specific to those aspects involved in the therapy and not to other, unrelated processes. This result was taken to reinforce the specific effects of the therapy.

Because the therapy focused on a procedure rather than on a set of structures or items, we planned for generalization through types of stimuli other than those being worked on in therapy. Because the patients were learning something about structuring sentences involving a specific type of verb, it should not matter which specific verbs within that class were being used, because they were learning not item-specific information but rather some procedures about combining nouns and verbs. We measured generalization of this kind. For example, in naming of action pictures, a subset of which had been used in therapy (not the specific pictures, but other pictures depicting the same actions as those in the assessment set), JG and AER showed improvement in naming all the pictures, and there was no difference between the treated and untreated items.

The predictions made about patterns of improvement again held good in these patients. Although we were working on aspects of sentence production in our patients, the therapy focused only on revealing to the patients aspects of predicate-argument structure, so we did not anticipate that there would be any increase in other aspects of production, such as the ability to produce closed-class items or to use obligatory determiners, for example. Indeed, these aspects of production did not improve as a result of therapy. This kind of finding strengthens the case for the efficacy of a specific therapy: If the positive outcome was a result of spontaneous or nonspecific improvement, then it is difficult to explain how predicate-argument structure could have improved spontaneously when closed-class items showed no improvement.

The premise of this paper is that theories about the nature of language deficits are a necessary precursor to developing therapies specifically addressed to a given language impairment. However, simply having a detailed analysis of the deficit does **not** by itself suggest the formulation of specific theraputic procedures to effect change. That is the province of theories of therapy. Three recent studies of therapy for people with naming problems show that knowing what the deficit is does not always entail knowing what to do about it. These three studies (Hillis, 1989; Jones, 1989; Marshall, 1989) describe three patients who had poor naming ability, despite having good comprehension of semantically related items as measured on picture-word matching tasks. Table 1 shows some features of the performance of the three people, with hypotheses about the locus of the naming deficit and the aim of the therapy in each case. Although the three studies employ slightly different descriptions, all three people have some deficit between the semantic system and the phonological output system. Given the inexplicit nature of current models, it is difficult to characterize the specific form that the deficits take, but the deficits seem approximate.

However, even the small amount of additional data provided in Table 1 makes clear that these three patients are not the same in many other respects. PC is more like a Wernicke's aphasic, whereas RS is more like a Broca's aphasic. These differences aside, however, one might suppose that *if* there is some direct link from the analysis of the naming deficit to therapeutic intervention, similar therapies might have been generated; this was not the case. On the basis of their spontaneous speech, Jones's and Hillis's patients sound like each other more than either sounds like Marshall's patient, yet the intervention strategies employed were quite different for all three.

Table 1. Comparison of Language Deficits of Three Aphasics Who Received Therapy for Naming Deficits

Descriptive and Evaluative Data	Subject/Study		
	Pt. 2 (Hillis, 1989)	PC (Jones, 1989)	RS (Marshall, 1989)
Speech characteristics	Fluent speech minus content words	Empty speech with omission of content words	Nonfluent, Broca's type aphasia
Word-picture matching	100%	94%	98%
Oral naming	66% (25% semantic errors)	0% (60% no response; 40% neologisms)	32% (few semantic errors)
Written naming	11%	0%	44%
Oral reading	67%	0%	good
Repetition	profoundly impaired	unable	probably good
Hypothesised mechanism of naming problems	an inability to retrieve the correct phonologic representation of the word oral naming	some of his problems in accessing the output form of words possibly arose because of weak semantic drive	a breakdown in the route linking semantics and phonology
Aim of therapy	to improve frequency and accuracy of their writing attempts	to improve picture naming as a measure of increased access to the phonological form due to enhanced access to semantic information	to rebuild the communication between RS's good semantic knowledge and his intact word phonology

Jones used a predominantly semantic strategy based on the idea of judging the relatedness of pictures or words to a central target item. After the judgment task, the patient ordered lettered tiles to form the target word; then, if he could say the name easily, he was encouraged to produce it, but no emphasis was laid on doing this. Hillis's therapy, which involved a cueing hierarchy to facilitate written naming, was devised by noting the sorts of stimuli that sometimes elicited correct names. After this therapy, a hierarchy for facilitating oral naming was introduced. Marshall's therapy for RS consisted of a three-stage procedure in which the patient first identified from a list of five related words one of the items that was being described. Then he "brainstormed" around a target picture, miming, drawing and giving as many words or ideas as he could related to the picture. Finally, he matched a printed word to the picture from a choice of five and read it aloud.

These three therapy procedures have some similarities, but it is hard to compare them directly because even the two semantically based procedures of Marshall and Jones have very different task demands. The precise formulation of each seems to result from the constellation of observed performance features, not just the identification of the deficit's approximate locus. For example, because her patient (RS) could read aloud well, Marshall incorporated production of the phonological form into the treatment of oral reading with a semantic task (matching of the printed word to a picture) to try to activate the impaired link between semantics and output phonology. Jones's therapy was designed to avoid as much auditory input as possible because single word auditory input was severely impaired for PC. In addition, the lettered tile component to the therapy was introduced to enhance the concept of phonological segmentation; this indirect introduction to the idea of a word being segmented into sounds served as a precursor to future work on phonological segmentation. Hillis's therapy derived from the observation that her patient was frequently able to write picture names when given scrambled anagrams.

The outcome of each of these therapies was, not surprisingly, quite different. The studies raise a number of questions about both the nature of the patients' deficits and the nature of the therapies, such as what it means to locate the naming deficit in the same place when each of the three patients studied clearly differs from the others in terms of many other aspects of language processing. Are the two semantically based therapies the same? Were the patients learning the same information from the therapies? Can we *assume* that the patients are getting the same information from similar therapies? If I were to try these therapies, would the way I implemented them be the same as the way they were implemented by these therapists?

It is clear that deficit analysis does not *by itself* suggest the formulation of specific therapeutic procedures. Because this is what therapy aims to do, theories about how to effect change through therapy must be derived from sources other than the analysis of the deficit. My position is that an analysis of the nature of the language impairment, rooted in a relationship to the normal language-processing system, should provide the most informative way for us to describe the deficit as a basis for therapy. We need to know more precisely how the language system is impaired, what impairments can be treated, what psycholinguistic variables should be controlled in therapy, and what we can predict the effects of the treatment to be. The decision about whether these impairments should be treated and how represents a different set of questions not addressed by the account of the deficit; that issue rests on the development of a theory of therapy. I consider what I have been describing to be just one of the prerequisites toward developing such a theory of therapy for language deficits, but it is clear that theories for therapy are as crucial as theories of the deficit if our treatments are to progress.

REFERENCES

Berndt, R. S. (1991). Sentence processing in aphasia. In M. T. Sarno (Ed.), *Acquired Aphasia* (2nd ed., pp. 223–270). New York: Academic Press.

Byng, S. (1988). Sentence processing deficits: Theory and therapy. *Cognitive Neuropsychology, 5,* 629–676.

Byng, S. (1992). Testing the tried: Replicating therapy for sentence processing deficits in agrammatism. *Clinics in Communication Disorders: Approaches to the Treatment of Aphasia, 1*(4), 34–42.

Byng, S. (in press). Hypothesis testing and aphasia therapy. In Audrey Holland and Margaret Forbes (Eds.), *World perspectives on aphasia.* Singular Publishing.

Byng, S., & Black, M. (1989). Some aspects of sentence production in aphasia. *Aphasiology, 3*(3), 241–263.

Coltheart, M., Patterson, K. E., & Marshall, J. (1980). *Deep dyslexia.* London: Routledge and Kegan Paul.

Coltheart, M., Sartori, G., & Job, R. (1987). *The cognitive neuropsychology of language.* Hove and London: Erlbaum.

Hillis, A. E. (1989). Efficacy and generalisation of treatment for aphasic naming errors. *Archives of Physical Medicine in Rehabilitation, 70,* 632–635.

Holland, A. L. (1991). Some thoughts on future needs and directions for research and treatment of aphasia. National Institutes of Health.

Howard, D., & Patterson, K. E. (1989). Models of therapy. In X. Seron and G. Deloche (Eds.), *Cognitive approaches in neuropsychological rehabilitation* (pp. 39–64). Hillsdale, NJ: Erlbaum.

Jones, E. V. (1989). A year in the life of EVJ and PC. *Proceedings of Advances in Aphasia Therapy in the Clinical Setting.* British Aphasiology Society.

Marshall, J. (1989). R. S.—Three specific treatment programmes. *Proceedings of Advances in Aphasia Therapy in the Clinical Setting.* British Aphasiology Society.

Nickels, L., Byng, S., & Black, M. (1991). Sentence processing deficits: A replication of therapy. *British Journal of Disorders of Communication, 26,* 175–199.

Schwartz, M., Linebarger, M., & Saffran, E. (1985). The status of the syntactic theory of agrammatism. In M. L. Kean (Ed.), *Agrammatism* (pp. 83–124). New York: Academic Press.

Clinical Aphasiology, Vol. 22, 1994, pp. 275–282

Cognitive Neuropsychological Theory and Treatment for Aphasia: Exploring the Strengths and Limitations

Audrey L. Holland

Cognitive neuropsychology generally, and cognitive-theory-driven approaches to treatment specifically, have been getting big press, with everyone from computational modelers to speech-language pathologists participating in the excitement and praise. From the perspective of clinical aphasiology, the source of this excitement is that cognitive neuropsychology provides a principled way of conceptualizing a language disorder, which thus can be related to a theoretical foundation and possibly even be tested by a number of approaches, including computer modeling (Hinton and Shallice, 1991). The processing models of cognitive neuropsychology have also shown clinicians the potential productivity of thinking about language as a number of processes and as a set of components. They have provided a logical way to proceed by allowing hypothesis testing about the way language is processed in the brain. This detailed study of deficits in aphasia can influence ways to treat aphasic and other cognitively impaired individuals. Nevertheless, I believe that the contributions that theory-driven therapy can make to treatment for aphasia are limited in both number and scope.

This limitation is primarily because cognitive neuropsychology has never pretended to be a theory of therapy and in fact has only indirect relationships to therapy. Caramazza (1989) has articulated this point well; he notes that "an informed choice [from among intervention approaches] cannot be made in the absence of an equally rich theory of the modifications that a damaged cognitive system may undergo as a function of different forms of intervention." What Caramazza is implying is that even after we get the deficit correctly nailed down by using a model that delineates the sources for any given functional impairment, it does not

275

necessarily follow that we know what to do about it. The theories that drive theory-driven treatment are not theories about how to fix deficits; rather, they are theories about how and why the deficits occur.

This is probably nowhere better illustrated than in Howard and Franklin's detailed case study, *Missing the Meaning?* (1988). Described on its cover as "a textbook example of how to do cognitive neuropsychology," this work concerns the single-word processing of MK, a patient who seems to have Wernicke's aphasia. Using a box-and-arrow processing model derived from Morton and Patterson (1986), Howard and Franklin present data that they gathered over a 3-year period, delimiting those aspects of the model that have apparently been rendered inaccessible (in MK's case, as a result of his brain damage) and those that have not. For some individuals, such as Gilbert (1992), this work is taken as a major contribution not only to cognitive neuropsychology but to the clinical enterprise as well.

> Howard and Franklin's interpretations of their results will be of continuing great value to SLP's [sic] who at times are convinced that a particular patient may have just about everything. Take heart, these authors will show you how to apply a model-based interpretation to aphasic problems, a useful way to approach both diagnosis and treatment. (p. 54)

But in their closing chapter, Howard and Franklin themselves make the following comment concerning therapy:

> We are both aphasia therapists, and one of our aims in interacting with MK was to "improve" his language, to try to lessen the limitations that his aphasia imposed on his life. Over the years that we have been seeing him, we have tried a number of different treatment approaches, partly in order to improve his language, but also as an experimental tool in trying to understand his problems. None have been particularly successful, and so no results seem worth reporting. We wonder, sometimes, whether our failures are the inevitable result of multiple and severe processing impairments. The difficulty that is the greatest impediment to communication is probably his severe problem in sentence comprehension. (p. 113)

In terms of clinical remediation, Howard and Franklin's *Missing the Meaning?* might be better titled *Missing the Boat*. But why does their work seem so irrelevant to their therapy? Part of the answer of course is that MK's major difficulty (i.e., sentence comprehension) was more encompassing than the single-word tasks that were the focus of the study. But there is another, substantially more important reason. Howard and Franklin never intended to deal with treatment in their work. Instead, they were interested in the precise description of a deficit. To make this or any similar aim relevant to treatment, another type of theory must be invoked.

My thesis is that relevant theories for such a goal are not cognitive neuro-psychological in nature; rather, they are theories about how one conducts aphasia therapy. The remainder of this paper will explore the theory of therapy and theory-driven treatment models.

WHAT DOES THERAPY DO TO A PATIENT?

An underlying assumption of theory-driven therapy as it relates to the clinical process is that deficits and therapeutic techniques will be straight-forwardly and unambiguously related. Isolating the functional deficit will directly entail a therapy technique to repair a broken or destroyed box. This *is* a theory concerning the nature of the therapeutic process; however, it is only one of many equally viable underlying assumptions and alternatives. It certainly is possible that theory-driven therapy may furnish data that is ultimately relevant to an "exercise the deficit" theory of therapy, but there are a number of other plausible contenders for Caramazza's *"rich theory of the modifications that a damaged cognitive system may undergo as a function of different forms of intervention."* What follows is a sampling from among them. Before beginning this discussion, however, it is necessary to point out that the experimental evidence for all of them is limited, despite the ease with which some of them are accepted.

Are cortical pathways being reorganized? This is an old idea, possibly best exemplified by Luria's approaches to the treatment of aphasia. Tech-niques such as pairing a relatively undamaged skill in hierarchical man-ner with a damaged one (e.g., "deblocking") or applying an unusual response form to a well-practiced skill (e.g., writing words in the sand with one's fingers) are said to result in some reorganization of brain function that facilitates the ability to perform deficient behaviors.

Are previously untapped capabilities of the undamaged areas of the brain being trained to take over some new functions (in the case of aphasia, language functions)? Melodic Intonation Therapy (MIT) (Helm-Estabrooks & Albert, 1991), is a pertinent example. It is built on the explicit hypothesis that functions associated with the intact right hemisphere may be exploited for purposes of rehabilitating speech in left-brain-damaged individuals.

Is the spontaneous recovery process being strengthened and sped along? This notion is to some degree answerable by research into the timing of treatment, including when to begin therapy and how frequently to provide it to a patient, regardless of the technique involved. The VA Cooperative study on the efficacy of treatment (Wertz et al., 1986) indi-cated that aphasic patients who began treatment later did as well as those who had begun earlier. And most of us have the clinical impression that aphasic patients who begin treatment later do not necessarily do worse, although it is possible that more gain might have been made if their treatment had begun earlier. Nevertheless, we all know patients who improve long after the spontaneous recovery period is over.

Are underlying deficits that block the aphasic patient's ability to communicate being mitigated? Should broader deficits than language problems, such as working memory, attentional deficits, perseveration, and the like, be a focus of management? Some examples of therapy approaches that result from this perspective are Helm-Estabrooks's TAP (Treating Aphasic Perseveration) and VAT (Visual Action Therapy) (Helm-Estabrooks & Albert, 1991). Both of these approaches, although linguistically relevant, carry with them the assumptions that some modifiable aspects of brain-damaged behavior, nonspecific to aphasia but nevertheless modulating it, can have fruitful payoff in language gains.

Are compensations or alternatives for bypassing damaged language components being provided? Just as most individuals with cerebellar disease learn quickly, usually without being told, that they can touch their index fingers to their noses a lot more efficiently if they lodge their elbows in their rib cages, one should expect aphasic patients to make adaptations to their disorders. Some clinicians, myself among them, believe that excellent therapy involves exploiting or training compensatory strategies and capitalizing on intact language components.

Are damaged language components being repaired, usually using a set of tools called language drills? Are these drills directed to the functions previously performed by the damaged components? Many researchers and clinicians share this underlying assumption concerning the nature of therapy for aphasia. In fact, it is a pervasive and almost thoughtlessly accepted belief about treatment. And one can hardly fault the neuropsychologists who are doing theory-driven therapy for buying into it. After all, many clinicians do. In essence, the clinical assumption is often that one practices what is hard to do, or cannot be done, until one gets it right.

Is some combination of the above going on, dependent on the extent and presentation pattern of the aphasia and usually coupled with counseling for the patients and their families as well? This is called the way to hedge one's bets, but in the ideal, it is a deliberate *choice*, not a default.

Before leaving the topic of how change is affected, which I believe is central to increasing our knowledge about the process of therapy, I wish to emphasize that theory-driven therapy cannot substitute for it. A theory about remediation can be *informed* by normal language-processing models, to be sure, but its core must be a concern with accomplishing repair and compensation. I would also note that in the ideal, it should contain some sound neurophysiological basis as well.

THE FOCUS OF TREATMENT FOR APHASIA

A second set of questions also impinges on what we can and cannot expect from theory-driven therapy. These questions focus on beliefs about what is the proper focus of the treatment. Unlike concerns with how therapy modifies language behavior, these questions do not particularly depend on other disciplines' contributions to the management of aphasia. Generally, they relate to the focus of clinical encounters in aphasia management. The notion of focus of treatment might seem transparent. An obvious answer is that aphasia management focuses on the aphasic patient and the context in which he or she operates. That is certainly true, but this focus also has subtler aspects that must be studied to develop strong treatment theories. I would like to suggest five of them, although there are probably many more.

Should the focus of treatment be the missing language? I agree with Byng, who elsewhere in this volume says that we need to know a great deal about the missing language (i.e., the deficit) if we intend to conduct knowledgeable aphasia treatment. Elsewhere, Byng (1990) suggests that the account must include information about the *nature* of the deficit; that is, whether the patient is exhibiting a capacity deficit, a problem in accessing representations, or a problem in inhibiting unwanted representations. Second, the *locus* of the deficit should be specified, not in neurostructural terms, but within the general architecture of a model or process, and it should be related to some understanding of the way in which that component or process normally functions. Finally, she suggests that some consideration must be given to the *relevance* of the deficit to the communicative needs of the aphasic person and to the rest of his or her language-processing system. For example, to understand the spelling process better, it is certainly interesting to attempt to remediate spelling deficits in aphasic patients. But because many Americans cannot spell very well in the first place, and most are tolerant of spelling errors, its remediation might be of questionable use to an aphasic person.

As a result of a deficit analysis, such as that which precedes theory-driven therapy, we should have a better idea of what variables need to be controlled, what procedures cannot be used, and what kind of information the therapy needs to convey. However, what should occur in treating these deficits is not necessarily clarified by such models. In fact, it is often not easy to see from the analysis how treatment should progress, or even that a direct attack on damaged or missing functions is preferable to an attempt to bolster intact ones. There is still room for clinical ingenuity. For example, some of Byng's very interesting earlier work on sentence processing in aphasia (1988) resulted from an initial deficit analysis. The treatment that was derived, however, was a creative approach to active linguistic problem solving centered on the patients' deficits. It is possible that this therapy's success resulted from what these tasks permitted the nondamaged parts of these patients' brains to do. In any event, once the deficit is clearly analyzed, it can be the focus of treatment, possibly by directly attacking it, but also possibly by devising provocative and engaging language activities in which the rest of the brain can become involved.

Should the focus of treatment be on the language that is preserved? Most clinicians use preserved language skills as the *background* for their clinical interventions with disordered aspects of language. Some smaller number put preserved language and communication in the *foreground*, focusing treatment there and exploiting what skills are left. Just as explicit analysis of the deficit should precede loss-centered approaches, specific inventories both of preserved processes of language and communication and of the contexts that maximize good performance should precede the treatment. It strikes me as entirely possible to derive a box-and-arrow model for treatment that parallels the processing models for deficits.

Potential treatments range from deblocking drills to coaching aphasic patients in the use of strategies that serve to minimize or even mask the extent of their deficits in language. It is interesting that positive changes occur in the deficits despite a focus on the preserved skills. There is practically no explanatory research on why this is so. One possibility is that such a focus reduces the amount of effortful processing, which itself often directly results from a deficit-centered struggle on the part of the patient. This in turn allows more automatic access to intact components of the language processor. For treatments of this genre, it seems particularly important to seek alternative and competing explanations of effects.

Should the focus be on the tasks that are used in treatment? One of the thorniest of issues in aphasia treatment is what appears to be a tendency on the part of many practitioners to confuse the *tasks* of treatment with the *process* of treatment. Thus, as Byng (1990) points out in a recent lecture, "PACE is viewed as a therapy technique, rather than the medium" through which the therapist teaches the patients a socially acceptable end run on a communication problem and gives them opportunities to communicate in a minimally complicated microcosm of communication. Davis (1983) refers to this tendency to treat tasks rather than patients as "pure task blindness." To legitimize the study of how good therapists go about doing what they do is a critical step in specifying adequate treatment for aphasia.

Should the focus be on the interaction between the person with aphasia and his or her environment? The patient with aphasia is not an invariant language deficit on (one or) two legs. The deficit almost always varies as a consequence of context, both linguistic and interpersonal. This variation must be accounted for in developing falsifiable theories of treatment, for one cannot escape expectations, setting, interpersonal skills, that enhance or impede communication. These are overarching concerns, affecting everything from generalizing treatment effects to modifying communication behaviors of others in the aphasic individual's environment. Not only language but also sociolinguistic and interpersonal skills should be legitimate concerns for treatment theory.

Should the focus reflect some balance of the above? In a recent paper, Byng (1990) defined the scope of aphasia treatment to include at least the following:

1. an account of the uses of language made by the aphasic patient before becoming aphasic;

2. a delineation of the nature and effects of the language deficit on the whole language system;

3. an attempt to remediate the deficit;

4. an attempt to increase the use of all other potential means of communication to support, facilitate, and compensate for the impaired language;

5. an enhancement of the remaining language;

6. an opportunity to use newly acquired and emerging language skills not only in a clinical environment but also in more natural communication situations;

7. the facilitation of adjustment to the loss of communication skills; and

8. an attempt to change the communication skills of those around the aphasic patient to accommodate the aphasia.

This is perhaps a disturbingly broad definition of aphasia treatment. Yet, if aphasic patients are to be served appropriately, each feature of this "work scope" needs to be accounted for. To do this, I have been trying to suggest that clinical intervention in aphasia will require a theory of therapy. The principles of **language therapy**, just as much as the principles of **language processing**, need to be delimited and clinically tested. Until that occurs, the motion of using a theory of the deficit to dictate the aphasia therapy offers many hints but few palliatives. No one can do this particular theoretical work for us. We have to do it for ourselves.

ACKNOWLEDGMENT

This work was supported in part by Research and Training Grant DC 01409 from the National Institute on Deafness and Other Communication Disorders.

Portions of this manuscript will appear the following publication: Holland, A., (in press). Future directions and research needs for treatment for aphasia. In Cooper, J. (Ed.), *Aphasia Therapy: Current Trends and Research Opportunities*. Bethesda, MD: NIH Monographs.

REFERENCES

Byng, S. (1988). Sentence processing deficits: Theory and therapy. *Cognitive Neuropsychology, 5*, 629–676.

Byng, S. (1990). The art and science of clinic practice in aphasia. Mary Law Memorial Lecture, London. (Unpublished.)

Caramazza, A. (1989). Cognitive neuropsychology and rehabilitation: An unfulfilled promise? In X. Seron & G. Deloche (Eds.), *Cognitive approaches in neuropsychological rehabilitation* (pp. 383–398). Hillsdale, NJ: Erlbaum.

Davis, G. A. (1983). *A survey of adult aphasia*. Englewood Cliffs, NJ: Prentice Hall.

Gilbert, J. (1992). Review of *Missing the Meaning? Journal of Speech-Language Pathology and Audiology, 16*, 54.

Helm-Estabrooks, N., & Albert, M. (1991). *Manual of aphasia therapy*. Austin TX: PRO-ED.

Hinton, G., & Shallice, T. (1991). Lesioning an attractor network: Investigations of acquired dyslexia. *Psychological Review, 98*, 74–95.

Howard, D., & Franklin, S. (1988). *Missing the meaning? A cognitive neuropsychological study of processing of words*. Cambridge, MA: MIT Press.

Morton, J., & Patterson, K. E. (1986). A new attempt at an interpretation or an attempt at a new interpretation. In M. Coltheart, K. E. Patterson, and J. C. Marshall (Eds.), *Deep dyslexia* (pp. 91–145). London: Routledge and Kegan Paul.

Wertz, R. T., Weiss, D. G., Aten, J. L., Brookshire, R. H., Garcia-Bunel, L., Holland, A., Kurtzke, J. F., LaPointe, L. L., Milianti, F. J., Brannegan, R., Greenbaum, H., Marshall, R. C., Vogel, D., Carter, J., Barnes, N. S., & Goodman, R. (1986). Comparison of clinic, home and deferred language treatment for aphasia: A Veterans Administration cooperative study. *Archives of Neurology, 43*, 653–658.

Clinical Aphasiology, Vol. 22, 1994, pp. 283–289

Model-Driven Treatment: Promises and Problems

Lee Ann C. Golper

THE "DECADE OF THE BRAIN"

Neuroscientists like to refer to the 1990s as the "Decade of the Brain." One television discussant recently described brain research in the 1990s as "the greatest intellectual guest of all time" because it promises to change the way we think about perception, learning, intelligence, and communication in the normal and damaged nervous system. Certainly, we can expect the next decade to bring continued advances in both physiologic imaging and models of brain activity. The technologies that enable us to see the brain in action, along with the application of nonlinear cognitive models, ought to lead to a more holistic and dynamic view of various cognitive processes.

In their comments at the 1991 Clinical Aphasiology Conference, McNeil, Odell, and Tseng noted the tendency for cognitive research to stay stuck within the functional architecture of the Wernicke-Lichthiem model. Cognitive-linguistic research generated in the previous two decades was preoccupied with linguistic validation for centers and pathways of the brain (McNeil, Odell, & Tseng, 1991). Those were the decades of CT scans, artificial intelligence, and neuropsychology. Cognitive-linguistic research reflected the technology and attitudes of the time—the brain was viewed with fixed images, and mental processes were discussed through analogies to computers. Psychological and neurolinguistic experimentation largely was applied to validate long-held, conventional notions about the brain's architecture.

We are now on the threshold of revolutionary changes in the neurosciences that will cause us to think differently about the brain. We are able to observe mass activity in the nervous system through computerized imaging of metabolic functions, neuroelectrical activity, blood flow, and other physiologic markers. Physiologic studies examining the brain when involved in exposure to different stimuli or involved in activities that require adaptation to experience now allow us to envision better the physical bases for cognition. Additionally, hypotheses are emerging to account for interactions in complex, dynamic brain systems using models that have what Gleick has referred to as the "right features" (Gleick, 1987, p. 299), that is, where the organizational structure itself has both stable and unstable features, and regions can be structured to have changeable boundaries.

In the February 1991 issue of *Scientific American,* Freeman illustrated neuroelectrical brain activity with what he called "phase portraits," based on computer replications of EEGs taken from a rabbit brain during the perception of odors. Freeman believed these electrical patterns demonstrated that brain activity, like other events in nature, can be studied as a system having *chaotic* properties. In science, *chaos* refers to complex behaviors or phenomena that seem random but actually have order. The formalisms of chaos theory, originated in physics and mathematics, have come to be applied to analyses of a full spectrum of natural events, from arrhythmic activity of heartbeats to changes in weather patterns. Chaos theory proposes that nature is organized with a dynamic, fluid geometry formed by the influences of "basins of attractions" (Gleick, 1987). Changeability is one of the prime characteristics of a chaotic system (Freeman, 1991). In brain research *changeability* has been demonstrated in neural patterns as a function of learning, in response to new inputs, and whenever the tendency for vast collections of neurons to shift abruptly and simultaneously from one complex activity pattern to another is observed (Freeman, 1991). The contour patterns described by Freeman demonstrate how one stimulus condition is changed following exposure to an intervening condition, thus providing evidence for how new experiences or contexts can affect subsequent perceptions. Freeman and his coworkers (Freeman, 1991; Skarda & Freeman, 1987) have suggested that chaos is what makes the brain different from artificial-intelligence machines.

If brain activity is indeed chaotic, then it is conceivable that brain damage disrupts the neurophysiologic balances, or basins of attraction, that need to be in place to maintain chaos. In a damaged state, regions that are normally active would have diminished reactivity once their interactions were disconnected, resulting in truly random, inefficient nervous system processes.

Along with the application of chaos theory to mental models, new hypotheses about the psychological side of cognition may also emerge from what Shallice (1989) called the "ultra-cognitive researchers," that is, research that has little interest in defining the neural basis of cognition (Margolin, 1992). One of the prime characteristics of the ultra-cognitive models is their proponents' stated neutrality on the issue of neuroanatomical architecture.

PROMISES

Each new piece added to the puzzle of human cognition contributes to the emerging picture of brain processes as dynamic activations that flow and change within and between multiple mental networks. We see a picture of the brain in which preserved processors, or attractors, could be manipulated and the brain "rehabilitated." Dynamic imaging and dynamic models of brain activities promise to provide both a picture and a schema of brain damage as a condition that compels rather than defies therapy.

TESTING THE MODELS

The Decade of the Brain is going to give us models of cognition and brain physiology that may or may not fit with the experiences of clinical aphasiology. Aphasia therapists need to conduct their tests or to challenge, defend, or explain treatment rationales within the context of one or another model. We are going to have to participate in shaping the framework if linguistic-cognitive models are going to come close to representing our experiences and our conceptions of aphasia and its treatment.

In his remarks in the *Archives of Neurology* regarding the future of cognitive neuropsychology, Margolin seemed to suggest that computational models, or computerized "lesion simulations," ultimately might provide a basis for cognitive rehabilitation techniques (Margolin, 1991). It is encouraging to see that a neurologist could perceive cognition to be treatable. However, theoretically-based therapeutic approaches that are equally valid and tested might be viewed as inadequate, or poor practice, if they could not be predicted by a computational model. There is a substantial amount of literature describing individuals with aphasia who improved their language performance as a function of treatment that was not model-driven (Loverso & Horner, 1991).

Fortunately, we have clinicians here and in Europe who are contributing a clinical perspective in cognitive research. At this juncture we have some hypotheses about how single words are processed, but there is a great deal of work to be done before we understand what the brain does when we speak, listen, read, and write to communicate our ideas with others.

PROBLEMS IN THE APPLICATION OF MODELS

In the past couple of years I have attempted to incorporate existing theoretical models of linguistic-cognitive processes into my clinical practice because the treatment studies built on these models are convincing. Processes and associations in theoretical models, such as those suggested by Patterson and Shewell (1987), have been helpful to me in focusing certain aspects of treatment with certain patients at certain times.

There is resistance to the use of group designs in model-based treatment reports; thus, information about some of the effects of variables one could typically examine from a large data base drawn from a heterogeneous sample is not available in their work. Additionally, the evidence for the modules and processes contained in models like Patterson and Shewell's is more substantive in some areas than in others; some parts of the map may be more accurate than other parts. Furthermore, having a map can help you find your way, but it cannot help you drive the car. Any positive outcome in aphasia treatment results partly from a fruitful focus of therapy and partly from the confidence and skills of the clinician who implements the therapy. The best outcomes probably come from clinicians who have confidence that they are doing the right things. They are sure that they are going to make a difference, and so they do.

A direct *frontal attack* on linguistic-cognitive deficits is only one aspect of the speech-language pathologist's therapy with a person with aphasia. In treatment studies we often ignore the simple truth that aphasia therapy, like aphasia, is multifaceted and has aspects that might more accurately be called psychotherapy and metacognitive or metalinguistic therapy. Treatment tasks, even those that are intended to develop automatic mental processes, frequently require getting the patients to understand why they are having the difficulties they are having, why they need to participate in what are sometimes tedious exercises, what they can consciously and routinely do to communicate better, and then getting them to do it. Also, at some point, with most patients with aphasia a prominent facet of therapy involves helping the patient work through the psychosocial adjustments necessary when living with a chronic communication impairment.

Model-driven therapy, as envisioned by its proponents, requires extensive *definitive assessment* across tasks that are balanced for control of certain variables, such as the frequency of occurrence of a given word in the language, the "wordness" of the word, the part of speech it represents, its regularity, and its concreteness. The assessment rarely uses published tests, so most of the tasks lack performance norms. Processing deficits are identified by computing the number or percent correct and then considering what chance performance might be for a given task. With the exception of rare agnosias, deficits tend to be partial losses. Consequently, this so-called definitive testing is open to a fair amount of subjective interpretation. Additionally, reading, writing, listening to, or speaking these long, balanced word lists, as well as undergoing assessment across multiple domains, can constitute an exhausting amount of testing. It is not easily or appropriately accomplished with all patients, nor is it within the constraints of some reimbursing agents.

Although I recognize that it is sometimes necessary, I find even cursory testing with an aphasic patient during the acute or early postacute period of recovery to be uncomfortable. Causing patients to focus too closely on their language deficits right after they have stared into the wide maw of their own mortality seems to be missing the point of the moment. Definitive testing may not be reasonable or appropriate in the early recovery stages.

Because processing deficits are usually partial and require an analysis of *relative* differences between areas of performance, we cannot ignore fatigue, order effects, or any other factor that might affect *reliability*. Reliability of performance and stability of the tests used should receive far more attention in the literature.

The timing of intensive, deficit-directed therapy also needs to be investigated, especially with the more severely impaired patient. Efficacy has been demonstrated with the stable, chronically aphasic patient, who may be several years post injury, but access to treatment is often determined by financial constraints, and for the majority of patients, access can diminish with chronicity, when there is a reduction of third-party payment for treatment once the patient has *recovered* from the neurological insult.

CONCLUSION

There is nothing novel about the idea that language therapy should be driven by theories about cognition. The writings and work of Head, Wepman, Goldstein, Schuell, and others support the notion that linguistic impairment results secondarily from a processing impairment (Martin, 1981). What we are discovering is evidence for what those impairments might be and how cognitive resources, or, perhaps chaos within the nervous system might serve to allow us and our patients to comprehend and express messages. In this decade and into the next millennium the best ideas coming from an array of neurosciences might ultimately map brain physiology to mental processes.

Over a decade ago, A. Damien Martin asked us to consider the role of theory in our therapy. In the September 1981 issue of *Topics in Language Disorders,* Martin said that language behavior can be described with reference to cognitive processing. In the model he proposed, cognition has an integrated, hierarchical organization that is cybernetic and interrelated in its nature and contains processes that occur in parallel with one another. He described how interrelated and parallel scanning processes might be involved in word retrieval. He suggested that we consider, for example, the ease or difficulty of lexical access when we design articulatory tasks for the patient with a phonological expressive disorder.

Martin said that language as a *code* is an artifact, and therefore, the code *itself* is not impaired by damage to the processing organism. He reminded us that aphasic speakers use language pretty much the same way as normal speakers do but in a reduced and less efficient manner. Finally, he suggested that the more detailed and explicit the model of cognitive processing, the more detailed and explicit the diagnostic hypotheses and the therapeutic goals may be. My own ideas and loosely conceived theory for aphasia treatment originally came in part from the writings and presentations made over a decade ago by Dr. A. Damien Martin. I continue to appreciate both his insight and his foresight. He, like Loverso and Horner (1991), pointed out that an absence of overt theory in our work and in our research is, at the very least, scientifically undesirable. Suggested models for aphasia treatment that are based on prevailing theories of linguistic-cognitive processes can provide an overt rationale for certain aspects of therapy. Treatment theories will always benefit from more clinical trials, more discussion and elaboration, and from constant input from clinicians. Treatment models should, and will, be drawn and redrawn in response to new information and influences so that we can continue to structure aphasia therapy for the best possible outcome.

ACKNOWLEDGMENT

This work was supported in part by the Mary and Mason Rudd Teaching Endowment, Jewish Hospital and the Department of Surgery, University of Louisville.

REFERENCES

Freeman, W. J. (1991, February). The physiology of perception. *Scientific American,* pp. 78–85.
Gleick, J. (1987). *Chaos: Making a new science.* New York: Penguin Books.
Loverso, F., & Horner, J. (1991). Models of aphasia theory in *Clinical Aphasiology.* In T. E. Prescott (Ed.), *Clinical aphasiology,* Vol. 20 (pp. 61–75). Austin, TX: PRO-ED.
Margolin, D. I. (1991). Cognitive neuropsychology: Resolving enigmas about Wernicke's aphasia and other higher cognitive cortical disorders. *Archives of Neurology, 48,* 751–765.
Margolin, D. I. (1992). *Cognitive neuropsychology in clinical practice.* New York: Oxford University Press.

Martin, A. D. (1981). The role of theory in therapy: A rationale. *Topics in Language Disorders, 1* (4), 63–72.

McNeil, M. R., Odell, K., & Tseng, C-H. (1991). Toward a theory of resource allocation into a general theory of aphasia. In T. E. Prescott (Ed.), *Clinical aphasiology,* Vol. 20 (pp. 21–39). Austin, TX: PRO-ED.

Patterson, K., & Shewell, C. (1987). Speak and spell: Dissociations and word-class effects. In M. Coltheart, R. Job, & G. Sartori (Eds.), *The cognitive neuropsychology of language.* London: Lawrence Erlbaum.

Shallice, T. (1989). *From neuropsychology to mental structure.* Cambridge: Cambridge University Press.

Skarda, C. A., & Freeman, W. J. (1987). How brains make chaos in order to make sense of the world. *Behavioral and Brain Sciences, 10*(2), 161–195.

Clinical Aphasiology, Vol. 22, 1994, pp. 291–305

The Use of Linguistic Theory as a Framework for Treatment Studies in Aphasia

Lewis P. Shapiro and Cynthia K. Thompson

This paper outlines the theoretical underpinnings of a linguistic-specific treatment program for aphasia. It opens with some introductory comments about why we think linguistic theory should be taken seriously as a possible framework for investigations of normal and disordered language. Then, it presents an overview of some current linguistic theory and briefly shows how linguistic constructs borrowed from such a theory appear to affect both lexical and sentence processing in normal and brain-damaged adults. Finally, it reviews some recent treatment literature and shows how linguistic theory can be used to devise treatment programs. Given the uniqueness of our treatment approach, however, we must initially offer only promissory notes and await some considerable data before our program can be fully evaluated. We have begun this data-gathering process (see Thompson, Shapiro, & Roberts, 1993; Thompson & Shapiro, 1992), and our initial results look promising.

Effective language research, including work in psycholinguistics, neurolinguistics, and language treatment studies, requires knowing as much as possible about the object of inquiry—language. The most proper characterization of language comes from formal linguistic theory. As a point of logic, if one discovers that certain constructs from linguistic theory have "processing reality"—that is, affect lexical and sentence processing in normal subjects—and assumes that a brain-damaged language system reflects an impaired version of the normal system, then one needs to control and manipulate in treatment those aspects of language that affect the normal system. The beauty of formal linguistic theory lies in its explicitness; it offers language scientists a way to understand the nature of the material used in their experimental manipulations.

This approach should be considered regardless of any concomitant theory of the language disorder in aphasia. For example, if you support the notion that an attentional impairment underlies the language disorder, you should probably manipulate those linguistic structures in your research that you hypothesize might tax sustained attention. Relatedly, if you support the notion that there is an underlying memory deficit in some language disorders, it appears necessary to understand how linguistic structures and parsing routines might affect *sentence memory*. This is the only way in which to understand the underlying memory requirements of the sentence processor (see, for example, Shapiro, McNamara, Zurif, Lanzoni, & Cermak, 1992). If you support the notion that agrammatic Broca's aphasia involves a parsing disorder, you must manipulate those structures relevant to your hypotheses (see, for example, Zurif & Swinney, in press). Finally, if you support a computational complexity deficit in Broca's aphasia (see, for example, Frazier & Friederici, 1991), then you need a theory of what it means for language to be computationally complex. The point is that if linguistic theory is not exploited in the work of language scientists undertaking treatment research, then explictness will give way to vague intuitions about language, and greater generalizations may be missed.

A BRIEF REVIEW OF SOME LINGUISTIC THEORY

Lexical Properties

Our approach borrows from the government-binding framework (Chomsky, 1986), but with some modifications, several other linguistic theories might be equally useful.[1] Critical to our approach are the *mental lexicon* and the kinds of information in a lexical entry that must be represented with the phonological form of a lexical item. For example, our grammatical intuitions tell us that the verb *hit* allows a direct object noun phrase (NP) to follow it; the verb *give*, if followed by a direct object NP, also requires a prepositional phrase (PP); and the verb *sleep* does not require a direct object NP. That is, when we acquire these labels (*hit, give,* and *sleep*) and what these labels refer to in the real world, we also acquire the knowledge that they

---

1. Government-binding theory contains several subtheories and modules, including x-bar theory (concerned with phrasal geometry); the theory of move-alpha (transformations); binding theory (antecedent-referent relations); bounding theory (constraints on movement); control theory (concerned with the controller of certain "empty categories"); case theory (abstract case); theta theory (the assignment of thematic roles); and the theory of empty categories (governing traces, etc.) In this paper we will summarize only those aspects of GB theory that are relevant to our present approach. For further information we refer the reader to Liliane Haegeman's (1991) *Introduction to Government and Binding Theory*.

can—and sometimes must—occur in particular structures. This phrasal (and clausal) information is known formally as *strict subcategorization*. Part of this subcategorization information is predictable from the real world contingencies of language use. For example, when you learn the label for the concept of *hit*, you also learn that the object of *hit* is *affected* by the "hitting"; when you learn the label for the concept of *give*, you learn that you have to give something to someone and that the action of giving something to someone entails a *path* along which the object metaphorically travels. This type of information is reflected in *lexical conceptual structure* (roughly, "semantics"). By some accounts (Jackendoff, 1990), the theory of lexical conceptual structure encompasses the notions of *thematic roles* (e.g., Agent-of-action, Theme-of-action, Goal-of-action, Experiencer, etc.) and *argument structure* (either a set of indices that relate the semantic/thematic roles to the syntax or an indication of the number of *logical arguments* or participants—usually described by NPs—entailed by a predicate). On other accounts, argument structure forms a level of representation separate from that of conceptual structure (Grimshaw, 1990). For our present purposes, we will use the term *argument structure* generically to describe the semantic/thematic information about a predicate.

The verb *hit*, for example, requires two participants, each occupying an *argument position* in the sentence. One of these arguments is assigned the role of Agent, and the other argument is assigned the role of Theme:

1. [Joelle$_{Agent}$] hit [the ball$_{Theme}$];

the verb *give* requires three arguments, the final argument having the role of Goal:

2. [Joelle$_{Agent}$] gave [the ball$_{Theme}$] to [Zack$_{Goal}$];

and the verb *sleep* requires only one argument, the subject:

3. [Joelle$_{Experiencer}$] slept.

With this argument structure information, the lexical representation for *hit*, for example, looks something like that in Example 4:

4. *hit* V: lexical category
  /HIT/: phonology
  [____ NP]: strict subcategorization
  (Agent/Theme): argument structure

The entry in Example 4 expresses both the syntactic and general semantic character of a sentence in which the lexical item is contained.

Let us now briefly consider how these lexical properties are reflected in the syntax. Again, the verb *hit* requires one and only one direct object NP. This lexical property is reflected in the sentences of Example 5:

5a. Joelle hit the ball.
  b. Joelle hit Zack.
  c. *Joelle hit.
  d. *Joelle hit the ball Zack.

Sentences 5a and 5b are acceptable and well formed because the verb *hit* is followed in both cases by one NP. Sentence 5c is unacceptable and ill formed because there is no NP following the verb. And Sentence 5d is unacceptable because there are two NPs following the verb. To be more specific, any adequate grammatical theory should be able not only to describe why any given sentence is grammatical in a language but also formally to rule out ungrammatical sentences. Much of this work is done by the interaction of the lexicon and the sentence via the *Projection Principle:* Lexical properties are observed at all levels of syntax.

Consider again the sentences in Example 5. The lexical entry in Example 4 reflects what we know about the verb *hit*, that it entails a direct object NP position to which the role of Theme can be assigned. The projection principle requires that this lexical property be syntactically represented. The verb *theta-marks* its arguments; that is, it assigns its thematic roles the argument positions in the sentence. Skipping the details, *hit* (and the VP it heads) has two thematic roles to assign—Agent to the subject argument and Theme to the object argument. Thus, Sentences 5a and 5b are well formed because there are two argument positions represented in the syntax. On the other hand, Sentence 5c is ill formed and rendered ungrammatical by the projection principle because the lexical properties for *hit* are not satisfied in the sentence; there is no direct object position in the sentence to which the role of Theme can be assigned. Sentence 5d also violates the Projection Principle because there are two NPs following the verb; the lexical properties of *hit* require only one. In this way, lexical information and the Projection Principle largely determine the syntactic structure of a sentence. We will show later that these linguistic properties indeed have processing and treatment significance.

Syntactic Properties

Consider now some wh-questions containing the verb *hit:*

6a. What did Joelle hit?
  b. Whom did Joelle hit?

c. *What did Joelle hit Zack?
d. *Who did Joelle hit the ball?

The sentences in Example 6 appear to present a problem. Note that our generalization about the sentences in Example 5 makes exactly the wrong predictions about the sentences in Example 6. That is, our knowledge of English has told us that a sentence containing the verb *hit* must have a direct object NP coming directly after the verb for that sentence to be grammatical, as in Sentences 5a and 5b. Sentences 6a and 6b do not seem to have direct object NPs after the verb, yet they seem well formed by any native English speaker's grammatical intuitions. Perhaps even worse, Sentences 6c and 6d do seem to have the required direct object NP position, yet they are ill formed. The theory is either wrong or needs to be extended to explain these grammatical facts.

One possibility is that our generalization about *hit*—that it must take a direct object—was simply wrong, but this possibility conflicts with what we know about *hit*, that there is always some affected object of the action. So let us assume that there is indeed a direct object position in Sentences 6a and 6b and that the wh-word originated in that position and moved to sentence-initial position by a *transformation*. The structure that exists before the wh-word is moved is called the *underlying* or *D(eep)-structure*, and that which exists after the wh-word is moved is called the *S(urface)-structure*.

A first approximation of the underlying structure in Sentence 6a is shown in Example 7:[2]

7.

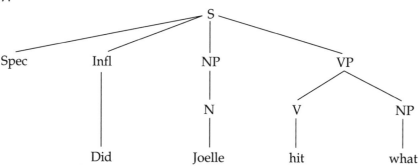

Note that this underlying structure is consistent with our generalization that the verb *hit* requires one and only one direct object NP position (occupied in the underlying structure by *what*). On most accounts, the-

---

2. The phrasal geometry shown in Examples 7 and 8 are simplifications; they have a flatter structure and contain node labels that are quite different from that proposed by more current theory. For present purposes we can ignore these differences.

matic role assignment takes place at D-structure, so that, again, the role of Theme is assigned to the direct object position and Agent is assigned to the subject NP. The *wh-movement* rule—a transformation—applies to the underlying structure in Example 7 and transforms it to the S-structure in Example 8:

8.

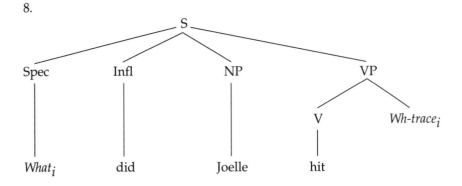

The structure in Example 8 shows that the NP *(what)* has moved from the postverb direct object position in the underlying structure to the sentence-initial position in S-structure. The moved constituent leaves behind a *trace* of its movement, which is *coindexed* with its *antecedent*, the wh-word. The trace serves as the direct object argument position, one that, again, is required by the lexical properties of *hit*. The trace and its antecedent form a *theta-chain* such that the moved constituent (in this case, *What)* inherits its thematic role (the Theme) from its trace. Now we can explain the grammaticality of Sentences 6a and 6b by claiming that both the under-lying- and surface-structure representations of the sentences contain the direct object positions required by the lexical properties of *hit* and the Projection Principle.

Passive sentences in the government-binding framework undergo simi-lar grammatical mechanics:

9. Zack was hit by Joelle.

Example 9, like the wh-questions in Example 6, does not have a phono-logically filled direct object NP position occurring after the verb. Addi-tionally, a general property of all sentences is that they must have subjects, regardless of the argument structure of the verb. This property, along with the stipulation that lexical information must be represented at all levels of syntax, is termed the *Extended Projection Principle (EPP)*. Given this principle and the lexical properties of *hit*, consider the D- and S-structures for Example 9, shown in Examples 10 and 11:

10. *e* was hit Zack by Joelle (D-structure)
11. Zack$_i$ was hit *NP trace$_i$* by Joelle (S-structure)

The *empty category (e)* in the underlying structure of Example 10 is required by the EPP. Skipping many details, the direct object NP *(Zack)* is forced to move into the empty category position (because of the lack of structural Case, which has been "absorbed" by the passive morphology), leaving behind an *NP trace.*

Thus, there are two kinds of movement subsumed under the general rule *move-alpha,* wh-, and NP-movement. Again, NP-movement occurs in the derivation of the passive (and in so-called NP-raising structures). NP-movement moves an NP from an argument position (in the passive, the direct object position) to another argument position (the subject position), leaving behind an NP-trace. In effect, both the site from which the constituent moves and its "landing site" are positions projected from the verb's lexical representation. Wh-movement derives wh-questions, relative clauses (e.g., "The man$_i$ that the bully hit *trace$_i$* was tall"), and relative clefts (e.g., "It was Popeye$_i$ that$_i$ Bluto hit *trace$_i$*"). Unlike NP-movement, wh-movement involves displacement of wh-phrases from argument positions (e.g., direct object) to *nonargument positions* (e.g., Specifier of COMP), leaving behind a wh-trace. Thus, unlike NP-movement, wh-movement involves a landing site that falls outside those positions projected by the verb's entry. Finally, another difference between NP-movement (specifically, the passive only) and wh-movement involves the distance between the trace and its antecedent. Consider the simplified structures in Examples 12 and 13:

12. [$_S$ [$_{NP}$ the boy]$_i$ was hit [$_{NP}$ *trace*]$_i$ by [$_{NP}$ the girl]]
13. It was [$_{NP}$ the boy]$_i$ [$_S$[who]$_i$ [$_S$ [$_{NP}$ the girl] hit [$_{NP}$ *trace*]$_i$]]

Note Example 12 shows that only one S node intervenes between the trace and its antecedent in the passive, yet in the object cleft (Example 13) both a more dominant S-bar node and an embedded S node intervene. We will show that this distinction between wh- and NP-movement derived structures has processing and treatment implications.

Arguments and Adjuncts

Related to the notion that verbs project their lexical properties onto syntax is the distinction between an argument of the verb and an *adjunct.* Again, an argument of the verb is entailed by the verb's meaning or conceptual structure; it is idiosyncratic to the verb and is thus represented with the verb's phonological form in the lexical entry. The argument position is assigned a thematic role by the verb or its VP. An adjunct, however, is not selected by the verb; it can appear with any verb in the language and thus need not be specified as part of the verb's lexical entry. Subsequently, the adjunct is not theta-marked by the verb. Consider, for example, the prepositional phrases in Examples 14 and 15:

14. Mitzi sent the car *to the garage.*
15. Mitzi fixed the car *in the garage.*

In Example 14, the verb *send* allows three arguments: Agent is assigned to the subject NP *Mizi,* Theme is assigned to the direct object NP *the car,* and Goal is assigned to the indirect object NP *the garage* that forms part of the PP. That is, you have to "send something to *someone* or *somewhere*," and thus the Goal is implied—and supplied—directly by the verb. In Example 15, however, the PP *(in the garage)* is considered a locative adjunct; it's meaning is not inherent in the verb's representation. Though you indeed have to "fix something somewhere," that fact cannot be inferred from the verb but instead is supplied by additional material in the sentence—the adjunct PP. Thus, an adjunct is always optional, whereas an argument can be either obligatory (e.g., "John gave the ball *to Mary,*" where "*John gave the ball" is ungrammatical if the third argument is omitted) or optional (e.g., "Mitzi sent the letter," where, though the third argument is omitted, it is still implied). Finally, an adjunct can be ambiguous, whereas an argument rarely is. In Example 15, for example, *in the garage* is structurally ambiguous; it can either modify the direct object NP *the car* (as in "it was the car in the garage [and not the car outside the garage] that Mitzi fixed"), or it can modify the VP *fixed the car* (as in "it was in the garage [and not in the driveway] where Mitzi fixed the car"). There are no interpretive or attachment ambiguities involving the PP *to the garage* in Example 14; it is the Goal of where the car was sent.

SENTENCE PROCESSING

Recent psycholinguistic and neurolinguistic work has shown that virtually all these theoretical constructs have lexical- and sentence-processing implications. For example, in a series of psycholinguistic studies, Shapiro and colleagues (Shapiro, Brookins, Gordon, & Nagel, 1991; Shapiro, Zurif, & Grimshaw, 1987, 1989) found that a verb's lexical properties (e.g., thematic representations/lexical conceptual structure) directly affect sentence processing. That is, as the verb becomes more complex in terms of number of different argument structure arrangements, processing load increases in the immediate temporal vicinity of the verb. For example, the verb *fix* allows only one two-place argument structure (Agent/Theme, as in "Rico fixed the toilet"), whereas the verb *send* allows both a two-place (Agent/ Theme, as in "Phil sent the message") and a three-place structure (Agent/ Theme/Goal, as in "Phil sent the message to Pepe"). When embedded in simple NP-V-NP structures, *send* yields a greater processing load than *fix*. In effect, all possible argument structures associated with a verb are momentarily and exhaustively activated when the verb is accessed.

In a more recent effort, Shapiro, Nagel, and Levine (in press) found that, given a verb with multiple argument structure possibilities, a subject's preferences for one of these possibilities might then be used to determine the initial course the parser takes after encountering the verb. In this study we also found some indications that adjuncts are more computationally expensive than arguments of the verb; that is, processing load increased in the immediate temporal vicinity of a preposition heading an adjunct PP (as in, for example "The old man sent the toy *in the box*") relative to a preposition heading a PP that contains an argument (as in "The old man sent the toy *to the girl*").

Agrammatic Broca's aphasic patients normally activate a verb's multiple argument structure possibilities in the immediate vicinity of the verb (Shapiro & Levine, 1990). This result implies that verb properties need to be controlled in language experiments, including treatment research, because these properties are projected from the lexicon to the syntax and indeed have direct consequences on online performance. Importantly, Broca's aphasic patients also seem able to use this lexical information as a way "into" the sentence production system (Canseco-Gonzalez, Shapiro, Zurif, & Baker, 1991). However, such patients appear to have difficulty with sentences where arguments have been moved out of their canonical positions (Grodzinsky, 1990; Schwartz, Linebarger, Saffron, & Pate, 1987), as in, for example, passives, wh-questions, and relative clause constructions.

There is also a large body of evidence suggesting that the antecedent to a trace (the moved NP, for example) is normally reactivated in the immediate vicinity of the trace, well after the moved constituent has appeared in the sentence (see, for example, Frazier, 1987, for a review). Again, however, in sentences with moved arguments, agrammatic Broca's patients may not reactivate the antecedent to a trace at the right time for normal thematic role assignment to occur (Zurif & Swinney, 1992). Finally, it also appears that wh- and NP-movement may each have its own processing routines: More "work" must be done to attach an antecedent to a wh-trace (i.e., in wh-questions or relative clauses) than to an NP trace (i.e., in a passive sentence) because a wh-trace and its antecedent are separated by clausal boundaries (see, e.g., Berwick and Weinberg, 1984). Indeed, such a distinction between the movement types shows up in aphasic performance (Caplan and Hildebrandt, 1988) and in the sentence production performance of amnesic patients and their controls (Shapiro et al., 1992). Better performance is observed on sentences derived from NP-movement relative to wh-movement.

These facts argue for using a principled account of grammatical representations when investigating normal and disordered sentence processing and, subsequently, when devising treatment programs. For example, fully specified lexical entries seem to be available at D-structure for some, if not all, Broca's aphasic patients; the problem for some of these patients lies either in the derivation of the S-structure representations (e.g., traces; see Grodzinsky, 1990) or in the sentence-processing routines computing these representations (see, for example, Prather, Shapiro, Zurif, & Swinney, 1991; Schwartz et al., 1987; Zurif & Swinney, in press). We exploit this obvious strength and purported weakness in our treatment experiments. We also consider the representational similarities and differences underlying the surface realizations of sentences used in our treatment program— similarities and differences that can be explained only by reference to linguistic theory (Thompson et al., 1993; Thompson and Shapiro, 1994).

With our linguistic and psycholinguistic perspective in mind, consider now a brief review of some recent treatment literature.

TREATMENT RESEARCH

Recent studies concerned with treatment of sentence-level disorders have begun to consider both the nature of aphasic language deficits and what is known about normal sentence processing (Byng, 1988; Jones, 1986; Loverso, Prescott, & Selinger, 1986, 1992; Mitchum, in press; Saffran, Schwartz, Fink, Meyers, & Martin, in press; Thompson, in press). For example, Byng (1988), Jones (1986), and Saffran et al. (in press) developed treatments for aphasia based on the "mapping hypothesis," which holds that agrammatic performance reflects an impaired mapping between grammatical constituents (e.g., subject, object) and thematic roles (e.g., Agent/Theme) (Schwartz et al., 1987). In these studies treatment was provided largely for chronic, long-term Broca's aphasic patients who were claimed to have a "mapping" deficit. Using color-coded materials corresponding to sentence constituents, patients were trained to recognize the thematic roles of noun phrases set around the verbs in sentences in both canonical (active NP-V-NP sentences) and noncanonical sentences by responding to questions of the form "Who did what to whom." Generalization both within and across sentence types was claimed for some subjects.

Though we fully agree with the intent of these studies, the experimental designs used fall short of those required in a controlled treatment study. That is, internal validity was not demonstrated. For example, Byng (1988) presented case studies for two subjects, reporting only pre- and posttreatment data, without control subjects or a controlled single-subject design. Saffron et al. (in press) attempted to incorporate a single-subject research design, but experimental control was lost when shifts in baseline performance were noted on untrained sentence types. In addition, subjects in both studies exhibited high performance rates prior to treatment, allowing little opportunity for changes to occur on the dependent measures; the lack of repeated measurement precluded examination of the variability within and across phases of the experiments; and, importantly, changes in the independent variables and in the manner by which the dependent measures were tested were made throughout the course of the experiments.

Further, in Saffron et al., a pretraining phase was instituted whereby patients were trained to understand wh-questions necessary for the subsequent training phase. As noted by the investigators, however, wh-questions are problematic for these patients. Indeed, according to the "mapping" hypothesis, the same deficit contributes to the problems these patients have in understanding both wh-questions and the sentences that were targets for treatment; that is, both sentence types are derived from noncanonical thematic role assignment. Nonetheless, to reap the benefits of the treatment the patients had to understand the wh-questions in the pretraining phase.

These design issues aside, none of the treatment studies of which we are aware has considered recent findings from the psycholinguistic literature. For example, though both Byng and Mitchum use Garrett's (1982) sentence production model as a base for treatment programs, the representations and processes underlying "functional" and "positional" frames in the model were never clearly specified. As we have claimed in this paper, the psycholinguistic literature is now rife with examples that such issues as lexical properties and their access and integration into the syntax, arguments versus adjuncts, phrasal density, inferential chains consisting of traces and their antecedents, and so on all affect normal and aphasic sentence processing to some degree. Such linguistic constructs have not been used to fill in the gaps of Garrett's model, nor have they been controlled or manipulated in treatment studies.

Finally, one recent treatment program has used linguistic theory as a guide. Loverso and colleagues' "cueing verb treatment" (CVT) (Loverso et al., 1986, 1992) uses case grammar (Fillmore, 1968) as a basis for a treatment program for producing simple sentence structures. Case grammar, whose constructs have found their way into more modern approaches to lexical representation (see, for example, Jackendoff, 1990), considers the verb as the "motor" of the sentence's propositional structure. Loverso et al. have designed a treatment program that first trains the verb and then, in a series of graduated steps, attempts to expand the verb to include both its subject and, depending on the type of verb, either its object or a location, adverbial of time, instrument, etc. The sentence expansion is produced by clinician controlled use of wh-words (e.g., "who run" written on index cards yields patient initiated "I run," "who run when" yields "I run yesterday," "who hit" yields "I hit," etc.). The investigators claimed generalization given increases in *Porch Index of Communicative Ability* (PICA) subtest scores. (So far as we are aware, however, generalization to untrained verb and verb-argument combinations was not assessed in their experimental design. Whether these subjects would show such generalization remains unanswered).

The generalization issue aside, from our present perspective Loverso and colleagues should be commended for devising perhaps the first treatment program that considered the influence of lexical properties on sentence generation. Their approach in its current status, however, is limited to the production of simple sentences, and, not unlike the Saffron et al. program, the use of *wh*-words to elicit the simple sentences may be problematic for some patients. Furthermore, though their materials were controlled for frequency of occurrence, imagery, and concreteness, the verbs themselves were not controlled for the number and types of arguments they entailed. These verbs included, for example, pure intransitives that do not allow direct object NPs, like *run* and *look*; "psychological" verbs like *think, feel,* and *like*; two-place transitive verbs like *hit* and *read*; datives like *write* and *buy*; and obligatory three-place verbs like *give*. Again, we know from the recent psycholinguistic literature that the lexical properties of verbs have direct consequences in sentence comprehension and production; thus it may be necessary to initially control for these properties when devising treatment programs.

To the best of our knowledge, the treatment literature thus contains few instances of studies that have seriously considered the linguistic and psycholinguistic underpinnings of sentence targets. In developing our present treatment approach, we considered, for example, the data derived by Wambaugh and Thompson (1989), who examined the effects of training *wh*-interrogative production in agrammatic patients. Questions like "What is he cooking?" (derived from "He is cooking *a steak,*" for example) and "Where is he sleeping?" (derived from "He is sleeping *in the park*") were trained because of their *surface* similarities. Results indicated that although generalization within *wh*-structures occurred (i.e., from trained *what* constructions to untrained *what* constructions), generalization across *wh*-structures (i.e., from *what* to untrained *where* constructions) was negligible.

Again, from our present perspective, generalization across wh-forms may not have occurred because the verbs *cook* and *sleep* have very different lexical properties. *Cook* is a transitive verb allowing a direct object NP argument to which the role of Theme is assigned (for example, you cook *the steak*); *sleep* is a pure intransitive verb not allowing a direct object NP. Indeed, the locative phrase *in the park* that is the focus of the *where* question is an adjunct of the verb, not an argument. Because these verbs differ in their underlying thematic properties, it follows that the sentence structures in which these verbs are contained will also have different D- and S-structure representations. We suggest therefore that these differences in *what* and *where* interrogatives—distinctions having to do with the lexical properties of verbs—were reflected in the lack of generalization noted by Wambaugh and Thompson. If this postulate is correct, *wh*-interrogatives that use verbs with *similar* lexical properties would be better candidates for generalization. For example, we would predict generalization from *what* interrogatives to *who* because verbs that enter into both of these can take a direct object NP to which the role of Theme can be assigned. *Wh*-movement would then apply, yielding *wh*-interrogatives with similar S-structure and surface realizations as in, for example, "She is fixing *the car*" yielding "*What* is she fixing?" and "She is hitting *the boy*" yielding "*Who* is she hitting?"

We have recently begun a treatment program that controls for just these variables, and we think our program of research, takes the investigation of generalization a big step further. Again, consider that in our linguistic framework there are two types of constituent movement: *NP*- and *wh*-movement. We are not only examining generalization patterns across different kinds of *wh*-questions, but we are also examining whether generalization occurs across different sentence structures that rely on the same rule for their derivations, *even though the surface realizations of these sentences will be very different* (see Thompson et al., in press; Thompson and Shapiro, 1992).

We have outlined a theoretical approach to treatment that takes linguistic theory seriously as the proper description of language. We have attempted to show that the constructs born from the minds of theoretical linguists have consequences for the production and comprehension of sentences in both normal and brain-damaged populations. Finally, we have claimed that it is time for these facts to be considered in treatment research, and we offer one such program as our initial attempt in this enterprise.

ACKNOWLEDGMENT

Some of the research reported here was supported by NIH Grants DC00494 and DC01809.

REFERENCES

Berwick, R. D., & Weinberg, A. (1984). *The grammatical basis of linguistic performance: Language use and acquisition.* Cambridge, MA: MIT Press.

Byng, S. (1988). Sentence processing deficits: Theory and therapy. *Cognitive Neuropsychology, 5,* 629–676.

Canseco-Gonzalez, E., Shapiro, L. P., Zurif, E. B., Baker, E. (1991). Lexical argument structure representations and their role in translation across cognitive domains. *Brain and Language, 40,* 384–392.

Caplan, D., & Hildebrandt, N. (1988). *Disorders of syntactic comprehension.* Cambridge, MA: MIT Press.

Chomsky, N. (1986). *Barriers.* Cambridge, MA: MIT Press.

Fillmore, C. J. (1968). The case for case. In E. Boch & R. T. Harms (Eds.), *Universals of Linguistic Theory,* 1–88.

Frazier, L. (1987). Sentence processing: A tutorial review. In M. Coltheart (Ed.), *Attention and performance XII.* Hillsdale, NJ: Lawrence Erlbaum.

Frazier, L. & Friederici, A. (1991). On deriving the properties of agrammatic comprehension. *Brain and Language, Vol. 40,* 151–166.

Garrett, M. (1982). The organization of processing structure for language production: Implications for aphasic speech. In M. S. Arbib & D. Caplan (Eds.), *Neural models of language processes.* New York: Academic Press.

Grimshaw, J. (1990). *Argument structure.* Cambridge, MA: MIT Press.

Grodzinsky, Y. (1990). *Theoretical perspectives on language deficits.* Cambridge, MA: MIT Press.

Haegeman, L. (1991). *Introduction to government and binding theory.* Cambridge, MA: Blackwell.

Jackendoff, R. (1990). *Semantic structures.* Cambridge, MA: MIT Press.

Jones, E. V. (1986). Building the foundations for sentence production in a nonfluent aphasic. *British Journal of Disorders of Communication, 21,* 63–82.

Loverso, F. L., Prescott, T. E., & Selinger, M. (1986). Cueing verbs: A treatment strategy for aphasic adults. *Journal of Rehabilitation Research, 25,* 47–60.

Loverso, F. L., Prescott, T. E., & Selinger, M. (1992). Microcomputer treatment in aphasiology. *Aphasiology, 6,* 155–163.

Mitchum, C. C., (1992). Treatment generalization and the application of cognitive neuropsychological models in aphasia therapy. In: NIDCD Monograph, *Aphasia treatment: Current approaches and research opportunities.* Bethesda, MD: National Institutes of Health/National Institute on Deafness and Other Communication Disorders.

Prather, P., Shapiro, L. P., Zurif, E. B., & Swinney, D. (1991). Real-time examination of lexical processing in aphasia. *Journal of Psycholinguistic Research, 23,* 271–281.

Saffran, E. M., Schwarz, M. F., Fink, R., Meyers, J., & Martin, N. (1992). Mapping therapy: An approach to remediating agrammatic sentence comprehension and production. In: NIDCD Monograph, *Aphasia treatment: Current approaches and research opportunities.* Bethesda, MD: National Institutes of Health/National Institute on Deafness and Other Communication Disorders.

Schwartz, M. F., Linebarger, M., Saffron, E. M., & Pate, D. (1987). Syntactic transparency and sentence interpretation in aphasia. *Language and Cognitive Processes, 2,* 85–113.

Shapiro, L. P., Brookins, B., Gordon, B., & Nagel, H. N. (1991). Verb effects during sentence processing. *Journal of Experimental Psychology: Learning, Memory, and Cognition, 17,* 983–996.

Shapiro, L. P., & Levine, B. A. (1990). Verb processing during sentence comprehension in aphasia. *Brain and Language, 38,* 21–47.

Shapiro, L. P., McNamara, P., Zurif, E. B., Lanzoni, S., & Cermak, L. (1992). Processing complexity and sentence memory: Evidence from amnesia. *Brain and Language, 42,* 431–453.

Shapiro, L. P., Nagel, H. N., & Levine, B. A. (In press). Preferences for a verb's complements and their use in sentence processing. *Journal of Memory and Language.*

Shapiro, L. P., Zurif, E. B., & Grimshaw, J. (1987). Sentence processing and the mental representation of verbs. *Cognition, 27,* 219–246.

Shapiro, L. P., Zurif, E. B., & Grimshaw, J. (1989). Verb representation and sentence processing: Contextual impenetrability. *Journal of Psycholinguistic Research, 18,* 223–243.

Thompson, C. K. (1992). A neurolinguistic approach to sentence production treatment and generalization research in aphasia. In: NIDCD Monograph, *Aphasia treatment: Current approaches and research opportunities.* Bethesda, MD: National Institutes of Health/National Institute on Deafness and Other Communication Disorders.

Thompson, C. K., & Shapiro, L. P. (1994). A linguistic-specific approach to treatment of sentence production deficits in aphasia. In M. L. Lemme (Ed.), *Clinical Aphasiology* (Vol. 22, pp. 307–323). Austin, TX: PRO-ED.

Thompson, C. K., Shapiro, L. P., & Roberts, M. (1993). Treatment of sentence production deficits in aphasia: A linguistic-specific approach to wh-interrogative training and generalization. *Aphasiology, 7,* 111–133.

Wambaugh, J., & Thompson, C. K. (1989). Training and generalization of agrammatic aphasic adults' wh-interrogative productions. *Journal of Speech and Hearing Disorders, 54,* 509–525.

Zurif, E. B., & Swinney, D. (In press). The neuropsychology of language. In M. A. Gernsbacher (Ed.), *Handbook of Psycholinguistics.* New York: Academic Press.

Clinical Aphasiology, Vol. 22, 1994, pp. 307–323

A Linguistic-Specific Approach to Treatment of Sentence Production Deficits in Aphasia

Cynthia K. Thompson and Lewis P. Shapiro

Over the years, a number of researchers have undertaken research concerned with treatment of sentence-level deficits in aphasic individuals (e.g., Byng, 1988; Doyle, Goldstein, & Bourgeois, 1987; Helm-Estabrooks, Fitzpatrick, & Barresi, 1981; Helm-Estabrooks & Ramsberger, 1986; Jones, 1986; Kearns & Salmon, 1984; LeDorze, Jacobs, & Coderre, 1991; Loverso, Prescott, & Selinger, 1987, 1992; Mitchum, 1992; Naeser, 1975; Saffran, Schwartz, Fink, Meyers, & Martin, 1992; Thompson & McReynolds, 1986; Wambaugh & Thompson, 1989; and others). Findings derived from these investigations have shown that aphasic subjects can rather easily be retrained to produce certain sentences noted to be difficult for them. Unfortunately, limited generalization to untrained sentence types results from this training. For example, training such selected sentences as imperative transitives, wh-interrogatives, and passives does not yield observed, generalization across sentences. With few exceptions (namely, Byng, 1988; Jones, 1986; Loverso et al., 1992; and Saffran et al., 1992), most of this work has focused treatment only on the surface realization of sentences, with little attention given to underlying representational and processing antecedents that might have resulted in the sentence production deficits noted.

Inasmuch as surface realizations result from an underlying linguistic representation (i.e., D[eep]-structure) (Chomsky, 1981, 1986), we postulate that treatment focused on this underlying form, in which the linguistic and psycholinguistic underpinnings of sentences targeted for treatment are controlled, may result in successful generalization across sentence structures sharing similar linguistic properties. That is, treatment designed to train access to linguistic or grammatical rules, processes, and representations used for more than single sentence types may potentially lead not only to improved production of trained sentences but also to generalization across linguistically related responses presumed to be influenced or subserved by similar linguistic rules and principles.

This paper presents our preliminary findings concerned with examining the effects of a *linguistic-specific* treatment on complex sentence productions—sentences in which noun phrases (NPs) have been moved out of their canonical positions. Using this treatment approach we have begun to study generalized sentence production within and across linguistically related sentences in Broca's aphasic subjects with agrammatism. We discuss here the results of two initial studies focused on wh-interrogative and object cleft sentence productions—sentences relying on wh-movement, one major type of movement subsumed under the rule *move-alpha*. The linguistic and psycholinguistic underpinnings of these sentence structures were considered in designing our treatment approach, which addressed verb predicate argument structure, thematic role assignment in the D-structure representation of targeted sentences, movement of NP sentence constituents, and trace formulation (see Shapiro & Thompson, 1994, where the authors discuss these linguistic constructs in more detail). Because we recognize that linguistic theories generally are not designed as processing/production models, the production treatment that we derive is several steps removed from the linguistic theories themselves; nevertheless, we use the representational constructs derived from linguistic theory to teach subjects to make contact with the linguistic representations involved in the sentences that we target.

In the first study, wh-interrogatives requiring wh-movement of a direct object NP to the *specifier* position of COMP phrase and using verbs with similar lexical properties and predicate argument structures were selected (*what* and *who*). We also explored the role of sentence complexity, with complexity defined in terms of the number of phrasal nodes in the D-structure representation of sentences. That is, we trained sentences with four phrasal nodes (NP-V-NP-PP) and assessed generalization to sentences derived from three (NP-V-NP). This experimental question was based on evidence from studies of acquisition of English as a second language (ESL) (Eckman, Bell, & Nelson, 1988) and of treatment of phonological disorders (Gierut, 1990); these studies indicated greater generalization when treatment began with more complex items rather than less complex ones.

The second study examined two separate sentence types that, though they take very different surface forms, have similar underlying linguistic representations and rely on wh-movement: wh-interrogative questions and object cleft sentences. In this second experiment another sentence type relying on NP-movement (passive sentences) was studied for generalization. Here we made a rather fine-grained prediction: Given that wh-interrogatives and relative clause sentences derive from a particular aspect of the move-alpha (wh-movement) rule that involves movement of a direct object from an argument position to a nonargument specifier position of a COMP phrase, we conjectured that generalization might occur between these two sentences. At the same time, we reasoned that our treatment would not influence passive sentences, which rely on a different aspect of move-alpha (NP-movement). As has been recently shown by Shapiro, McNamara, Zurif, Lanzoni, and Cermak (1992), wh- and NP-movement-derived sentences yield distinct sentence production patterns, perhaps because producing sentences derived from wh-movement may impose a greater processing load than producing some sentences derived from NP-movement—the former but not the latter requires linking a trace to its antecedent across clausal boundaries. Indeed, object relative sentences have been shown to be more difficult for aphasic subjects to comprehend than passive sentences (Caplan, Baker, & Dehaut, 1985).

The experimental questions of interest concerned (a) the acquisition effects of treatment, (b) the generalization patterns occurring from more to less complex sentence structures, (c) the generalization patterns occurring from one wh-interrogative form to another, and (d) the generalization patterns occurring from wh-interrogatives to object cleft sentences and vice versa.

METHOD

Subjects

The study investigated five aphasic adults who exhibited deficit patterns consistent with a diagnosis of nonfluent aphasia with agrammatism. Two subjects (one male and one female) participated in the first study, and three subjects (one male and two females) participated in the second. Although of differing etiologies, all subjects were between 13 and 40 months post onset of aphasia symptoms at the time of the study. Both subjects in the first study had suffered a single left cerebrovascular accident (CVA), whereas in the second study, one subject had sustained a left CVA, one had suffered a gunshot wound, and a third carried a diagnosis of primary progressive aphasia of the nonfluent type (Duffy & Petersen, in press) with no evidence of infarction noted on SPECT scan. All subjects were native English speakers, were premorbidly right-handed, and had completed high school.

Testing of the subjects' language behavior using the *Western Aphasia Battery* (WAB) (Kertesz, 1982) revealed performance patterns consistent with nonfluent (Broca's) aphasia. Aphasia Quotients (AQs) of 56 and 62, respectively, were derived for the subjects in Study 1, whereas higher-level subjects were selected for the second study, with AQs ranging from 75 to 93. Additional testing concerned with lexical-semantic processing, reading comprehension, auditory sentence comprehension, and sentence production was undertaken using a series of published and unpublished tests. Results indicated that all subjects sustained mild to moderate disruptions of lexical-semantic processing but had relatively intact reading comprehension and oral reading, at least for simple sentences.

Study 1 tested auditory sentence comprehension and production using wh-interrogatives, active and passive nonreversible sentences, and active and passive reversible sentences; the results indicated somewhat compromised comprehension of wh-interrogatives and reversible sentences. Comprehension of passive sentences was the most difficult for both subjects. Additionally, both subjects were completely unable to produce grammatically correct wh-interrogative or passive sentences. Subjects in the second study were administered the *Philadelphia Comprehension Battery for Aphasia* (Saffran & Schwartz, unpublished), which, among other things, tests comprehension of active, passive, and object relative sentences. All subjects evidenced good comprehension of active sentences, and a reversibility effect was noted for all subjects (i.e., near-perfect performance was noted on semantically nonreversible sentences and poorer performance was noted on semantically reversible ones). However, comprehension difficulty was apparent for all subjects on both passive and object relative sentences. Interestingly, object relative sentences were more difficult than passives across subjects—a finding consistent with linguistic predictions, in that object relatives are more computationally complex than passive sentences.

Experimental Stimuli

Study 1. Ninety sentences were prepared to elicit *what* and *who* question productions (45 items for each) and printed in large upper-and lowercase letters on cards. Each set of 45 items was further divided into three sets of 15. The first and most complex set consisted of sentences with the D-structure form of NP-V-NP-PP (e.g., "The man is giving money to the boy"); Set 2 consisted of sentences using transitive verbs taking a direct object with the D-structure form of NP-V-NP (e.g., "The man is fixing the car"), and Set 3 consisted of sentences using the copula with the D-structure form of NP-V(copula)-NP (e.g., "A dictionary is a book"). Using the linguistic principles and rules described by Shapiro and Thompson (1994) for deriving the surface form of these sentences from their underlying linguistic representation, the following target *what* questions could be formulated, respectively: What$_i$ is the man giving$_{ti}$ to the boy? What$_i$ is the man fixing$_{ti}$? What$_i$ is a dictionary$_{ti}$? For treatment purposes, the words of each sentence were individually displayed on 3-1/2-x-5-in. cards, as were *who*, *what*, and a question-mark.

Study 2. Twenty-five target sentences (e.g., "The girl hit the boy") were prepared to represent the D-structure of three separate sentence types—

wh-interrogatives, object cleft, and passive sentences—and an additional 25 foil sentences representing the reversed action were prepared (e.g., "The boy hit the girl"). Pictures also were prepared to coincide with both target and foil sentences. All sentences were printed in large upper-and lowercase letters on cards. Using the linguistic principles and rules described by Shapiro & Thompson (1994) for deriving the surface form of wh-interrogative, object cleft, and passive sentences from their underlying linguistic representation, the following sentences could be formulated: "Who did the girl hit?" (wh-interrogative); "It was the boy who the girl hit" (object cleft); or "The boy was hit by the girl" (passive). For treatment purposes, individual sentence elements of the target sentences again were displayed on 3-1/2-in. × 5-in. cards, together with other elements required to produce the S-structure sentence forms (e.g., *who, did, it, was*).

Design

Combined single-subject experimental designs were used in both studies to examine the effects of treatment. These designs were selected for a number of reasons concerned with experimental control, examination of variability and other issues that have been discussed elsewhere (Kearns, 1986; McReynolds & Thompson, 1986). An additional, compelling reason for selecting this experimental strategy was to examine explicitly the covariance among and between linguistically related structures. Single-subject experiments allow design components to be arranged such that this covariance can be systematically examined through measurement of generalization while experimental control is maintained (Connell & Thompson, 1986). We believe that carefully designed research in which the lexical and syntactic properties of sentences selected for treatment are manipulated and controlled may lead not only to improved production of certain sentences but also to generalization across sentences relying on the same processes. Therefore, by examining generalization within and among theoretically related behaviors using single-subject design strategies, we may—in addition to discovering effective interventions strategies—derive important data relative to the formal characterization of mental structures and operations that subserve language. That is, we may be able to use the evidence gathered from carefully controlled experiments evaluating the effects of treatment to further develop sentence-processing and sentence production models (for a complete discussion of this use of single-subject designs, see Thompson, 1992).

Single-subject multiple baseline designs across behaviors and subjects were used in the present studies. Treatment was applied to one sentence type at a time, and untrained sentence types were tested continuously. If generalization did not occur across sentences, treatment was applied to them. In cases in which generalization did occur, experimental control was demonstrated across subjects, with treatment being applied to each subject following baselines of increasing length. In the first study, the two interrogative types (*what* and *who*) provided the multiple baseline across behaviors. Production of both wh-constructions was examined using all experimental stimuli during the baseline phase, followed by application of treatment to the most complex form (Set 1 sentences) of either *what* or *who* interrogatives, counterbalanced across subjects. Treatment then was extended to the other interrogative if generalization across interrogatives did not occur. In the second study, three sentence types provided the behaviors of interest: wh-interrogatives, object cleft, and passive sentences. During baseline, production of all sentence types was tested, followed by application of treatment to either wh-interrogatives or object cleft sentences, counterbalanced across subjects. Passive sentences were held in baseline throughout the study to examine the relation between wh-and NP-movement-derived sentences.

Baseline and Treatment Probes

Baseline testing was accomplished using the following procedures. These probe procedures also were applied prior to each treatment session to measure the effects of treatment.

Study 1. Production of *what* and *who* questions was assessed using the 90 experimental stimuli. A randomly selected written stimulus sentence was presented for the subject to read, repeat, or both (e.g., "The man is reading a book"). Next, with the full sentence in view, the examiner said, "You want to know *the thing* that the man is reading, so you ask . . .?" The word *thing* was emphasized, rising inflection was used, and a question mark was placed above the sentence. For *who* question elicitation, for example, using the stimulus sentence "The father is protecting his son," the examiner said, "You want to know *the person* the father is protecting, so you ask . . .," again emphasizing the word *person*, using rising inflection and placing a question mark on the table above the stimulus sentence. A 10-sec. response time was provided following each stimulus presentation. Response contingent feedback was not provided. Each response was scored for both lexical and grammatical accuracy. All sessions were videotaped for reliability purposes.

Study 2. Production of the three sentences types (wh-interrogatives, object cleft, and passives) was assessed using the 25 experimental stimuli. Each stimulus was randomly presented three times each during each baseline session—once to elicit production of a wh-question, once to stimulate production of an object cleft sentence, and once for production of a passive sentence. To elicit each sentence type a modeling paradigm was used. Two written sentence stimuli (one target sentence and one foil) were presented together with corresponding pictures, and the subject was instructed to read/repeat both sentences (e.g., "The girl hit the boy," and "The boy hit the girl"). The examiner then instructed: "Here are two pictures. One shows a girl [pointing to the girls] and the other shows a boy [pointing to each boy]." The examiner asked the following questions to elicit each of the three response types:

> *Wh-Interrogatives:* "In this picture [pointing to the foil], if you wanted to know the person the girl hit, you would ask the question 'Who did the girl hit?' In this picture [pointing to the target], if you wanted to know the person the boy hit you would ask . . ."
> *Object Cleft Sentences:* "In this picture [pointing to the foil], it was the girl who the boy hit. But in this picture [pointing to the boy in the target] . . ."
> *Passivization:* "In this picture [pointing to the foil], the girl was hit by the boy, but in this one [pointing to the boy in the target picture] . . ."

Treatment

Subjects were trained to recognize the verb, its argument structures, and their thematic role assignments using the D-structure representation of target sentences. Instructions concerned with movement of D-structure sentence constituents to derive target surface forms were then provided. Treatment protocols for wh-interrogative sentences and object cleft sentences are presented in Tables 1 and 2, respectively.

Reliability

An independent observer coded responses for reliability on a randomly selected 30% of videotaped baseline and treatment probe sessions, and point-to-point agreement was calculated. In addition, randomly selected treatment sessions were coded for reliability on the independent variable. Overall reliability was greater than 90% across the two studies for both the dependent and independent variables.

RESULTS

Study 1

Results of Study 1 are displayed in Tables 3 and 4, for Subjects 1 and 2, respectively. Examination of these data indicated some differences in the

Table 1. Treatment Protocol: Wh-Interrogatives

Step 1: E presents d-structure sentence printed in upper- and lowercase letters on large card (3 in. x 18 in.) with instructions to read/repeat it (e.g., *"The man is sending flowers"*). E presents instructions for S to produce a question response as in baseline. A 5-sec response interval is provided.

Step 2: E presents d-structure sentence elements on individual cards. "What," "Who," and "?" cards also are presented (e.g., *"The man is sending flowers"* *"What" "Who" "?"*). E instructs S to produce a question response as in baseline. A 5-sec response interval is provided.

Step 3: E identifies the verb, the subject NP, and the object NP of the sentence. E then explains (a) that the object NP is either "the thing" (for *what* questions) or "the person" (for *who* question) receiving the action of the verb and (b) that it is replaced by *What* or *Who*, respectively. E replaces the object NP with the appropriate wh-morpheme, by selecting either the "What" or "Who" card, and places the "?" card at the end, forming an echo question (e.g., *"The man is sending What ?"*). The echo question is read/repeated by S.

Step 4: E demonstrates subject/auxiliary verb inversion by physically moving the subject NP cards and the auxiliary verb card (e.g., *"Is the man sending What ?"*).

Step 5: E demonstrates movement of the wh-morpheme to the sentence initial position. The correct question is read/repeated by S (e.g., *"What is the man sending ?"*).

Step 6: Sentence element cards are rearranged in their d-structure order. "What," "Who," and "?" cards are presented. Steps 3, 4, and 5 are repeated with S replacing/selecting/moving cards. E provides assistance at each step if needed. Once formed, the correct question is read/repeated by S.

Note: E = examiner; S = subject; NP = noun phrase.

generalization patterns observed across subjects. During baseline, neither subject produced correct wh-interrogative sentences of any type—most responses were produced with rising inflection; wh-morphemes were infrequently produced; and no attempts at movement were demonstrated. When treatment was applied to the most complex *what* interrogative constructions (NP-V-NP-PP) for Subject 1, acquisition of target question responses was noted (see Table 3). Additionally, throughout this training, generalization to less complex *what* interrogative constructions was noted (both to NP-V-NP structures and to NP-V (Copula)-NP structures). Interestingly, correct production of the less complex structures actually preceded that of the trained structures (see probe sessions 16–20 on Table 3). However, during this treatment period, generalization to untrained *who* constructions was not seen. Therefore, treatment was extended to *who* questions (NP-V-NP-PP), resulting in acquisition patterns of *who* interrogative productions similar to those noted for *what*. In addition, general-

Table 2. Treatment Protocol: Object Cleft Sentences

Step 1: E presents d-structure sentences (target and foil) printed in upper and lower case letters on large card (3 in. x 18 in.) with instructions to read/repeat as in baseline testing (e.g., *"The girl hit the boy," "The boy hit the girl"*). E presents stimulus for S to produce a question response as in baseline. A 5-sec response interval is provided.

Step 2: E presents d-structure sentence elements (of target sentence only) on individual cards. "It," "Was," and "Who" cards also are presented (e.g., *"The girl hit the boy" "It" "Was" "Who"*). E instructs S to produce an object cleft sentence as in baseline (using a foil sentence that is removed before the subject responds). A 5-sec response interval is provided.

Step 3: E identifies the verb, subject NP, and object NP in the sentence and explains that (a) the object NP is the object of the sentence (e.g., *"This is the person who the girl hit"*) and that (b) the "Who" card is placed next to the person who was hit (e.g., *"The girl hit the boy" "Who"*)

Step 4: E explains that "to make the new sentence, the object NP and "Who" cards are moved to the beginning of the sentence" (e.g., *"The boy Who the girl hit"*). E demonstrates movement and reads the newly formed utterance.

Step 5: E instructs that to make the sentence grammatically correct, the elements "It was" are added in the sentence initial position. The correct sentence is read/repeated by S (e.g., *"It was the boy who the girl hit"*).

Step 6: Sentence element cards are rearranged in their d-structure order. "It," "Was," and "Who" cards are presented. Steps 3, 4, and 5 are repeated with S replacing/selecting/moving cards. E provides assistance at each step if needed. Once formed, the correct question is read/repeated by S.

Note: E = examiner; S = subject; NP = noun phrase.

ization patterns to the less complex, untrained *who* interrogative constructions again emerged.

Treatment effects similar to those noted for Subject 1 also were seen for Subject 2, as shown in Table 4. Following baseline, when treatment was applied to the most complex *who* interrogative constructions (NP-V-NP-PP), correct wh-movement was noted on some responses by session 14, and by session 24 most *who* questions were produced not only with perfect syntax but also with accurate production of word labels. Additionally, during this training, production was generalized not only to less complex *who* sentences but also across interrogatives to all *what* forms. That is, for this subject, training only a small subset ($N = 15$) of *who* interrogative productions resulted in correct production of a large portion of the total 90 target sentences. This generalization included that to less complex forms, which again preceded acquisition of the most complex forms (see probe sessions 14–18 for *who* structures and sessions 20–24 for *what* structures).

Table 3. Number of Grammatically Correct *What* and *Who* Interrogative Sentence Productions Across Sentence Complexity Levels During Baseline and Treatment Phases of Study 1 (Subject 1 Data)

What Interrogative Sentence Productions

Probe sessions	1	2	4	6	8	10	12	14	16	18	20	22	24	26	28	30	32	34	36	38	40	42	44	46	48	50
	Baseline								*Treatment*															*Maintenance*		
NP-V-NP-PP (trained)	0(3)	0(0)	0(1)	0(3)	0(1)	0(3)	0(1)	0(1)	0(1)	1(12)	3(12)	5(10)	4(11)	9(6)	10(5)	4(9)	7(8)	3(12)	2(13)	2(8)	3(10)	7(8)	9(6)	10(4)	10(4)	10(4)
	Generalization Probes																									
NP-V-NP	0(0)	0(0)			0(0)			0(0)	12(3)		9(6)		12(3)		14(1)			12(2)			9(6)			7(5)		
NP-V(Cop)-NP	0(2)	0(1)			0(1)			0(0)	11(4)		11(4)		12(3)		8(6)			8(6)			12(3)			11(3)		

Who Interrogative Sentence Productions

Probe sessions	1	2	4	6	8	10	12	14	16	18	20	22	24	26	28	30	32	34	36	38	40	42	44	46	48	50
	Baseline																			*Treatment*						
NP-V-NP-PP (trained)	0(3)	0(0)	0(0)	0(0)	0(0)	0(0)	0(0)	0(0)	0(0)	0(0)	0(0)	0(0)	0(0)	0(0)	0(0)	0(0)	0(0)	0(0)	0(0)	0(1)	2(1)	3(8)	6(9)	8(6)	6(3)	10(3)
	Generalization Probes																									
NP-V-NP	0(0)	0(0)	0(0)					0(0)				1(0)			0(0)			0(1)			2(3)			8(6)		
NP-V(Cop)-NP	0(0)	0(0)	0(0)					0(0)				0(0)			0(0)			0(3)			2(4)			5(8)		

Note: NP = noun phrase, V = verb, Cop = copula, PP = prepositional phrase. Numbers in parentheses refer to the number of grammatically, but not lexically, correct sentences produced per probe.

Table 4. Number of Grammatically Correct *Who* and *What* Interrogative Sentence Productions Across Sentence Complexity Levels During Baseline and Treatment Phases of Study 1 (Subject 2 Data)

Probe sessions	1	2	3	4	6	8	10	12	14	16	18	20	22	24	26	28	30	32	34	36
	Baseline				*Treatment*															
Who Interrogative Sentence Productions																				
NP-V-NP-PP (trained)	0(0)	0(0)	0(0)	0(0)	0(0)	0(0)	0(0)	0(1)	2(5)	4(8)	4(7)	7(6)	4(8)	13(2)	12(2)	10(5)	11(4)	11(3)	10(3)	
Generalization Probes																				
NP-V-NP	0(1)	0(0)	0(0)			1(0)			11(3)			12(3)			11(2)			13(0)		
NP-V(Cop)-NP	0(0)	0(0)		0(1)			0(1)			8(5)				11(2)			8(4)			7(5)
What Interrogative Sentence Productions																				
Generalization Probes																				
NP-V-NP-PP	0(0)	0(0)	0(0)	0(0)	0(0)	0(0)	0(0)	0(0)	0(0)	1(0)	0(1)	0(1)	2(8)	2(5)	6(3)	10(4)	3(5)	8(3)	9(4)	
NP-V-NP	0(3)	0(1)	0(0)			0(0)			1(0)			13(0)			10(1)			14(0)		
NP-V(Cop)-NP	0(0)	0(1)		0(0)	0(0)		0(3)				0(7)			5(8)			8(6)			9(2)

Note: NP = noun phrase, V = verb, Cop = copula, PP = prepositional phrase. Numbers in parentheses refer to the number of grammatically, but not lexically, correct sentences produced per probe.

Study 2

Results of Study 2, summarized in Table 5, again revealed somewhat different findings across subjects, with Subjects 2 and 3 showing greater generalization than Subject 1. Although successful acquisition of targeted sentences was seen when Subject 1 was trained to produce each sentence type, no generalization was noted across forms, from who-interrogative to object cleft sentences. For Subjects 2 and 3, however, acquisition and generalization across forms were noted (i.e., from object cleft sentences to who-interrogatives and vice versa). Interestingly, this is the direction in which generalization was predicted based on the underlying linguistic representation of the sentences under study (i.e., both wh-interrogatives and object cleft sentences require wh-movement). The predicted clear distinction between wh-movement structures and NP-movement structures (passives), however, was noted only for Subject 2. That is, Subject 1 evinced some change in passive sentence production during who-interrogative training, although an inconsistent trend was noted across probe sessions. This covariance was not expected. Because Subject 3 produced passive sentences at a high level prior to treatment, examination of the relation between wh- and NP-movement structures was not possible in her case. However, for subject 2, treatment of object clefts clearly influenced who-interrogatives, but not passive sentences—a predicted finding, in that passives require NP-movement but not wh-movement.

DISCUSSION

The data derived from these two sentence production studies indicated that for all subjects under study, the linguistically based treatment facilitated acquisition of trained sentences. In addition, for both subjects in the first experiment, generalization to less complex sentences was noted when treatment was applied to the most complex forms of the same type, and for three of the five subjects studied across the two experiments, generalization to untrained sentence types was evident.

That generalization was enhanced with treatment *first* being applied to the most complex forms of sentences is in keeping with findings reported by Eckman et al. (1988) and Gierut (1990) concerned with generalization from more to less complex language forms in teaching English as a second language (ESL) and phonologically disordered children. The present findings with aphasic subjects support this treatment approach and stand in contrast to the aphasia treatment literature recommending that treatment programs begin with elicitation of the easiest responses of a particular type and advance to more difficult ones.

Table 5. Percent Grammatically Correct Productions of *Who* Interrogative, Object Cleft, and Passive Sentences During Baseline and Treatment Phases of Study 2 Across Subjects

Probe sessions	1	2	3	4	5	6	7	8	9	10	11	12	13	14	15	16	17	18	19	20	21	22
	Baseline			*Treatment*																*Maintenance*		
																				Treatment		
Subject 1																						
Who interrogative (trained)	0	12	20	88	88	100	92	88	100	88	88	88	88	88	100	88	88	92	100	100	96	100
						Generalization Probes																
Object Clefts (trained)	12	0		0					0	0	0	0	0	8	12	0	8	40	72	28	72	
Passives	12	12	20		24	20	20		20		44		40		56		20		12		12	
Subject 2																						
	Baseline			*Treatment*																		
Object Cleft (trained)	8	12	8	0	8	0	16	16	24	28	32	48	56	56	48	68	68	56	76	68	68	76
										Generalization Probes												
Who interrogatives (trained)	0	0	0	4		4		0		8		8		16		56		48		56		8
Passives	16	20	16		8		4		4		8		8		12		12		8		8	
Subject 3																						
	Baseline					*Treatment*																
Who interrogatives (trained)	0	18		8		32	56	76	68	76	88	92	88	92	100							
							Generalization Probes															
Object Cleft	0	0	0	0		4	4	4	48	48	68	68	76	56								
Passives	44	84	76	64	64		88		92		64		76		64							

The generalization noted *across* sentence types (from *who* to *what* questions in the first experiment, and from *who*-questions to object clefts and vice versa in the second) also is a novel finding. We suggest that this generalization was observed because the sentences selected for treatment and for generalization involved similar underlying forms and because they relied on similar linguistic processes for deriving surface representations. Further, the generalization patterns noted suggest that disrupted production of some complex sentences seen in aphasia may result, in part, from disrupted grammatical or linguistic processes and representations involved in the translation of D-structure representation to surface realizations, including the assignment of thematic roles of verbs to argument positions, empty category representation, and coindexing of the trace to its proper antecedent. That generalization occurred to sentences relying on wh-movement in both experiments—and did not occur from wh-movement structures to NP-movement structures (at all for Subject 2 or as strongly for Subject 1)—is of theoretical interest in terms of language representation and processes involved in sentence production. Because the generalization patterns noted were in keeping with those predicted from formal linguistic theory, these data provide some experimental verification of the relation between the sentence structures studied. That is, the covariance noted between trained and generalized structures suggests that the various structures are governed by the same linguistic principles. Further, these findings support the arguments advanced by Grodzinsky (1990) in favor of the "breakdown compatibility" of Government-Binding (GB) theory. In the present experiments we have shown that, at least for some subjects, the processes expected to influence certain sentence productions based on our working theoretical model did in fact influence them as predicted.

Our enthusiasm for this approach, however, must be tempered by the apparent discrepant findings noted *across* subjects in both experiments. For one subject in each experiment, generalization was not seen beyond that reported in earlier studies in which linguistically based treatments were not provided. These results are difficult to explain. Because not all subjects conformed to hypotheses based on linguistic theory, it could be suggested that our use of GB theory to explain the nature of sentence production deficits in agrammatic individuals is not entirely appropriate. However, we feel that this conclusion is premature, especially in light of the interesting generalization patterns noted for some of our subjects. Indeed, a number of variables need to be considered when examining discrepant results across subjects, including the nature of the subjects' language disruptions as well as other subject variables, both neurological (e.g., site of lesion, etiology) and psychosocial (e.g., motivation, depression, adjustment to disability).

In fact, some differences in language behavior across subjects in the present studies have been noted that are beyond the scope of discussion here (see Thompson, Shapiro, & Roberts, 1993, for a more complete profile of one subject who participated in our first experiment). Important neurological differences (i.e., etiological disparity) across the subjects in Study 2 also may have influenced our findings. Recall that, in that study, Subject 1's language disruption stemmed from a gunshot wound; therefore, his lesion was *more diffuse* than those of the other subjects. However, the extent to which this variable influenced responses cannot be gleaned from the present study. It is equally likely that other unknown variables may have influenced this subject's response patterns and that etiology alone may not adequately explain the discrepant finding. In terms of etiology, it is most interesting to note that Subject 3 (who carried a diagnosis of primary progressive aphasia) demonstrated linguistically predicted generalization patterns, suggesting a lawfulness, even in progressive language decline, that may be described along linguistic lines.

The data derived from these initial experiments are encouraging and support our continued endeavors in this direction. Replication of the present findings across additional subjects is needed, and many questions remain to be answered. However, we believe that further research using theory-driven, linguistic-specific approaches to treatment in which neurolinguistic models of language representation and processing are considered holds promise for developing effective treatments and for furthering understanding of aphasic sentence production deficits.

ACKNOWLEDGMENT

The work reported here was supported in part by NIH (NIDCD) grants DC01809 and DC00494.

REFERENCES

Byng, S. (1988). Sentence processing deficits: Theory and therapy. *Cognitive Neuropsychology, 5*, 629–676.

Caplan, D., Baker, C., & Dehaut, F. (1985). Syntactic determinants of sentence comprehension in aphasia. *Cognition, 21*, 117–175.

Chomsky, N. (1981). *Lectures on government and binding.* Dordrecht: Foris.

Chomsky, N. (1986). *Knowledge of language: Its nature, origin, and use.* New York: Praeger.

Connell, P. J., & Thompson, C. K. (1986). Flexibility of single-subject designs. Part III: Using flexibility to design or modify experiments. *Journal of Speech and Hearing Disorders, 51*, 214–225.

Doyle, P. J., Goldstein, H., & Bourgeois, M. (1987). Experimental analysis of syntax training in Broca's aphasia: A generalization and social validation study. *Journal of Speech and Hearing Disorders, 52*, 143–155.

Duffy, J. R., & Petersen, R. C. (in press). Primary progressive aphasia. *Aphasiology.*

Eckman, F. R., Bell, L., & Nelson, D. (1988). On the generalization of relative clause instruction in the acquisition of English as a second language. *Applied Linguistics, 9,* 1–20.

Gierut, J. (1990). Differential learning of phonological oppositions. *Journal of Speech and Hearing Research, 33,* 540–549.

Grodzinsky, Y. (1990). *Theoretical perspectives on language deficits.* Cambridge, MA: MIT Press.

Helm-Estabrooks, N., Fitzpatrick, P. M., & Barresi, B. (1981). Response of an agrammatic patient to a syntax stimulation program for aphasia. *Journal of Speech and Hearing Disorders, 46,* 442–427.

Helm-Estabrooks, N., & Ramsberger, G. (1986). Treatment of agrammatism in long-term Broca's aphasia. *British Journal of Disorders of Communication, 21,* 39–45.

Jones, E. V. (1986). Building the foundations for sentence production in a nonfluent aphasic. *British Journal of Disorders of Communication, 21,* 63–82.

Kearns, K. P. (1986). Flexibility of single-subject designs. Part II: Design selection and arrangement of experimental phases. *Journal of Speech and Hearing Disorders, 51,* 204–213.

Kearns, K. P., & Salmon, S. (1984). An experimental analysis of auxiliary and copula verb generalization in aphasia. *Journal of Speech and Hearing Disorders, 49,* 152–163.

Kertesz, A. (1982). *The Western Aphasia Battery.* New York: Grune & Stratton.

LeDorze, G., Jacobs, A., & Coderre, C. (1991). Aphasia rehabilitation with a case of agrammatism: A partial replication. *Aphasiology, 5,* 63–85.

Loverso, F., Prescott, T., & Selinger, M. (1987). Cueing verbs: A treatment strategy for aphasia adults. CVT. *Journal of Rehabilitation Research and Development, 15,* 47–60.

Loverso, F., Prescott, T., & Salinger, M. (1992). Microcomputer treatment applications in aphasiology. *Aphasiology, 6,* 155–163.

McReynolds, L. V., & Thompson, C. K. (1986). Flexibility of single-subject designs. Part I: Review of the basics of single-subject designs. *Journal of Speech and Hearing Disorders, 51,* 194–203.

Mitchum, C. E. (1992). Treatment generalization and the application of cognitive neuropsychological models in aphasia therapy. In: NIDCD Monograph, *Aphasia treatment: Current approaches and research opportunities.* Bethesda, MD: National Institutes of Health/National Institute on Deafness and Other Communication Disorders.

Naeser, M. (1975). A structured approach teaching aphasics basic sentence types. *British Journal of Disorders of Communication, 10,* 70–76.

Saffran, E. M., Schwartz, M. F., Fink, R., Meyers, J., & Martin, N. (1992). Mapping therapy: An approach to remediating agrammatic sentence comprehension and production. In: NIDCD Monograph, *Aphasia treatment: Current approaches and research opportunities.* Bethesda, MD: National Institutes of Health/National Institute on Deafness and Other Communication Disorders.

Shapiro, L. P., & Thompson, C. K. (1994). The use of linguistic theory as a framework for treatment studies in aphasia. In M. L. Lemme (Ed.), *Clinical Aphasiology* (Vol. 22, pp. 291–305). Austin, TX: PRO-ED.

Shapiro, L. P., McNamara, P., Zurif, E., Lanzoni, S., & Cermak, L. (1992). Processing complexity and sentence memory: Evidence from amnesia. *Brain and Language, 42,* 431–453.

Thompson, C. K. (1992). A neurolinguistic approach to sentence production treatment and generalization research in aphasia. In: NIDCD Monograph, *Aphasia treatment: Current approaches and research opportunities.* Bethesda, MD: National

Institutes of Health/National Institute on Deafness and Other Communication Disorders.

Thompson, C. K., & McReynolds, L. V. (1986). Wh-interrogative production in agrammatic aphasia: An experimental analysis of auditory-visual stimulation and direct-production treatment. *Journal of Speech and Hearing Research, 29,* 193–206.

Thompson, C. K., Shapiro, L. P., & Roberts, M. (1993). Treatment of sentence production deficits in aphasia: A linguistic-specific approach to wh-interrogative training and generalization. *Aphasiology, 7,* 111–133.

Wambaugh, J., & Thompson, C. K. (1989). Training and generalization of agrammatic aphasic adults' wh-interrogative productions. *Journal of Speech and Hearing Disorders, 54,* 509–525.

Clinical Aphasiology, Vol. 22, 1994, pp. 325–333

Contextual Influences on Judgments of Emotionally Ambiguous Stimuli by Brain-Damaged and Normally Aging Adults

Connie A. Tompkins, Kristie A. Spencer, and Richard Boada

Contextual influences on normal perception are pervasive and powerful; our interpretation of sensory information depends on the environment in which it is embedded (Ashcraft, 1989). Some literature suggests that adults with right hemisphere brain damage (RHD) have difficulty processing contextual cues that contribute to drawing intended interpretations (Joanette, Goulet, & Hannequin, 1990; Myers, 1991), whereas other evidence has identified contextual-processing capacities that are spared after RHD. For instance, priming studies (Tompkins, 1990, 1991) have shown that RHD adults profit from prior linguistic contextual information in certain situations, even when judging materials in domains that are typically problematic (e.g., metaphor or emotional prosody). However, it is important to note that the experimental materials in those studies had a single, unambiguous interpretation.

The study described in this paper examined the influence of linguistic context on RHD adults' judgments of moods conveyed prosodically by ambiguous emotional stimuli. Ambiguous stimuli should provide a more sensitive test of RHD subjects' ability to profit from context. In addition, because most human exchanges are ambiguous to a certain extent (Russell & Fehr, 1988), ambiguous materials should be more ecologically valid than messages having a single, straightforward interpretation.

Our prediction for non-brain-damaged listeners was based on literature demonstrating that emotional inferencing, like other perceptual processing, is relative. Verbal statements of context have been found to influence the perception of emotional expressions among psychiatric patients and normal adults (Knudsen & Muzekari, 1983), and the same facial expression is seen as conveying different types and degrees of emotion, depending on what other faces are seen before it (Russell & Fehr, 1987). On the basis of these data, we expected normal adult listeners' judgments of ambiguous emotional target stimuli to shift according to the mood conveyed by the linguistic context preceding them.

Predictions for brain-damaged listeners were less certain. However, because the task was designed to tap relatively automatic processes (see Tompkins, 1990, 1991), brain-damaged subjects were expected to perform similarly to non-brain-damaged individuals.

METHOD

Subjects

Sixty adults participated in this study. Twenty were control subjects without known neurologic impairment and 40 were stroke patients (20 each with unilateral right hemisphere damage [RHD] or left hemisphere damage [LHD]). Subjects met strict inclusion criteria concerning radiologic documentation of lesion, hearing acuity, reading ability, and premorbid right-handedness (see Tompkins, 1991, for details from a related study). Descriptive data are summarized in Table 1. The groups did not differ in sociodemographic attributes, but clinical characteristics distinguished LHD and RHD groups in expected ways.

Stimuli and Tasks

Target stimuli came from a pool of semantically neutral phrases (e.g., "I can't believe it") that had been read by female speakers to convey one of four moods (happy, angry, afraid, no emotion) through prosody (see Tompkins & Flowers, 1985, for details). After several validation sessions we identified eight target phrases that conveyed more than one mood both across normally aging subjects and in repeated presentations to the same subjects. These ambiguous targets were used in three experimental tasks in which subjects judged how the speaker "sounded."

In Task 1, subjects judged target phrases presented in isolation. Three blocks of trials (given in two sessions) each consisted of two presentations of the eight targets and of five nonambiguous fillers. Thus, subjects made six judgments of the mood conveyed by each ambiguous target phrase in isolation.

Table 1. Descriptive Data for Three Subject Groups

Patient Characteristics	RHD (N = 20)	LHD (N = 20)	Control (N = 20)
Age (years)	64 (51–75)	64 (49–77)	66 (52–77)
Education (years)	12.4 (8–21)	13.3 (8–20)	12.9 (8–17)
Gender	11 male/ 9 female	10 male/ 10 female	10 male/ 10 female
Estimated IQ[a]	105 (92–127)	108 (88–125)	108 (94–119)
Auditory comprehension[b] (overall BDAE %ile)	95 (86–98)	90* (32–98)	97 (94–98)
Percent literal concepts[b] ("Cookie Theft" sample)	63 (44–81)	58 (31–92)	61 (5–75)
Judgment of line orientation[c]	17** (5–28)	23 (17–30)	24 (15–30)
**Contralateral neglect (medical records)	9 = Yes**	0 = Yes	N/A
*Aphasia (medical records)	0 = Yes	16 = Yes*	N/A
Etiology	13 thromboembolic	13 thromboembolic	N/A
Months post onset	26 (8–40)	23 (9–48)	N/A

Note: Data are means (with ranges) unless otherwise indicated. RHD = Right-hemisphere-damaged; LHD = Left-hemisphere-damaged. [a]Wilson, Rosenbaum, & Brown (1979). [b]From *Boston Diagnostic Aphasia Examination,* (Goodglass & Kaplan, 1983). [c]Benton, Hamsher, Varney, & Spreen (1983). *LHD significantly poorer than other groups. **RHD significantly poorer than other groups.

For Task 2, each target phrase was combined with four versions of five different prior linguistic contexts (see example in Table 2). The events in each version had been validated to represent one of the four mood choices, but the stories were read with neutral intonation (see Tompkins, 1991). Each story-target pair was presented twice, along with 32 fillers (four blocks of 24 trials each). Subjects judged the mood of the target phrases after the stories were presented.

Several manipulations were made to discourage subjects from adopting a conscious strategy of "matching" target responses to mood information in the stories. First, subjects performed a distractor task (monitoring for the occurrence of the words *he* or *she*) to keep them from focusing on the stories' emotional content. Second, target phrases followed the stories

Table 2. Sample Story Context in Four Versions

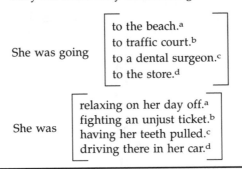

Amy left home early one morning.

She was going
{ to the beach.[a]
to traffic court.[b]
to a dental surgeon.[c]
to the store.[d] }

She was
{ relaxing on her day off.[a]
fighting an unjust ticket.[b]
having her teeth pulled.[c]
driving there in her car.[d] }

[a]Version for "happy." [b]Version for "angry." [c]Version for "afraid." [d]Version for "no emotion."

after a brief interval (550 ms) to reduce the opportunity to form expectancies. Third, through instruction, demonstration, and practice, subjects were informed that the mood of the story would not "go with" the speaker's voice much of the time, so they should ignore the story and try to judge the target phrase as if it had occurred by itself. Twenty of the 32 fillers contained nonambiguous target phrases, paired in incongruent trials with stories of different moods, to reinforce these instructions. Finally, although response-time data were not collected, subjects were encouraged to respond as quickly as possible.

For Task 3, each version of the five story contexts (20 trials total) was presented in isolation. Subjects were asked to select the mood label that indicated how the main character would feel in the situation described.

Subjects also performed two preliminary emotion recognition tasks (see Tompkins, 1991). For the first, they chose the mood label (*happy, angry, or afraid*) that was synonymous with each of 18 emotion words presented singly on index cards (e.g., *delighted, furious, anxious*). For the second, they selected the mood label that described each of 12 orally described emotional situations (e.g., "Your brakes don't work on the freeway").

Test Procedures

Experimental stimuli were tape-recorded for consistency of production. Trials within each block were pseudorandomly ordered: a filler always occurred first, and no more than three trials of each type (experimental vs. filler) or emotion occurred in sequence. The order of presentation of various blocks of trials was counterbalanced. Subjects responded manually to the experimental tasks by pressing one of four labeled buttons on a custom-built response-time apparatus (see Tompkins, 1991). Experimental tasks were interspersed with tasks from a related study and with the clinical descriptive tasks reported in Table 1. The blocks of the isolated target judgment task (Task 1) were separated as much as possible, and the isolated story judgment task (Task 3) was given last. Most subjects completed the study in two sessions, 5–10 days apart.

Scoring Procedures

Because the experimental target phrases were intended to be ambiguous, there was no standard by which to describe performance as correct or incorrect. We developed a scoring system that captured the extent to which the mood judgment of a single target phrase in Task 2 *shifted* from one interpretation to another when it was preceded by linguistic contexts describing situations associated with differing emotional reactions.

Before any scoring was done, we assessed the accuracy of judgments for stories presented in isolation (Task 3). When a story context was assigned a mood different from that intended, we substituted the subject's judgment for our own before examining the influence of prior context on target judgments in Task 2. This occasionally occurred when subjects, especially males, indicated that our female characters would be afraid in situations that had been validated as creating anger.

"Shift" point values were assigned to each target phrase when it matched the mood of its prior context in Task 2. Scoring rules depended on whether the moods selected for a target phrase in Task 2 had also been selected when that target phrase was judged in isolation (Task 1), or whether the mood selected in Task 2 had never been chosen in the isolation task. The scoring procedures for each occasion will be described separately.

When a mood choice had been made *in isolation* for a particular target phrase, conservative scoring procedures were applied. Two criteria had to be met before a target phrase was evaluated for scoring. First, that target phrase must have been judged as portraying two or three different moods when presented in isolation. To illustrate, Target A, variously identified as "happy" and "afraid" in Task 1, would qualify for a shift score in Task 2. Target B, always judged as "happy," and Target C, for which all four mood choices were made over six presentations, would not be scored in Task 2. The second criterion for assigning shift scores was that both occurrences of a single target phrase had to be judged with the same mood as that conveyed by the prior context in Task 2.

After selecting qualifying target phrases in this manner, we gave more weight to shifted target moods that were selected less often in isolation, and vice versa. To accomplish this, we determined the proportional frequency with which each mood choice occurred for these targets in the isolation task (e.g., four judgments of "happy" and two of "afraid" for Target A represent a 0.67–0.33 split). The shift point value awarded was the inverse of the ratio calculated for that mood's occurrence in isolation (e.g, when an "afraid" judgment followed an "afraid" story on *both* occurrences of Target A, 0.67 points were awarded, the inverse of the relative occurrence for "afraid" in Task 1).

For target moods that were *never chosen in isolation* (e.g., an "angry" judgment for Target A, above), scoring was much more liberal. Here, a full point was given any time the target judgment in Task 2 matched the mood of its prior context, capturing the strong influence exerted by the story on the target judgment.

All points were summed to create the shift scores shown in Table 3. Because individual scores were based on different numbers of qualifying targets, each element of the shift score (points for choices made in isolation plus points for choices not in isolation) was divided by the number of targets contributing to its score and summed to provide an adjusted shift score (see Table 3). Finally, Table 3 reports the number of incongruent, nonambiguous filler trials for which story mood and target judgments matched. This provides an indication of the extent to which subjects' shift scores might have been due to the previously mentioned simple matching strategy.

Table 3. Experimental Task Performance for Three Subject Groups

Scores	RHD (N = 20)	LHD (N = 20)	Control (N = 20)
Shift score			
Mean	8.1	7.5	7.4
(Range)	(3–20)	(1–23)	(0–24)
SD	4.8	5.8	5.7
Adjusted shift score[a]			
Mean	1.2	1.0	1.0
(Range)	(0.5–2.7)	(0.2–3.0)	(0.0–3.0)
SD	0.7	0.8	0.7
Story-target "matches"[b]			
Mean	4.4	4.5	3.7
(Range)	(2–8)	(1–9)	(2–6)
SD	2.1	2.5	1.3

Note: RHD = Right hemisphere-damaged; LHD = Left hemisphere-damaged
[a]Shift score adjusted for number of targets contributing to its computation; score reflects extent of shifting per target. [b]For nonambiguous filler targets, paired with incongruent stories (maximum possible = 20).

RESULTS

Preliminary analyses indicated that there were no gender differences in shift scores (t for each group < 1.5). The groups did not differ in the number of targets contributing to the adjusted scores (M from 6.5 to 7.0 for choices made in isolation and from 6.9 to 7.7 for choices not made in isolation), so raw shift scores were used in subsequent analyses. In addition, the groups did not differ in the number of fillers for which story and target mood judgments "matched" [F (2, 57) = 2.3; p > .05; see Table 3].

One-way ANOVA on the three groups' shift scores (Table 3) was not significant [F (2, 57) = 0.91; p > .05]. Table 3 shows that the range of scores for brain-damaged subjects overlapped completely with the range for non-brain-damaged listeners. Pearson correlations indicated that shift scores were positively associated with the number of "matched" filler judgments for each group r_{LHD} = .70; r_{RHD} = .51; $r_{Control}$ = .49), with the strength of correlation similar for RHD and control groups. For the LHD group, the shift score was also correlated with overall auditory comprehension scores (r = –.57) and with the preliminary task involving mood recognition for emotional situations (r = –.58). There were no other meaningful correlations (r > .50) with shift scores for RHD or control subjects.

DISCUSSION AND IMPLICATIONS

Results of this study indicate that the perception of emotionally ambiguous target phrases was influenced by prior linguistic context to a comparable extent for all three subject groups: Listeners shifted their judgments of a single target phrase as the moods conveyed by its associated contexts changed. Although nonsignificant results can be difficult to interpret, the complete overlap in group distributions increases our confidence that our brain-damaged adults appraised emotionally ambiguous signals just as non-brain-damaged control subjects did. Of course, subtle group differences might have been detected with more sensitive response-time methods.

These results, together with those from previous priming studies (Tompkins, 1990, 1991), suggest that adults with RHD can process linguistic context sufficiently to influence judgments of intended meanings, even in domains (e.g., emotion or prosody) that tend to cause them difficulty. The findings extend results obtained with stimuli that conveyed mood information in a clear-cut, nonambiguous way.

Given the task manipulations incorporated to discourage extensive reliance on strategies, the contextual benefit for RHD adults probably reflects, at least in part, nonconscious spreading activation through an affective network (see Blaney, 1986; Gilligan & Bower, 1984; Tompkins, 1991). The correlations between shift scores, however, and the number of matched filler judgments suggest that all subjects probably did adopt a strategy to manage ambiguity by choosing moods for target phrases based on the emotional information implied by the prior context.

All groups resorted to this type of strategy on a similar proportion (about 20%) of the nonambiguous filler trials, but the strategy was more strongly related to LHD adults' shift scores than to either RHD or normal controls' shift scores. Apparently, RHD subjects were no more likely than normal controls to base target judgments on a simple matching strategy. Shift scores for LHD subjects were negatively correlated with auditory comprehension performance on the *Boston Diagnostic Aphasia Examination* (Goodglass & Kaplan, 1983) and with mood judgments of emotional situations. These correlations suggest that those LHD subjects who performed more poorly in task-relevant domains (e.g., auditory comprehension or emotional recognition) were more likely to adopt a matching strategy, relying on their understanding of the linguistic context to assist with judgments of emotional ambiguity. This pattern is frequently observed in studies of context effects on cognitive processing in normally aging individuals (e.g., Stine & Wingfield, 1987; Tompkins, 1991) and brain-damaged adults (e.g., Pierce & Wagner, 1985; Tompkins, 1991). Cohen and Faulkner (1983) suggest that this situation arises because listeners coping with a deterioration in stimulus quality or representation rely more heavily on available contextual cues.

In any case, the results call for continued investigation of conditions under which RHD adults exploit contextual information successfully. The conventional wisdom suggesting that RHD adults do not appreciate context needs to be carefully examined, as these sorts of data have implications for designing stimulus materials and conditions that may facilitate performance in treatment.

ACKNOWLEDGMENTS

Preparation of this manuscript was supported by grant DC00453 from the National Institute on Deafness and Other Communication Disorders, awarded to C.A.T. We appreciate the cooperation of Harmarville Rehabilitation Center and the Mercy Hospital of Pittsburgh, as well as the invaluable assistance of Kathrine McGarry and Maura Mullane Timko.

REFERENCES

Ashcraft, M. H. (1989). *Human memory and cognition*. Glenview, IL: Scott, Foresman.

Benton, A. L., Hamsher, K. deS., Varney, N. R., & Spreen, O. (1983). *Judgment of Line Orientation*. New York: Oxford University Press.

Benton, A. L., Hamsher, K. deS., Varney, N. R., & Spreen, O. (1983). Judgment of Line Orientation (pp. 44–54). *Contributions to neuropsychological assessment*. New York: Oxford University Press.

Blaney, P. H. (1986). Affect and memory: A review. *Psychological Bulletin, 99*, 229–246.

Cohen, G., & Faulkner, D. (1983). Word recognition: Age differences in contextual facilitation effects. *British Journal of Psychology, 74*, 238–251.

Gilligan, S. G., & Bower, G. H. (1984). Cognitive consequences of emotional arousal. In C. E. Izard, J. Kagan, & R. B. Zajonc (Eds.), *Emotions, cognition and behavior* (pp. 547–588). New York: Cambridge University Press.

Goodglass, H., & Kaplan, E. (1983). *Assessment of aphasia and related disorders* (2nd ed.). Philadelphia: Lea & Febiger.

Joanette, Y., Goulet, P., & Hannequin, D. (1990). *Right hemisphere and verbal communication*. New York: Springer-Verlag.

Knudsen, H., & Muzekari, L. H. (1983). The effects of verbal statements of context on facial expressions of emotion. *Journal of Nonverbal Behavior, 7*, 202–212.

Myers, P. S. (1991). Inference failure: The underlying impairment in right-hemisphere communication disorders. In T. Prescott (Ed.), *Clinical aphasiology*, Vol. 20 (pp. 167–180). Austin, TX: PRO-ED.

Pierce, R. S., & Wagner, C. (1985). The role of context in facilitating syntactic decoding in aphasia. *Journal of Communication Disorders, 18*, 203–214.

Russell, J. A., & Fehr, B. (1987). Relativity in the perception of emotion in facial expressions. *Journal of Experimental Psychology: General, 116*, 223–237.

Russell, J. A., & Fehr, B. (1988). Reply to Ekman and O'Sullivan. *Journal of Experimental Psychology: General, 117*, 89–90.

Stine, E. L., & Wingfield, A. (1987). Process and strategy in memory for speech among younger and older adults. *Psychology and Aging, 2*, 272–279.

Tompkins, C. A. (1990). Knowledge and strategies for processing lexical metaphor after right or left hemisphere brain damage. *Journal of Speech and Hearing Research, 33*, 307–316.

Tompkins, C. A. (1991). Automatic and effortful processing of emotional intonation after right or left hemisphere brain damage. *Journal of Speech and Hearing Research, 34*, 820–830.

Tompkins, C. A., & Flowers, C. R. (1985). Perception of emotional intonation by brain-damaged adults: The influence of task processing levels. *Journal of Speech and Hearing Research, 28*, 527–538.

Wilson, R. S., Rosenbaum, G., & Brown, G. (1979). The problem of premorbid intelligence in neuropsychological assessment. *Journal of Clinical Neuropsychology, 1*, 49–53.

Clinical Aphasiology, Vol. 22, 1994, pp. 335–343

Labeling of Novel Stimuli by Aphasic Subjects: Effects of Phonologic and Self-Cueing Procedures

Robert C. Marshall, Donald B. Freed, and David S. Phillips

A large number of studies have examined the effectiveness of cueing aphasic subjects during episodes of word-finding difficulty (Barton, Maruszewski, & Urrea, 1969; Brown, 1972; Goodglass & Stuss, 1979; Li & Canter, 1983, 1987; Li & Williams, 1989; Love & Webb, 1977; Pease & Goodglass, 1978; Podraza & Darley, 1977; Rochford & Williams, 1962; Weidner & Jinks, 1983). Overall, these studies have clearly shown that immediate word retrieval can be significantly enhanced by cues that provide additional phonologic or semantic information about the target stimulus. Of the different cueing methods examined in these studies, the first-phoneme cue was frequently cited as one of the techniques that provided the highest immediate naming accuracy (Goodglass & Stuss, 1979; Li & Canter, 1983, 1987; Li & Williams, 1989; Love & Webb, 1977; Pease & Goodglass, 1978).

As its name implies, the first-phoneme cue provides additional phonologic information to the aphasic patient. Several authors have offered reasons why the first-phoneme cue is such an effective prompt. Luria (1970) and Bensen (1979) suggested that phonemic cueing supplies information needed to initiate articulation of the target word. Li and Canter (1991) suggested that it supplements the functioning of an "inadequate semantic system" by providing the additional information needed to trigger the target word.

Although the first-phoneme cue is undoubtedly successful in providing immediate help to aphasic subjects during instances of word-finding difficulty, studies have shown that its effectiveness is usually quite short-lived (Howard, Patterson, Franklin, Orchard-Lisle, & Morton, 1985a; Patterson, Purell, & Morton, 1983). For example, Patterson et al. found that the benefits of a phonemic cue disappeared 30 minutes after its presentation. The transitory nature of the phonemic cue would, therefore, suggest that its value as a therapy tool may be limited, for the ultimate goal of aphasia rehabilitation is to increase speech and language functioning outside of therapy.

The effectiveness of a cue to assist aphasic patients' naming at some later time has been defined as "facilitation" (Howard et al., 1985a). Studies have suggested that the strongest facilitation of naming, ranging from 24-hours to slightly over one year, is obtained when therapy tasks require the activation of semantic representations of target words (Howard et al., 1985a, 1985b; Marshall, Neuburger, & Phillips, in press; Marshall, Pound, White-Thomson, & Pring, 1990; Pring, White-Thomson, Pound, Marshall, & Davis, 1990). The semantic training tasks used in these studies include pointing on auditory command to one of four pictures and making semantic judgments about the stimuli (e.g., answering a question like, "Is a car something you drive?").

The study presented in this chapter compared the effects of two training procedures on a delayed-naming task. The first procedure used repeated presentations of first-phoneme cues to teach aphasic subjects the labels of novel symbols. The second procedure used repeated presentations of subject-created self-cues on the same labeling task. No previous studies have directly compared the effectiveness of these two training procedures on delayed naming. It was hypothesized that the self-cue procedure would result in superior labeling performance because it required the subjects to semantically analyze the stimuli. In contrast, the procedure using the first-phoneme cue would require the subjects to attend only to the phonologic features of the stimuli. As a consequence, later naming performance would not be as accurate.

METHOD

Experimental Design

This study was designed as a repeated measures comparison with two experimental conditions: phonemic cue (PC) and self-cue (SC). Each experimental condition consisted of one pre-experimental probe, eight training trials, and three labeling probes. All sessions were conducted with individual subjects seated in a quiet therapy room. Table 1 illustrates the study's design.

Table 1. Sequence of Training Trials and Labeling Probes

First experimental condition

First session
Preexperimental probe

Second session
(Four days after preexperimental probe)

1. Training trial 1	5. Training trial 5
2. Training trial 2	6. Training trial 6
3. Training trial 3	7. Training trial 7
4. Training trial 4	8. Training trial 8
Midtraining probe	Posttraining probe

Third session
24-hour follow-up labeling probe

Second experimental condition

The second experimental condition was begun approximately one week after the first condition had been completed. The training and probe sequence was identical to that used in the first condition.

Subjects

Eight chronic aphasic subjects were recruited from the Portland Veterans Administration Outpatient Clinic for participation in the study. All were right-handed males. The mean age was 59 years (range, 49–69 years). Time post onset ranged from 30 to 72 months (mean, 51 months). Mean years of subject education was 13 (range, 11–20 years). All subjects demonstrated mild to moderate language deficits as measured by the *Porch Index of Communicative Ability* (PICA), (Porch, 1981) and the *Token Test* (Spreen & Benton, 1977). Each subject was informally screened for any visual, auditory, or oral-motor deficits that would interfere with his ability to complete the study.

Experimental Stimuli

Different but balanced sets of 12 words and 12 abstract symbols were assigned to each of the two experimental conditions. Each word was paired to one of the symbols. Each set contained six nouns and six verbs of no more than three syllables. All words were matched for their degree of picturability. Abstract black-and-white symbols were used as visual stimuli to control for the effects of prior learning and to minimize the variable naming performance so characteristic of people with aphasia. The symbols, which were identical to those used by Marshall et al. (in press), were Blyssymbols (Hehner, 1983) that had been modified to ensure a totally noniconic appearance. Even so, care was taken not to pair a word to a symbol that had any subtle characteristics of the object or action represented by the word. Each symbol was printed on a white 4-x-4-in. square card. To ensure that all subjects had the same randomized symbol presentation order during training, separate packets of the 12 word-symbol pairs were created for each of the eight training trials within an experimental condition.

Procedures

Preexperimental Probe. The preexperimental probes measured the subjects' ability to recall the word-symbol pairs prior to training. Probe administration was divided into two parts. In the first portion, the examiner presented the symbols singly and verbally provided the matched target word. The subjects were given 15 to 20 seconds to study the symbol. The word was repeated once if requested by the subjects. After approximately a 1-hour interval, the examiner presented the symbols again in random order and asked the subjects to provide the correct labels. All responses were recorded as either correct or incorrect. Minor articulatory errors that did not affect the intelligibility of the responses were ignored. The examiner did not provide any training, cues, or feedback to the subjects during these probes.

Phonemic Cue Training Trials. The initial portion of the PC training trials oriented the subjects to the word-symbol pairs and the phonemic cue. In this first step, the examiner presented a symbol to subjects and verbally provided three pieces of information: (a) the word paired to that symbol, (b) the number of syllables in the word, and (c) the first phoneme of the word. The first-phoneme cue was a verbal production of the target word's initial phoneme followed by a neutral vowel. Words that began with consonant blends were presented as the first two phonemes and a neutral vowel, and those beginning with a vowel used the vowel as the cue. The cues were repeated once if requested by the subjects. After all 12 word-symbol pairs were presented, the subjects began the first PC training trial.

In the training trials, the examiner presented the first symbol and told the subjects (a) the number of syllables in the target word and (b) the initial phoneme. The subjects were then asked to label the symbol with the correct target word. If the response was correct, the examiner verbally indicated the accuracy of the answer. If the subjects were unable to recall the word, the examiner provided the correct label and repeated the phonemic cue. The responses were recorded as either correct or incorrect. The first PC training trial was completed when the subjects had attempted to label all 12 symbols. Each subsequent PC training trial followed the same training procedure; however, the order of symbol presentation varied from trial to trial.

Self-Cue Training Trials. Before beginning the SC training trials, the subjects were asked to create the self-cues for each of the word-symbol pairs. The examiner presented the first symbol and verbally provided its paired word. The subjects were then requested to develop a personalized self-cue to aid in the later recall of that word. They were told to attend to the meaning of the target word and the perceptual characteristics of the symbol when formulating the cue. In those instances when the subjects could not create a self-cue, the examiner offered an example of what might be appropriate for that particular symbol. In most instances, one example from the examiner was sufficient to help the subjects develop their own self-cues. The final self-cues were almost always short phrases or sentences, five to six words in length. Once the self-cues were created, the first SC training trial began. All training steps in this condition were identical to those in the PC condition except that the subjects used self-cues instead of phonemic cues.

Labeling Probes. Three labeling probes were completed within each experimental condition: (a) a midtraining probe, (b) a posttraining probe, and (c) a 24-hour follow-up probe. In each of these probes, the examiner presented the 12 symbols from the appropriate experimental condition one at a time and asked the subjects to label the symbol. No cues or feedback regarding the accuracy of the responses was provided by the examiner.

RESULTS

The results were analyzed in two sections: training data and labeling probe data. Two-way Analysis of Variance (ANOVA) with repeated measures was used to evaluate the data. In the analysis of the training trials, the effect of the cue (SC vs. PC) was not a significant factor in the subjects performance during the training trials ($F = 2.40$; $df = 1, 7$; $p = 0.16$). The effect of the trials was significant ($F = 72.45$, $df = 8, 56$; $p = .0001$), indicating that subject performance improved as the number of training trials in both cueing conditions increased. The cue by trial interaction was not significant ($F = 72.45$, $df = 8, 56$; $p = .28$), indicating that the subjects' rates and levels of improvement across training trials did not differ for the two cueing conditions. Overall, the analysis of training data revealed improved subject performance during the training trials but no significant distinctions between the two cueing conditions (see Figure 1).

In contrast to the training data, the probe data demonstrated significant differences between the PC and SC conditions. The cue effect was significant ($F = 12.95$; $df = 1, 7$; $p = .0088$), with mean group recall of the target words consistently higher in the SC probes than in the PC probes. The trial effect showed significant increases ($F = 38.35$, $df = 3, 21$; $p = .0001$) in subject labeling performance from the preexperimental probe to the 24-hour follow-up probe, indicating that probe scores increased for both conditions over time. Most importantly, the cue by trial effect revealed a significant difference ($F = 9.99$; $df = 3, 21$; $p = .0001$) between the two cueing conditions across time, with subject performance highest in the SC condition (see Figure 2).

An analysis of simple effects was conducted to examine differences between the two cueing conditions during each of the labeling probes. The results indicated that there was a significant difference ($p < .01$) between the two conditions on the midtraining, posttraining, and 24-hour follow-up probes. For these three probes, group mean performance was consistently higher in the SC condition. The difference between conditions during the preexperimental probe was not significant, which is an important finding because it suggests that the differences in subject performance were probably not due to unbalanced sets of experimental stimuli.

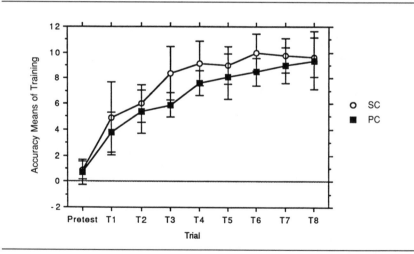

Figure 1. Group mean accuracy scores for training trials in the self-cue (SC) and phonemic cue (PC) conditions.

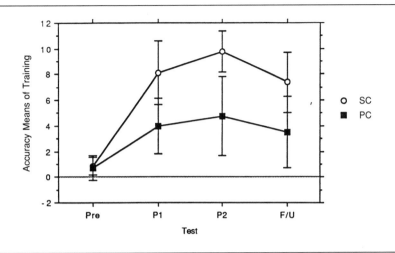

Figure 2. Group mean accuracy scores for preexperimental (Pre), midtraining (P1), posttraining (P2), and 24-hour follow-up (F/U) probes in the self-cue (SC) and phonemic cue (PC) conditions.

DISCUSSION

The findings of this study indicate that a training procedure requiring aphasic subjects to access semantic representations of target stimuli results in more accurate later naming than does a procedure that focuses only on phonologic representations. Overall, the results show that both the self-cue and the phonemic-cue training procedures were successful in teaching the labels of the novel symbols. On the labeling probes, however, subject naming performance was significantly more accurate in the self-cue condition, even after a 24-hour delay.

These findings are consistent with other studies that have examined the effects of semantic processing on word finding (Howard et al., 1985a, 1985b; Marshall et al., 1990; Marshall et al., in press; Pring et al., 1990) and may have clinical implications for aphasia therapy. They suggest that the quality of stimulus presentation may be more important than the quantity, especially when working to generalize aphasic subjects' word-finding skills to situations outside of therapy. This point is perhaps best illustrated by a brief examination of one of the techniques used in stimulation aphasia therapy. A hallmark of this therapy approach has been the use of "auditory bombardment" to enhance word finding in aphasic subjects (Schuell, Jenkins, & Jimenez-Pabon, 1964). This activity consists of presenting the subject with many verbal repetitions of a target word; Schuell et al. recommended as many as 20 repetitions per word. In essence, such a procedure supplies only phonologic information to the subject and requires little, if any, semantic processing of the stimuli. As demonstrated in the present study, such an activity may successfully elicit the target word at the time of cue presentation, but it might not significantly enhance later naming performance. In contrast, a therapy activity that requires aphasic patients to analyze the semantic features of target words slowly and carefully may be a more effective method of generalizing the naming skills learned in therapy to other settings. Such an approach would differ significantly from the frequent presentations of phonological information currently used in much of traditional therapy.

REFERENCES

Barton, M., Maruszewski, M., & Urrea, D. (1969). Variation of stimulus context and its effect on word-finding ability in aphasics. *Cortex, 5,* 351–365.

Bensen, F. (1979). Neurologic correlates of anomia. In H. Whitaker & H. Whitaker (Eds.), *Studies in neurolinguistics.* New York: Academic Press.

Brown, J. W. (1972). *Aphasia, apraxia, and agnosia: Clinical and theoretical aspects.* Springfield, IL: Charles Thomas.

Goodglass, H., & Stuss, D. T. (1979). Naming to picture versus description in three aphasic subgroups. *Cortex, 15,* 199–211.

Hehner, B. (1983). *Blyssymbols for use.* Toronto: Blyssymbolics Communication Institute.

Howard, D., Patterson, K., Franklin, S., Orchard-Lisle, V., & Morton, J. (1985a). The facilitation of picture naming in aphasia. *Cognitive Neuropsychology, 2,* 49–80.

Howard, D., Patterson, K., Franklin, S., Orchard-Lisle, V., & Morton, J. (1985b). Treatment of word retrieval deficits in aphasia. *Brain, 108,* 817–829.

Li, E., & Canter, G. J. (1983) Phonemic cueing: An investigation of subject variables. In R. Brookshire (Ed.), *Clinical aphasiology conference proceedings.* Minneapolis, MN: BRK Publishers.

Li, E., & Canter, G. J. (1987). An investigation of Luria's hypothesis on prompting in aphasic naming disturbances. *Journal of Communication Disorders, 20,* 469–475.

Li, E., & Canter, G. J. (1991). Varieties of errors produced by aphasic patients in phonemic cueing. *Aphasiology, 5,* 51–61.

Li, E., & Williams, S. E. (1989). The efficacy of two types of cues in aphasia patients. *Aphasiology, 3,* 619–626.

Love, R. J., & Webb, W. G. (1977). The efficiency of cueing techniques in Broca's aphasia. *Journal of Speech and Hearing Disorders, 42,* 170–178.

Luria, A. R. (1970). *Traumatic aphasia.* The Hague: Mouton.

Marshall, J., Pound, C., White-Thomson, M., & Pring, T. (1990). The use of picture/word matching tasks to assist word retrieval in aphasic patients. *Aphasiology, 4,* 167–184.

Marshall, R. C., Neuburger, S. I., & Phillips, D. S. (in press). Effects of facilitation and cueing on labeling of "novel" stimuli by aphasic subjects. *Aphasiology.*

Patterson, K., Purell, C., & Morton, J. (1983). Facilitation of word retrieval in aphasia. In C. Code and D. J. Muller (Eds.), *Aphasia therapy* (pp. 76–87). London: Edward Arnold.

Pease, D., & Goodglass, H. (1978). The effects of cueing on picture naming in aphasia. *Cortex, 14,* 178–189.

Podraza, B. L., & Darley, F. L. (1977). Effects of auditory prestimulation on naming in aphasia. *Journal of Speech and Hearing Research, 28,* 669–683.

Porch, B. E. (1981). *Porch Index of Communicative Ability.* Palo Alto, CA: Consulting Psychologists Press.

Pring, T., White-Thomson, M., Pound, C., Marshall, J., & Davis, A. (1990). Picture/word matching tasks and word retrieval: Some follow-up data and second thoughts. *Aphasiology, 4,* 479–483.

Rochford, G., & Williams, M. (1962). Studies in the development and breakdown of the use of names. *Journal of Neurology, Neurosurgery, and Psychiatry, 25,* 222–223.

Schuell, H., Jenkins, J., & Jimenez-Pabon, E. (1964). *Aphasia in adults: Diagnosis, prognosis, and treatment.* New York: Hoeber.

Spreen, O., & Benton, A. L. (1977). *Neurosensory center comprehensive examination for aphasia.* Victoria, BC: University of Victoria.

Weidner, W. E., & Jinks, A. F. (1983). The effects of single versus combined cue presentation on picture naming by aphasic adults. *Journal of Communication Disorders, 16,* 111–121.

Clinical Aphasiology, Vol. 22, 1994, pp. 345–356

An Investigation of the Communicative Use of Trained Symbols Following Multimodality Training

Mary H. Purdy, Robert J. Duffy, and Carl A. Coelho

Several studies have addressed the ability of people with aphasia to use trained nonverbal means of communication spontaneously to circumvent their verbal deficits. For example, Calculator and Luchko (1983) attempted to train subjects to use communication boards. Other researchers, such as Coelho and Duffy (1985, 1987), Coelho (1991), and Bellaire, Georges, and Thompson (1988), trained aphasic subjects to acquire manual gestures. The results of these studies have been tempered because subjects often acquired the target signs or symbols but did not use them for functional communication.

More recently, Garrett, Beukelman, and Low-Morrow (1989) used a multimodal approach in developing an augmentative communication system for a subject with a Broca's type aphasia. These authors suggested that a multimodal approach can potentially increase the efficiency of the communication efforts because it increases the opportunity for the subject to access residual capabilities.

Given aphasic subjects' reduced ability to retrieve symbols, the idea of multimodal training for them is worthy of study. If aphasic individuals fail to communicate in one modality, they could switch to a different modality. Therefore, if subjects were trained to acquire symbols in multiple modalities, overall communicative performance might be more successful.

The purpose of this study was to examine aphasic subjects' communicative use of trained symbols following multimodality training. The following specific questions were addressed:

1. Do aphasic subjects use trained symbols on structured communication tasks?

2. Do aphasic subjects improve their performance with cueing?

3. Which modalities do aphasic subjects use?

4. Do aphasic subjects spontaneously switch between modalities to communicate when an initial attempt fails?

METHOD

Subjects

Fifteen nonfluent aphasic subjects participated in this study. Subjects were right-handed, were native speakers of English, had normal estimated premorbid intelligence, and passed screening tests for vision and hearing. A summary of subject characteristics is listed in Table 1. Only subjects living at home with active communicative partners were selected; these subjects were believed to be most likely to succeed on functional communication tasks because they had the opportunity for meaningful, daily communicative interactions. Because the focus of this study was on symbol usage, subjects who were likely to be trainable were selected. Therefore, only aphasic patients with a *Porch Index of Communicative Ability* (PICA) (Porch, p. 81) overall percentile of 25 or greater were selected. This cutoff point was suggested by Coelho and Duffy (1985), who found subjects below this point were unable to acquire manual signs.

Symbol Acquisition

Twenty target symbols were trained in three different tasks representing three distinct modalities: communication board, gesture, and verbal. For

Table 1. Descriptive Information and Test Data for 15 Aphasic Subjects

Values	AGE	ED	IQ	MPO	PCOA	CADL
Mean	61.9	13.8	111.1	39.7	40.4	84
SD	9.6	2.9	9.9	51.1	10.7	16.4
Range	43–76	9–20	102–141	4–156	25–63	57–115

Note: ED = years of education; IQ = estimated premorbid intelligence quotient (Wilson, Rosenbaum, Rourke, Whitman, & Grisell, 1978); MPO = months post onset; PICA = *Porch Index of Communicative Ability* overall percentile; CADL = *Communicative Abilities of Daily Living* total score (number possible = 136).

the purpose of this study, a symbol is defined as a picture, sign, or word that represents a given concept. Seven symbols that commonly function as nouns, seven as verbs, four as adjectives, and two as adverbs were trained. All symbols were drawn from the *Communicative Abilities of Daily Living* (CADL) (Holland, 1980) and were judged to be representative of everyday communicative activities. See Appendix A for specific symbols trained.

A multiple baseline across behaviors design was used to train the 20 target symbols in three different communicative modalities. Initial baseline measures were taken over a 3-day period. The mean baseline was 80% on the communication board task (range, 45–100). All subjects had a stable baseline (< 5% variance between measures) on the board. The mean baseline performance for the gesture task was 34% (range, 0–60). Thirteen of the subjects had a stable gesture baseline. Mean baseline performance for the verbal task was 28% (range, 0–65). Eleven of the subjects had a stable verbal baseline. Training was then initiated.

Communication Board. Training began with an introduction to the symbols on the communication board. The 8 1/2-by-11-in. board was divided into a 4-by-6-in. grid that contained black-and-white line drawings representing the 20 target concepts. The word for each concept was printed above the appropriate picture. The examiner stated the concept and pointed to the corresponding picture on the communication board. All 20 symbols were introduced in this manner. During training trials, the symbol was stated and used in a sentence (e.g., "pencil—I write with a pencil"), and the subject was then required to point to the appropriate picture. If the subject was unsure of the correct response, a gestural cue was provided. If an error was made, the examiner showed the subject the accurate response and provided repetitions of the verbal and gestural stimuli. One to four training trials were run during each session. Testing trials were conducted at the conclusion of each training session. Again, the subject was asked to point to a picture when given an auditory stimulus. Responses were scored as accurate or inaccurate. To progress to the next training task, subjects must have attained 80% accuracy on three consecutive testing sessions.

Gesture. Training began with an introduction to the task. The examiner showed the subject a picture (as on the communication board) and demonstrated the corresponding gesture. Training proceeded to an imitative level. The subject was shown the picture stimulus and asked to imitate the gesture demonstrated by the examiner. A verbal explanation accompanied the gesture for the more abstract target concepts (e.g., "You're in a hurry so you go *fast*"). After successfully imitating all gestures, the subject began the formal training trial, in which the subject was expected to provide the correct gesture in response to the picture presentation only. Errors were corrected by giving the subject a verbal explanation (to ensure knowledge of the concept to be expressed) and demonstrating the correct gesture. When necessary, the examiner manipulated the subject's hand to form the correct gesture. The testing trial was conducted in the same manner as the training trials. The subject was expected to provide the correct gesture in response to a picture (without verbal input). Responses were scored as accurate or inaccurate. Training moved to the final task when the subject attained 80% accuracy on three consecutive testing sessions.

Verbal. Target responses were introduced by having the examiner show a picture to the subject and stating the appropriate word. Training for verbal responses began at an imitative level. Subjects were shown the same stimulus picture and asked to imitate the word. Phonemic, semantic, and visual placement cues were provided to facilitate verbal production. The subject was given three tries for each target, with feedback, before proceeding to the next item. Once a subject produced the word imitatively or in response to the cueing, formal training trials were conducted. The training trials consisted of eliciting the word in response to the picture only. Training ended when subjects reached 80% accuracy or after 20 training trials.

Baseline and Maintenance Probes. During training of the communication board task, baseline measures continued to be taken on the gesture and verbal tasks during each testing session. Once criterion was met for the communication board task, baseline measures continued to be taken on the verbal task, and maintenance of the communication board performance was probed every session. During training of the final task, performance maintenance was probed on the communication board and gestural tasks every testing session.

Overall Criterion. To participate in the current study, subjects had to maintain 80% accuracy in at least two of the three modalities trained. The mean accuracy was 91% on the communication board task (range, 80–100%), 90% on the gestural task (range, 80–100%), and 49% on the verbal-naming task (range, 0–80%). All subjects met the 80% criterion on the communication board and gestural tasks; only four subjects met criterion on the verbal task. All subjects acquired every symbol in at least one of the two nonverbal alternative modalities (communication board or gesture), and 9 of the 15 subjects had every symbol in both nonverbal modalities. Therefore, if subjects failed with their verbal attempts, they all had the potential means to communicate nonverbally with 100% accuracy on each functional communication task.

Functional Communication Tasks

Following training, subjects' use of the trained symbols was tested. Two functional communication tasks were designed to assess whether subjects spontaneously used trained symbols accurately to communicate specific information. These two tasks provided multiple opportunities to use the trained symbols. In addition, the two tasks represented different genres of communication, thus allowing examination of the similarities and differences in performance on different communicative activities. All tasks were recorded on audiotape and videotape for later analysis.

Structured Conversation. The first functional communication task simulated a conversation about common daily activities (e.g., driving and shopping). The communication board was placed on the table to the subject's left side, and the subjects were told to use it whenever they needed to. The examiner followed a highly structured script designed to elicit the trained symbols. All stimuli in the script were one to two sentences in length. One repetition was allowed at the subject's request. If the target symbol was not elicited following the stimulus, a standard cue was provided. Each cue consisted of a single sentence intended to elicit the target symbol (e.g., for the symbol "car," the cue was, "How do you get around town?").

Six variables were defined to describe subjects' performance on the structured conversation task. Three variables addressed successful symbol usage (the total number of correctly used target symbols emitted *spontaneously*, following a *cue*, and in each *modality*), and three variables addressed subjects' spontaneous attempts to switch to an alternative modality when the initial attempt failed (the ratio of the number of *successful*, *unsuccessful*, and *total* attempts to switch modalities to the number of opportunities to switch).

Referential Communication Task. The second task was a referential communication task consisting of 15 picture descriptions. Each picture contained two to three of the target symbols. Some symbols were used in more than one picture, so the total number of symbols targeted in the 15 pictures was 33. To demonstrate that the target concepts were accurately and clearly represented in the pictures and could be easily elicited, six non-brain-damaged adults were shown the pictures and asked to describe them. These subjects responded with all the target symbols in a given picture on the first attempt 87% of the time. All the remaining target symbols were identified on the second attempt. Message receivers were able to identify the target picture with 98% accuracy.

The communication board was placed on the aphasic subject's left side, and the subject was told to use it whenever necessary. The aphasic subject (sender) was then shown a target picture and required to communicate the contents of the picture to a receiver using whatever means the subject chose. The receiver—someone with whom the subject was very familiar—then attempted to select the target picture from four pictures. The receiver was allowed to make one request for additional information from the sender, if needed. If the receiver was unable to make a correct picture selection, the examiner then cued the subject by pointing to the target symbol in the picture and requesting, "Tell us about this."

The same six variables defined for the conversation task were used on the referential communication task. Again, three variables pertained to the number of target symbols correctly used by the aphasic subjects (spontaneously, following a cue, and in each modality), and three variables addressed aphasic subjects switching behavior (successful, unsuccessful, and total).

Intraexaminer Reliability

Intraexaminer reliability was determined for all variables by rescoring the videotaped performance of the first 10 subjects. Point-to-point agreement ranged from 80–90%.

RESULTS

Structured Conversation

The percentage of correctly used target symbols elicited spontaneously and with cueing are listed in Table 2. Spontaneous use averaged 49% for the group (9.8 symbols). When subjects were cued, usage increased by an average of 34% (6.4 symbols). Paired t-tests demonstrated a significant difference between the total number used spontaneously and following a cue ($t = -8.51$, $df = 14$, $p < .001$).

The percentage of target symbols used correctly in each modality (communication board, gestural, verbal) can also be found in Table 2. A repeated measure multivariate analysis of variance (MANOVA) demonstrated significance F (2,28) = 13.05, $p < .001$. Post hoc t-tests demonstrated that subjects spontaneously used the verbal mode significantly more than the gestural mode (34% versus 10%) ($t = 3.34$, $df = 14$, $p < .01$) or the communication board (34% versus 5%) ($t = 4.20$, $df = 14$, $p < .01$). There was no significant difference between use of gesture and the communication board ($t = -1.4$, $df = 14$, $p = .18$). The same pattern of usage was found following a cue. Again, a MANOVA revealed significance F (2,28) = 12.96,

Table 2. Percent of Symbols (N = 20) Correctly Used on a Structured Conversation Task

Values	Spontaneous				Cued				Spontaneous + Cued
	CB	Gest.	Verb.	Total	CB	Gest.	Verb.	Total	
Mean	5	10	34	49*	4	7	23	34	83*
SD	8.2	9.2	22.6	16.5	6.1	10.3	12.4	12.2	13.3
Range	0–30	0–25	0–65	20–70	0–20	0–40	0–45	0–55	45–100

Note: Spontaneous = symbols used spontaneously; Cued = symbols used with a cue; CB = communication board; Gest. = gesture; Verb. = verbal.
*Difference between the means is significant ($p < .001$).

$p < .001$. Post hoc t tests showed that subjects correctly used the verbal mode significantly more than the gestural mode (23% versus 7%) ($t = 3.31$, $df = 14$, $p < .01$) or the communication board (23% versus 4%) ($t = 4.85$, $df = 14$, $p < .01$). Again, there was no significant difference between use of gesture and the communication Board ($t = -1.05$, $df = 14$, $p = .31$). Subjects' first responses generally were verbal. Thus, the pattern of symbol usage was opposite that of symbol acquisition during the training task; that is, subjects used least frequently the modalities with which they were most successful during training (communication board and gesture). Subjects were least successful with the verbal modality during training (only four subjects reached the 80% criterion), yet this was the most frequently used modality.

Next, the ratio of the number of times each subject spontaneously attempted to switch between modalities to the number of opportunities present to switch was calculated (see Table 3). The results demonstrated that when subjects' first attempts to communicate failed, they attempted to switch to an alternative only 41% of the time that an opportunity was present ($N = 280$). Because most initial communicative attempts were verbal, the switch was almost always made from the verbal to a nonverbal modality. Of the total number of attempts made to switch ($N = 115$), 67% were successful ($N = 77$) and 33% were unsuccessful ($N = 38$). Although training apparently had provided subjects the means to use alternative modalities when their initial communicative attempt failed, they did not switch to these modalities as frequently as was expected.

Referential Communication Task

The percentage of target symbols correctly used spontaneously and with cueing (33 possible) can be found in Table 4. Subjects spontaneously used

Table 3. Number of Spontaneous Modality Switches on a
Structured Conversation Task

Values	Opportunities to Switch		Switches (N = 115)	
	Available	Taken	Successful	Unsuccessful
Total	280	115	77	38
Mean	18.7	7.7	5.1	2.5
SD	8.3	5.9	4.1	2.2
Range	8–35	0–19	0–13	0–7

53% (17.5) of the symbols. Usage increased by 23% following a cue. Paired t-tests demonstrated a significant difference between the number of symbols used spontaneously and following a cue ($t = -8.6$, $df = 14$, $p < .001$).

In terms of the mode of response, a pattern similar to the structured conversation task was demonstrated. For spontaneous symbol usage, a MANOVA demonstrated significance F (2,28) = 9.15, $p < .001$. As can be seen in Table 4, subjects correctly used the verbal mode most frequently both spontaneously and following a cue (34% and 12%), followed by the gestural mode (16% and 8%), and finally the communication board (3% and 3%). Post hoc t-tests showed that the differences in spontaneous symbol usage were significant between verbal and communication board ($t = 4.16$, $df = 14$, $p = < .01$). There was no significant difference between verbal and gesture ($t = 2.05$, $df = 14$, $p = .05$) or gesture and communication board ($t = 2.7$, $df = 14$, $p = .02$). For usage following a cue, a MANOVA revealed significance F (2,28) = 4.4, $p < .02$. Post hoc t-tests showed significant differences between verbal and communication board ($t = 2.86$, $df = 14$, $p < .01$). There was no significant difference between verbal and gesture ($t = -1.06$, $df = 14$, $p = .30$) or gesture and communication board ($t = 2.45$, $df = 14$, $p = .03$). As was found with the structured conversation task, the communication board and gesture were used less frequently than the verbal mode despite a high degree of accuracy with these modalities on the training task.

An analysis of subjects' switching behavior can be found in Table 5. Of the total number of opportunities present ($N = 494$), subjects attempted to switch modalities only 37% of the times an opportunity was present. Of the total number of times a subject switched ($N = 183$), 80% ($N = 147$) of the attempts were successful and 20% ($N = 36$) were unsuccessful. This pattern is similar to that found with the structured conversation task. That is, subjects did not typically initiate switching between modalities, but when they did, they were usually successful.

Table 4. Percent of Symbols (*N* = 33) Correctly Used on a Referential Communication Task

Values	Spontaneous				Cued				Spontaneous + Cued
	CB	Gest.	Verb.	Total	CB	Gest.	Verb.	Total	
Mean	3	16	34	53*	3	8	12	23	76*
SD	5.6	14.7	25.4	19.3	4.5	6.9	9.9	10	17.1
Range	0–15	0–45	0–73	21–82	0–12	0–27	0–30	6–42	36–97

Note: Spontaneous = percentage of symbols used spontaneously; Cued = percentage of symbols used with a cue; CB = communication board; Gest. = gesture; Verb. = verbal.
*Difference between the means is significant ($p < .001$).

Table 5. Number of Spontaneous Modality Switches on a Referential Communication Task

Values	Opportunities to Switch		Switches (N = 183)	
	Available	Taken	Successful	Unsuccessful
Total	494	183	147	36
Mean	32.9	12.2	9.8	2.4
SD	15.1	8.2	6.5	2.3
Range	11–57	0–25	0–18	0–8

DISCUSSION

This study demonstrated that multimodality training was successful in that all subjects were able to maintain a minimum of 80% of the symbols in at least two of the three modalities. However, though the subjects did correctly use the symbols in structured communication tasks, they did not use as many as the groups' high performance on the training tasks might have suggested. As a group, subjects spontaneously used only approximately 50% of the symbols on both communication tasks. It should be noted that correct symbol usage increased to 85% following a cue. This suggests that subjects did have the symbols available but that they could not always access them until the additional structure of the cued condition was provided.

The results also showed that the verbal modality was the most frequently used modality both spontaneously and following a cue, even though this was the modality with which subjects had the least success during training. In fact, the number of verbal symbols used correctly correlated significantly with the number of verbal symbols acquired (conversation, $r = .87$; referential communication, $r = .92$). It is likely that the verbal modality was used most frequently because it is the most natural or automatic means of communicating. Communication by gesture or a communication board is less automatic, and thus these modalities were used infrequently.

It is reasonable to hypothesize that ability to switch between modalities could affect successful use of trained symbols. If subjects attempted to switch to alternative modes, even if they were not successful, this would be evidence that they at least recognized their failure and the need to change approaches or try another alternative. Their lack of success may be because they could not access or produce the appropriate symbol. However, if subjects did not even attempt to switch, this would be evidence that some other factor was involved that interfered with the subjects' ability to recognize their failure or plan an alternative approach.

Aphasic subjects as a group switched modalities only 39% of the time. When they did switch, however, they were usually successful (73% of the time). Thus, even though they appeared to have adequate alternatives available to facilitate their communication, the communication attempt often failed because subjects did not switch to these means when their verbal attempts failed. There are several possible reasons why subjects did not spontaneously switch modalities. Perhaps it was because they were not trained to do so. The intent of this study was to examine what subjects did on their own, so it did not attempt to train the concept of switching between modalities. Future research could address whether specific training of switching behavior might enhance communicative use of trained symbols.

It may also be that specific subject variables may influence performance, including premorbid communicative style, personality variables, or psychological motivation to perform the task. However, these variables are difficult to control in group studies and would be more appropriately addressed in individual case studies.

Finally, switching behavior may be related to certain aspects of cognition for which aphasic subjects may experience deficits. Kraat (1990) has suggested that deficits in cognition could influence and limit subjects' use of alternative communication strategies. In describing aphasic subjects' performances, she noted that "it was as if the aphasic subjects did not think to turn to these alternative forms, could not shift strategies to use them, or somehow could not integrate them into real communicative contexts (p. 324)." More research is needed to identify the cognitive variables that may influence aphasic subjects' ability to use alternative communicative strategies.

REFERENCES

Bellaire, L., Georges, J., & Thompson C. (1988). Acquisition and generalization of gestures in aphasia: An experimental study. Paper presented at the Annual Conference of the American Speech-Language-Hearing Association, Boston.

Calculator, S., & Luchko, C. (1983). Evaluating the effectiveness of a communication board training program. *Journal of Speech and Hearing Disorders, 48,* 281–287.

Coelho, C. (1991). Manual sign acquisition and use in two aphasic subjects. In T. E. Prescott (Ed.), *Clinical aphasiology,* Vol. 19 (pp. 209–218). Austin, TX: PRO-ED.

Coelho, C., & Duffy, R. (1985). Communicative use of signs in aphasia: Is acquisition enough? In R. H. Brookshire (Ed.), *Clinical aphasiology conference proceedings* (pp. 222–228).

Coelho, C., & Duffy, R. (1987). The relationship of the acquisition of manual signs to severity of aphasia. A training study. *Brain and Language, 31,* 326–345.

Garrett, K., Beukelman, D., & Low-Morrow, D. (1989). A comprehensive augmentative communication system for an adult with Broca's aphasia. *Augmentative and Alternative Communication, 5,* 55–61.

Holland, A. (1980). *Communicative Abilities in Daily Living.* Austin, TX: PRO-ED.

Kraat, A. (1990). Augmentative and alternative communication: Does it have a future in aphasia rehabilitation? *Aphasiology, 4* (4), 321–338.

Porch, B. (1981). *The Porch Index of Communicative Abilities.* Palo Alto, CA: Consulting Psychologists Press.

Wilson, R., Rosenbaum, G., Rourke, D., Whitman, D., & Grisell, J. (1978). An index of premorbid intelligence. *Journal of Consulting and Clinical Psychology, 46,* 1554–1555.

APPENDIX A

Nouns	Verbs	Adjectives	Adverbs
car	move	flat	fast
tire	push	mad	slow
gas	break	blind	
shoelace	hit	cold	
boy	smoke		
fan	stop		
pencil	hurt		

AUTHOR INDEX